D0987275

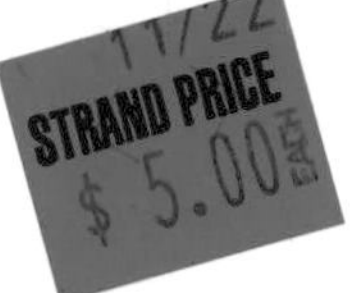
11/22
STRAND PRICE
$ 5.00
EACH

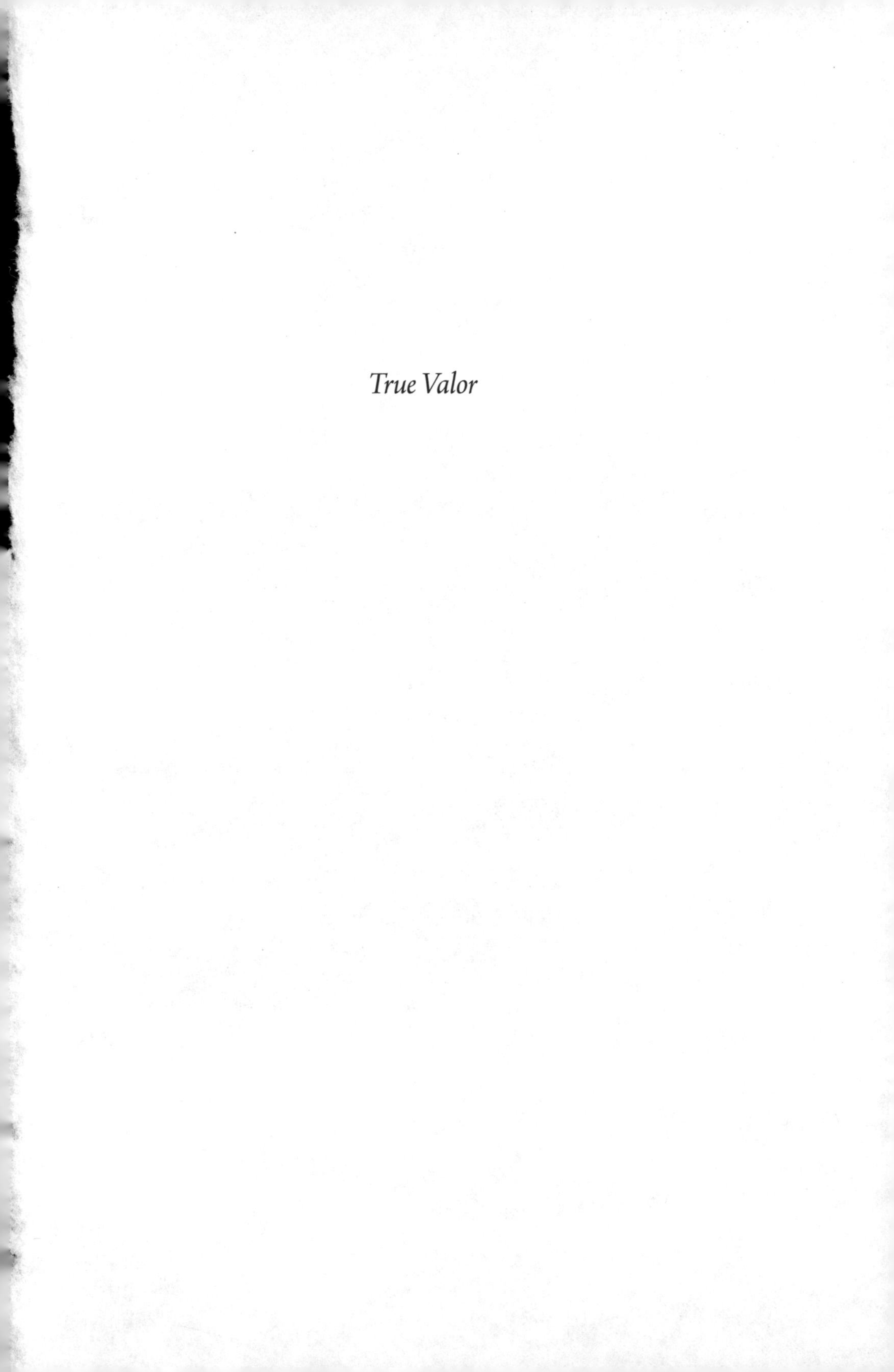

True Valor

TRUE VALOR

Barney Clark and the Utah Artificial Heart

Don B. Olsen

The University of Utah Press
Salt Lake City

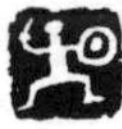

The Defiance House Man colophon is a registered trademark of the University of Utah Press. It is based on a four-foot-tall Ancient Puebloan pictograph (late PIII) near Glen Canyon, Utah.

19 18 17 16 15 1 2 3 4 5

LIBRARY OF CONGRESS CATALOGING-IN-PUBLICATION DATA

Olsen, Don B. (Donald B.), author.
True valor : Barney Clark and the Utah artificial heart / Don B. Olsen.
p.; cm.
Barney Clark and the Utah artificial heart
Includes bibliographical references and index.
ISBN 978-1-60781-391-0 (hardback : alk. paper) — ISBN 978-1-60781-392-7 (Ebook)
I. Title. II. Title: Barney Clark and the Utah artificial heart.
[DNLM: 1. Clark, Barney B., 1921–1983. 2. Heart, Artificial—history—Utah. 3. History, 20th Century—Utah. WG 11 AU8]
RD535.8.O45
617.4'12092—dc23
[B]

2014049409

Printed and bound by Sheridan Books, Inc., Ann Arbor, Michigan.

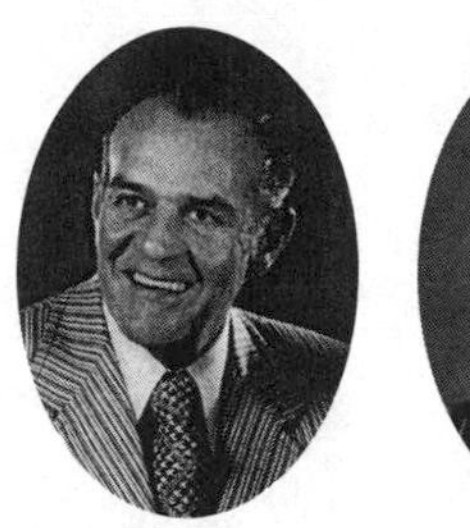
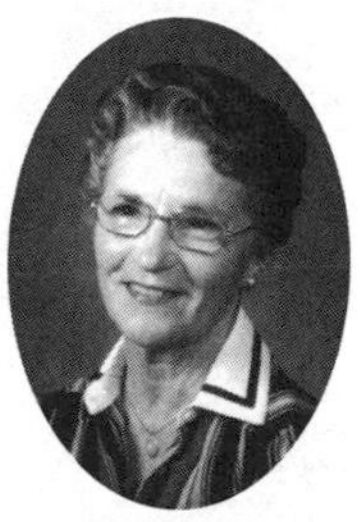

To

Dr. Barney B. Clark,

who courageously sacrificed the last days of his life

to become the first person to receive a permanent total artificial heart.

And to his wife, Una Loy Clark,

without whose love, support, and dedication

the experiment would have been impossible.

Contents

Acknowledgments

The way this book got written is a story in itself. Shortly after the artificial heart was surgically implanted in Dr. Barney Clark, some publishers contacted his family offering to purchase the publication rights to his story. The Clarks signed a contract with a very reputable publisher, which employed a Pulitzer Prize–winning author, Earl Selby, and his wife, Miriam, to write the story. They arrived in Salt Lake City to begin assembling the information for the book approximately two weeks after the landmark surgery. They were given office space in the research building and permission to interview everyone associated with the development of the artificial heart. They sometimes interviewed together, but most often Earl asked the questions, and Miriam transcribed the tapes of the sessions.

The Selbys also followed the television and newspaper coverage of the case and read virtually everything that was published about Barney Clark and the artificial heart, including articles in scientific journals. They frequently used this information to generate their next round of questions. During extensive interviews with Una Loy Clark, Barney's wife, they learned the names and addresses of Barney's relatives, friends, former high school and Brigham Young University classmates, and military comrades. They also interviewed many of these people. Within eighty days of Barney's death, the Selbys had completed all their interviews and transcriptions.

The Selbys even wrote an introduction to the book:

> We were not in the University of Utah's Medical Center that snowy night in December, but we were there on the night 112 days later, when Barney Clark died after his artificial heart had beaten 12,912,499 times. And we were there for many of the days in between and for several months thereafter.
>
> In the many pages of our interviews are the stories of Pim Kolff and his heart, Barney Clark and Una Loy, Chase Peterson and his "Utah team," and nearly all that went on to bring them to Barney's appointment in Samarra.[1]
>
> Death is here, but this is about those who treasure life, those who laugh and cry, bleed real blood, love and triumph, try and fail and rise to try again. These are heroes and winners who had the audacity to look up from everyday existence and see the vision of tomorrow, who learned what it is to challenge the unknown and let history be the judge of what they accomplished.

What we found you may find: that those in this book who chose to have the courage to persist hold up a looking glass to all of us.

When we know their stories, we can hold up this mirror and ask ourselves, if we would, if we could, do what they did. And ask ourselves if we, too, have their true valor.

Barney Clark died on March 23, 1983, and the Selbys were still conducting interviews in mid-June when they came into my office with tears running down their cheeks. "Oh dear, what has happened?" I asked.

They took a few minutes to compose themselves before telling me, "The publisher called and is canceling the project."

I was astounded. "No, no, you have amassed more data about the artificial heart than has ever been or is likely to be done. Please ask the company if I can archive the files."

Later that afternoon the Selbys returned and informed me that the publisher considered the research to be its property and insisted that it be shipped to the home office. I immediately called Una Loy and asked her to call the publisher and request that the information be left in Utah. I feared that in a very few years, some young accountant would enter the warehouse, see these boxes labeled Barney Clark, and scrap them.

Nearly two years later, I received a telephone call from Una Loy. She asked, "What do I do with all of these boxes shipped from the publisher?"

After I had caught my breath, I said, "Don't do anything; I will take care of it." I had been assisting the J. Willard Marriott Library at the University of Utah to archive many of Dr. Willem J. Kolff's papers so I knew whom to call. Responding to my high-pressured sales pitch, the library sent a panel truck to Seattle and hauled the material back.

The library policy was that it would not store, catalog, or index materials unless it owned them. A purchase agreement was signed, and Una Loy was allowed to place restrictions on what became known as the Barney B. Clark Collection. First, anyone was welcome to read any of the documents, but they could not make copies. The second provision was that Dr. Olsen could read and copy any of the documents because he was going to consider writing the Barney Clark book.

Initially I was not aware that I had such an assignment. Periodically Una Loy asked how the Barney Clark book was progressing. In 2008 I finally decided that I should begin work.

I gained access to the mass of materials known as the Barney B. Clark Collection. The interviews made up about four thousand double-spaced typed pages and sixty-nine tapes that had not been transcribed. There were also boxes of unindexed papers as well as numerous photos. I immediately decided that this was way beyond what I could handle—or even wanted to try. I said as much to a longtime friend. He asked if I remembered what President Kennedy had once said: "If not me, who, and if not now, when?" This question plagued me. I could find no suitable answer except that it had to be me and it had to be now.

My Medforte Research Foundation offered financial assistance if I needed it and even the funds to hire a ghost writer to help me. I first attempted to locate the Selbys to see if they might be willing to write the book after so many years. Their oldest son, a practicing attorney, informed me that his mother had died from breast cancer nearly fifteen years earlier and that his father had been killed in an automobile accident about five years later. I asked if he had found anything about Barney Clark when he had cleaned out their apartment. He said he had not, but he remembered that his parents had spoken about me and had been devastated when the publisher had cancelled the project.

In the library archives, I found an outline for some chapters of the book that the Selbys had begun. It was very helpful, and I used it as a basis for some of my chapters.

I am deeply indebted for the help of Twila Van Leer, a recently retired reporter from the *Deseret News.* She meticulously covered the early development of the artificial heart in the laboratory and the Barney Clark story in the newspaper. She read and edited nearly all of this book's chapters and corrected the grammar. She often questioned dates and made me double-check the sequence of various events.

I was fortunate to have access to our extensive laboratory records, as well as my personal experiences, notes, and records. These materials enabled me to verify dates and add details to this long chain of events.

Carol A. Rice began working as a secretary for Dr. Kolff in 1970—even before he hired me in 1972. Through the years, she has been invaluable in typing and editing my many NIH grant proposals, private contracts, and manuscripts for publications, as well as the reports generated by our international staff. For this project, Carol typed, further edited, formatted, and retyped various versions, incorporating both Twila's suggestions and my repeated rewording and rearranging.

I am also indebted to Shellie Dietrich for all her support with artificial-heart animal research over nearly twenty-eight years. After graduating as a dental assistant, she began assisting in assembling a wide variety of blood pumps. When my surgical assistant moved on, Shellie accepted the challenge of learning to assist with surgical procedures. She earned her master's degree in accounting at the University of Utah and has tracked millions of dollars annually from grants and research contracts.

Joyce, my wife of sixty-one years, tells me that she has seen enough of the Barney Clark book scattered across her kitchen counters every weekend and many evenings. That's because most of my writing took place outside my usual workweek. I thank her for her patience.

Dr. Lyle Joyce was the surgical assistant and valued consultant to first surgeon William C. DeVries throughout the 112 days of Barney's life on the artificial heart. He has remained active in both cardiac replacement and heart care utilizing ventricular-assist devices. He graciously provided much-appreciated encouragement and direction and helped verify and amplify some of the events in the book.

I am grateful to Dr. Kevin Murray, one of my junior colleagues who worked in the laboratory implanting artificial hearts in animals and later in humans. He contributed part of a chapter and encouraged and advised me on improving the book.

Thanks also to Don Isaacs, vice president of communications at SynCardia Systems, Inc., and Janelle Drumwright, senior marketing coordinator, for responding to my request for an update on the status of the SynCardia total artificial heart. I am honored to acknowledge this device, which helps put our many years of work into perspective. It is becoming the standard of care for end-stage biventricular-failure patients. Since SynCardia is pursuing both 70-cubic-centimeter and 50-cubic-centimeter sizes, the SynCardia total artificial heart will fit most adults and many adolescent patients needing biventricular replacement. The company has also developed a portable heart driver to enable patients to leave the hospital and live and travel more easily.

Several personal friends offered to read early drafts of the book and encouraged me to continue, even when the project seemed overwhelming. I greatly appreciate their support.

Finally, I want to acknowledge the immeasurable help offered by the University of Utah's J. Willard Marriott Library in giving me easy access to the Barney B. Clark Collection in the archives. The librarians' careful preservation and cataloguing helped me greatly.

Note

1. *Appointment in Samarra,* published in 1934, was the first novel by John O'Hara. It concerned the self-destruction of Julian English. He hurries to Samarra to escape death and finds it waiting there for him.

PART ONE

Prologue

Who would true valour see,
Let him come hither;
One here will constant be,
Come wind, come weather.

There's no discouragement
Shall make him relent
His first avow'd intent
To be a pilgrim.

—John Bunyan, *The Pilgrim's Progress*

First Warning

At dusk on December 1, 1982, while a blizzard swirled around the University of Utah's Medical Center, an electrocardiogram suddenly warned that there was trouble in Room 4 of the Cardiac Intensive Care Unit (CICU).

Nurse Jean Gonzales, twenty-four, a spirited, blue-eyed blonde who thrived on the excitement of crisis medicine, had been carefully monitoring signals on the central nursing-station screens. She ran to the room. Twice she called the patient's name. He glanced at her, seeming dazed. All the lights in the room were on. Technicians assigned to take blood samples had just finished tightening an arm tourniquet and spreading their tubes and equipment. It was the kind of maximum tension guaranteed to stimulate a patient's heart.

"Out!" Gonzales commanded. "You have complaints, see my supervisor." Hastily the technicians left. Gonzales looked at the EKG wall monitor connected to five sensors on the patient's arm and chest. Instead of the usual wave signals of a normally beating heart, a picket fence of spikes was shooting to the top of the screen. That was the mark of ventricular tachycardia (V-tach). The patient's heart was racing at breakneck speed, in too many cases the prelude to cardiac arrest and death.

Gonzales did what she had been trained to do in such cardiac emergencies. Placing her elbow level with the patient's chest, she let her fist fall hard over his heart, hoping the precordial thump would jar the heart's natural pacemaker back into a regular rhythm. The thump failed. The electrocardiogram still showed a picket fence.

Earlier in the day, the patient had shown occasional bursts of V-tach, but they had lasted only four to five seconds. Gonzales estimated this burst had continued for forty to fifty seconds. She was about to administer another thump when the V-tach abruptly ended. Worried that the sustained episode could have interrupted blood flow to the brain, causing cerebral harm, she called the patient's name again. "Are you with us?" she asked.

"Yes," a weak voice replied.

"Do you know where you are?"

"In a hospital."

"Remember my name?"

"Jean."

"Are you having any pain?"

"No."

"Did you feel that you were going to pass out?" The patient stared at her. Though his eyes were now focused, Gonzales realized he did not know what she was talking about.

"Do you remember my thumping your chest?"

"No," he said. "Did you?" Gonzales reached for a phone to alert doctors, using the word "stat"—the code for "status: emergency."

1

The Media Gathers

Through the battle, through defeat,
Moving yet, and never stopping.
Pioneers! O pioneers!

—Walt Whitman, "Pioneers, O Pioneers"

A Medical Odyssey

The patient in Room 4 of the CICU, the man struggling to stay alive just a while longer, was awaiting a unique surgery. A team of highly specialized medical experts was assembling to perform that surgery. And technology decades in the making was awaiting its first official trial in a human patient.

How this patient, these medical experts, and this technology converged on this night in this medical center is the story of a medical odyssey unmatched in modern times—the saga of the artificial heart.

As the clock ticked toward the appointed time for the surgery, some 25 newspeople, the vanguard of more than 150 media representatives who ultimately followed all or part of the implant story, were in the auditorium in Skaggs Hall, another building at the medical center. Among them were Christine Russell of the *Washington Post*; Jerry Bowen of CBS in Los Angeles; Dr. Larry Altman, medical/science writer for the *New York Times*; and Robert Bazell, the chief science and health correspondent for NBC News. The out-of-towners who had managed to get to Salt Lake City despite the heavy winter storm joined a bevy of local reporters who had followed the story for years and were excited that an innovation born and bred locally was to be in the international spotlight. Throughout the night, dozens of other reporters dribbled in as travel arrangements were finagled to circumvent the dwindling storm.

The Father of Artificial Organs

The man at the microphone on the Skaggs Hall podium wore a brown suit, white shirt, and red tie. He was seventy-one with white hair, a crooked nose, and a straight back. No one in the world was better suited to tell the story of the artificial heart than Dr. Willem Johan Kolff (known as Pim, the equivalent of Bill in his native Holland). Now head of the University of Utah's artificial-organs program, he had lived this story in intimate detail from the first tentative discussions of whether an artificial heart was a possibility to this moment when the mechanical device was to be permanently implanted in a human patient.

Godfather to the vision of a "bionic man"—one whose dying body organs could be replaced with man-made substitutes—he had earned the sobriquet "father of artificial organs." His early convictions had been confirmed when he had developed the first functional artificial kidney, working with spare parts and seat-of-the-pants ingenuity under the watchful eyes of World War II Nazi occupiers in Holland.

This December night he reminded the newspeople in his audience that the kidney he had jury-rigged in the Netherlands was the precursor to technology that by 1982 was saving or prolonging the lives of some quarter of a million patients throughout the world. Why not believe that the same life-saving success could ultimately be enjoyed by the artificial heart?

Kolff talked indirectly of the patient awaiting surgery elsewhere in the medical center. The man's name, as yet, had not been disclosed. He was, Kolff said, the victim of a mysterious killer known as idiopathic cardiomyopathy, incurable and inoperable. For unfathomed reasons, the muscle of the man's heart was gradually dying, losing its power to pump blood.

The patient had explored other options, Kolff said, including a possible heart transplant. However, he was beyond the age limit for a transplant, even if a donor heart could be found. Nostrums and knives no longer offered any options. Death appeared to be the only possible result. But, Kolff said, this patient had not been content just to wait for death when he felt that by participating in this unique medical experiment, he might contribute something helpful to others.

Kolff described the man as a pioneer, someone willing to go beyond the limits of science's frontiers. He was not going blindly into the surgery, Kolff assured the media. The patient had spent a couple of years carefully gleaning all the information he could about the artificial heart. When he had been admitted to University Hospital forty-eight hours earlier, he had signed the most exhaustive informed-consent form ever required from a patient. In chilling detail, the form

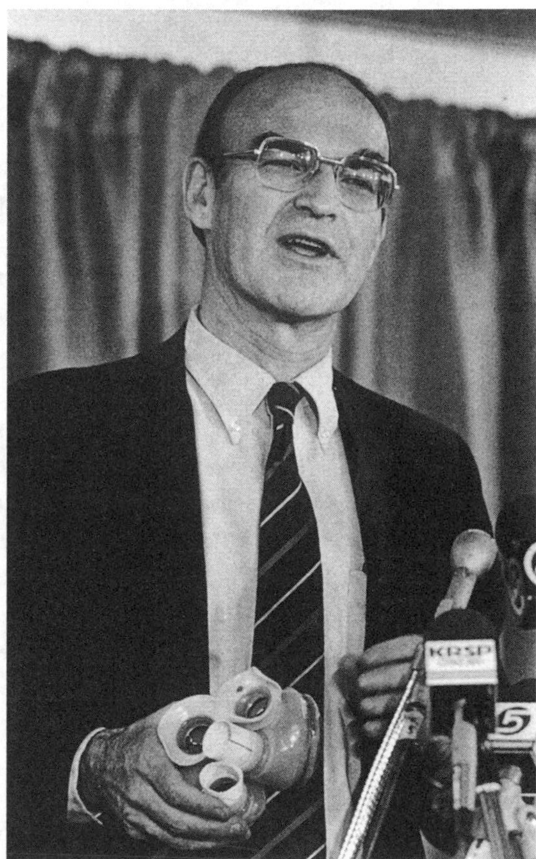

Dr. Chase N. Peterson, then University of Utah vice president for health sciences.

pinpointed all the disasters that could stem from the implant. It promised nothing. He had to sign the form again after twenty-four hours.

For Kolff, who had performed his early kidney experiments using himself, the patient, and sometimes family members as the screening committee, the current consent procedure was overwhelming. He told reporters that his European colleagues "would all run out of the hospitals in fear if they were exposed to even a third of this consent form." This patient, he emphasized, "is as well informed as any patient can ever be."

What were the chances for survival? Even Kolff could not answer that question. He might have recalled at that point the initial sixteen kidney patients who had died before one lived with an artificial kidney. But he was guardedly optimistic. "This man has a chance," he said. "How large a chance depends to a great extent on luck. How long the heart will last, we do not know. Whether there will be complications, we do not know. I hope the experiment will go well."

Dr. Chase N. Peterson, the University of Utah's vice president for health sciences and the designated spokesman for the heart implant, also addressed the Skaggs Hall audience. He had held positions as dean and vice president at Harvard University before returning to his native Utah. He was recruited by then-President James M. Gardner, who had ambitions to make the Utah school a world competitor in several science areas, including the development of a workable artificial heart.

Peterson took up the gauntlet of dealing with the complexities of volatile academia, where scientists and surgeons cherished their right to independence, where egos clashed and a galaxy of support systems, technicians, nurses, and therapists clamored for their share of recognition. He was among those who carefully molded what became the Utah heart team. It was Peterson who made the decision that the media would receive an "unvarnished play-by-play of the heart experiment." There were skeptics. An eastern colleague warned him that, "if you fail, you'll look like a fool on television."

Peterson was last to face the media during the Skaggs Hall news conference. He noted he had listened carefully to those who had preceded him. "I have not heard overstatements," he said. "But I have heard many understatements." In that context, he said,

> You should have one other: one other modest notion. Namely that this man, Barney [the first official mention of the patient's name], and these people, the team, are on the threshold of something as exciting and thrilling as has ever been accomplished in medicine. This man and his family share that. The team shares it. I share it. It is a moment of great human hope, and this man is no different than Columbus or a pioneer who might have settled this valley.

Peterson wanted everyone in the room, and every person to whom the words and pictures would be relayed around the world, to be aware of what was, to him, at the core of this heart implant: the daring, ingenuity, courage, and love that flows from the human spirit operating at its very best: true valor.

2

When to Operate

That which ordinary men are fit for,
I am qualified in, and the best of me is diligence.

—William Shakespeare, *King Lear*

V-Tach: Potential Demise

The media in the Skaggs Hall auditorium was being prepared for a heart implant that was scheduled for the following morning, but in the CICU, there were serious concerns that the patient would not live to meet that schedule. The V-tach episodes he was experiencing were cogent manifestations that his heart was on a serious downhill trend that could result in death at any time.

Dr. Fred Anderson, the medical center cardiologist who had admitted the patient, picked up the ringing phone in the catheter lab some fifty yards from the CICU. "The patient had a sustained burst of V-tach," the CICU resident reported. "He recovered spontaneously. His blood pressure's low but stable."

"Sit tight," Anderson responded in his flat, calm voice. "I'm on my way." At forty-five, the cardiologist was still trim at five feet, eight inches. He played weekly pickup basketball games, scrapping at any position that needed filling.

He hurried back to the CICU. Integral to any modern hospital, these units care for the sickest of the sick. Visitors, when they are permitted, automatically drop their voices. Few patients have extended CICU stays. Either their emergencies are quickly reversed, or they die.

On this night, because of the special patient in Room 4, there was an added feature—a security guard screened everyone entering the rectangular unit devoted to the care of those experiencing critical heart problems. Six patient rooms, each bristling with the technology hospitals employ to stave off death, clustered around a central nursing station. The carpeting was blue, the two long counters, green. Elaborate monitors reported each patient's heart activity, noting electrical waves, blood pressure, and heartbeat rate. Five outlets for oxygen, timers, respirators, suction aspirators, and a foot-wide clock were part of the array of equipment critical to this specialized unit. For some patients, the sight of that clock—tolling the seconds and minutes—was their last glimpse of the world they were leaving.

The complexities of the CICU were familiar to Anderson. He strode past the guard at the door, requesting a printout of the patient's V-tach volley while simultaneously reaching for his medical chart. The chart's cover sheet read,

> Clark, Barney Bailey. Age 61. Height 6'3". Weight 215.
> Occupation: self-employed; retired dentist.
> Residence: Des Moines, Wash.
> Presenting symptom: cardiomyopathy.

The printed sheet listing the following day's surgeries was also at the station. Alongside Clark's name was a notation identifying the upcoming surgery as TAHI: a total artificial heart implant. In the entire world, no hospital had ever used such a notation.

Anderson concentrated on the record of Clark's prolonged V-tach episode, considering what might have triggered it. The lights, the blood-sample technicians, the plethora of equipment—any of these could have put stress on an already-damaged heart, he thought. There also was the factor that no previous patient had ever had to contend with—the realization that the time was inexorably advancing when a team of doctors would remove his diseased heart and replace it with a man-made device.

"I'd be a little on edge if I were facing the prospect of what he's going to go through," Anderson acknowledged.

Jean Gonzales was still keeping an eagle eye on the patient, who was awake and alert. "How're you feeling?" Anderson asked Barney.

"Fine," he responded. He seemed puzzled by all the attention he was getting. "What's everybody so concerned about?" he asked.

"There's been a run of abnormal heartbeats," Anderson said. "But things seem to have quieted down." Referring to an earlier examination, during which Anderson and Barney had talked about dentistry and possible mutual acquaintances in the Seattle area, Anderson put into his log, "Patient looks much the same as he did earlier today. He is very calm and in control of feelings and conversation."

Despite his positive report, Anderson was aware that Barney Clark's condition was very precarious. The side effects of the steroids prescribed for his heart disease had left their mark. His abdomen was swollen into a huge mound; his cheeks were puffed out like a chipmunk's. His neck was so enlarged that he could not button a size-17 collar. For almost thirty years, he had kept his weight a lean 180 pounds. The medication-induced lardiness was offensive to him. It made him "look like hell," he complained.

One feature still stood out, though: his eyes—enormous and blue green with long dark lashes and thick, expressive brows. And even in sickness, his voice commanded respect. His wry sense of humor was also intact. "Wish we'd met him before he was sick" was a general comment by those caring for him. "He's a real man's man."

The person best acquainted with Barney, his wife of thirty-eight years, Una Loy, was on the other side of the CICU in a room made available to the family. She couldn't see into her husband's room unless she walked to the nursing station, and even then he was usually shielded behind opaque curtains.

On their arrival at the hospital, Una Loy had been told that the medical center's development and community-relations staff "is here to protect you." She was baffled. She called a daughter-in-law in Bellingham, Washington, and said, "Terry, I don't know what they're expecting with Barney. I have a public-relations person; I have a security person."

"You've got to be kidding," Terry laughed. They had expected the implant to generate a small item on page 10 of the *Salt Lake Tribune*. In a few weeks' time, Una Loy became less naïve, more confident, and the darling of the press. Even media hard noses recognized her as a genuine lady. At this point, people—each with a new request—were besieging her. There were doctors, nurses, social workers, psychiatrists, and hospital officials. Dr. Kolff came in briefly. When he introduced himself, his bearing reminded her of Barney. Hospital personnel remarked how unruffled she was, how cheerful and refreshingly down to earth.

Una Loy's ability to deal with every challenge was packaged in a tidy 108 pounds that fit nicely into a size-6 dress. She was sixty-one, the mother of three and grandmother to five, and a good listener with a ready laugh. She looked people in the eye, answering questions with directness. Like Barney, she had been born in Utah.

No one had told her of the distressing V-tach incident that afternoon, but she sensed from the flurry of medical personnel in the CICU that something had developed. "I wish I could go in," she said to her brother-in-law. "Now, Sis," he replied. Don't go worrying yourself. They say everything's okay for the morning."

"I don't know. I've been watching their faces," Una Loy replied.

Over the past three years, she had grown accustomed to watching doctors' faces. Cardiomyopathy had become the uninvited guest in the family. She had come to think of it as a stalker: now visible, now invisible, but always there. She had also accepted Barney's evaluation: "It just means that whenever this heart decides, it's going to quit." No one in their circle of family and friends took that to mean Barney was giving up. As one of their sons reminded the other, "Dad never participates in anything for the sheer joy of it. He wants to win." Throughout his illness, Barney had been more challenged than depressed. When doctors had suggested a new approach to his disease, he was willing to try.

It was this attitude, no doubt, more than any other factor that had ultimately brought the Clarks to Salt Lake City and to a closer relationship with the artificial heart technology that was blossoming there.

The Clarks Learn of the Artificial Heart

Like millions around the world, the Clarks had learned during the 1970s from the media that a marvelous new remedy for failing hearts might be on the horizon. They filed the information away under "items of interest" but not of great importance. Barney's heart disease was not advanced enough to look beyond what medicine then had to offer. Once or twice—in the spirit of two people talking about what it would be like to land on the moon—they discussed it. Barney broached the subject with his local cardiologist. "Instead of being the first to try that, I'd rather be the five-hundredth," the physician proclaimed.

In early 1982, the Clarks heard of a highly experimental drug that was being tested by cardiologists at LDS Hospital in Salt Lake City. Barney volunteered. The drug failed, and he was put on another drug regimen. The cardiologist, Dr. Jeff Anderson, scheduled him for another appointment in January of the next year. Then, almost as an afterthought, he mentioned, "You know, up at the university, the doctors are working with an artificial heart. While you're in Salt Lake, it might be fruitful to go talk with them. Maybe you could be a candidate for receiving one."

Only one cardiothoracic surgeon in the country was authorized to implant the artificial heart—Dr. William Castle DeVries—who was on the university medical staff. "I know him," Anderson said. "I have confidence in him."

Later, DeVries described the way he and Barney had come to meet: "I spoke with Jeff Anderson in July or August, and we talked at the time about what kind of patient we were looking for. Jeff said he had such a patient that he had seen in the spring. The man was not yet sick enough for the artificial heart, but Anderson thought he might eventually be an ideal candidate." DeVries told Anderson he would be interested in talking with his patient.

A couple of months later, Anderson told DeVries that Barney Clark was coming to town in October for another assessment. "He is doing fine but slowly

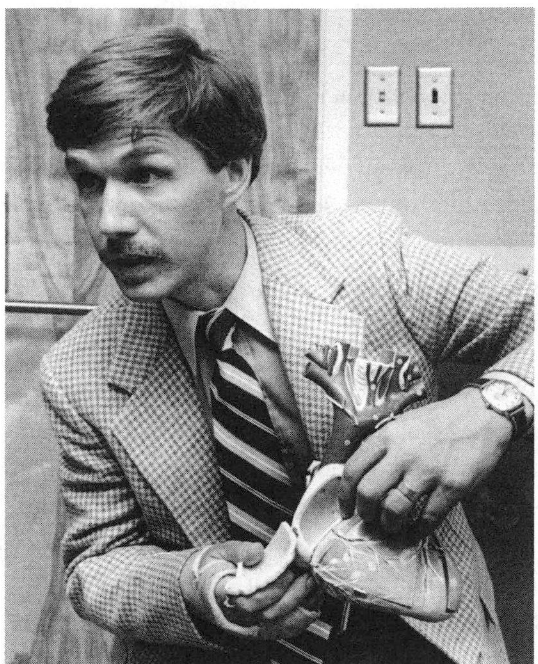

LDS Hospital cardiologist Dr. Jeff Anderson.

going downhill," Anderson said. DeVries later recalled, "I didn't even know his name at that time; I only knew that he was a dentist from Seattle and he had end-stage cardiomyopathy."

In October the Clarks arrived as expected and made arrangements to call on the surgeon. Immediately they ran into a chronic problem at the medical center. There was no parking near the entrance. Barney and Una Loy finally found an open space in the lot's far corner. They had to walk the length of about two football fields just to get to the door. In Salt Lake's 4,700-foot-high altitude, the trip was exhausting for Barney. He had to stop often, exhaling hard through pursed lips to force additional oxygen into lungs clogged with fluid by his failing heart, compounded with emphysema. Una Loy offered to get him a wheelchair.

When he said, "No," she was not surprised. Resorting to a wheelchair, for him, was tantamount to saying he was giving in to the disease. Fortunately elevators were nearby, but then it was another six hundred feet down a long corridor to the cardiothoracic unit. Grit in slow motion, Barney made his way, halting frequently to rest wherever a chair was available.

It took a half hour to get from the Clarks' parked car to DeVries's suite. His secretary, Renee Thomas, had booked the appointment and was astounded. She had pictured Barney arriving on a stretcher. "Do you mean you walked all that way?" she marveled.

DeVries was not in. A common joke in the medical center had it that the surgeon was late for everything except surgery. An hour passed, and Barney became visibly uncomfortable. "Honey," said Una Loy, "I think we had better go."

"Well, I would, except it was so hard to get here..." Barney replied. They came that close to giving up any thoughts of an artificial heart. They had decided to leave when a man walked in wearing a doctor's white coat. He saw Una Loy's distressed expression and asked if he could help. She told him they'd had an appointment with Dr. DeVries to talk about the artificial heart.

"I'm Dr. Lyle Joyce, Dr. DeVries's assistant," he told them. "Let's go in here and talk." He explained that earlier in the day, he had performed cardiac bypass surgery on DeVries's stepfather and he supposed the surgeon had forgotten the appointment in his concern for his family member.

Joyce gave the Clarks a bare-bones outline of the heart project. He was intimately familiar with the experimentation that was going on, having served as DeVries's or Dr. Don Olsen's second in many of the animal implants. Earlier in his career, he had worked as a student for a summer in the artificial-heart laboratory of another researcher, Dr. Michael DeBakey, in Houston, Texas. This experience had convinced him that the artificial heart had no prospects for success, but his faith was restored when he joined the Utah research group. He was eager to assist DeVries in the first trial with a human being if the right patient became available. He invited the Clarks to return the next day to visit with DeVries.

The Clarks retraced the half-hour walk to their car. The following day, they ignored a "restricted area" sign to park close to the medical center's entrance "Let 'em give me a ticket," Barney said. "I'll pay the fine."

DeVries was in his office. At six feet, five inches, he was rail thin and laid back, gaunt as Lincoln with deep-set eyes and high cheekbones. At thirty-nine, his youthfulness was accentuated by a clump of sandy hair. Like one of Norman Rockwell's rural family doctors who graced old *Saturday Evening Post* covers, he worked at a rolltop desk. Because of his height, he did not so much sit in his swivel chair as drape himself in it.

DeVries was well aware of the less-than-scholarly picture he presented. In one instance, when he was lavishly introduced during a Kiwanis meeting, he responded, "It's like taking the family pig to the fair. You can wash him up and put a ribbon on him, but he's still just a pig." It was easy to be fooled by what his mother called his "Clem Kadiddlehopper" image. Behind it, however, was a fierceness to excel in both mind and spirit. Being average was not good enough for DeVries. He hungered to be the best and was not afraid to travel to medicine's horizon—and beyond—if the opportunity presented itself.

He told the Clarks about the years of animal experimentation that had prepared the Utah team for the ultimate test of the device they had nurtured. He pointed to a picture on his office wall of one of his sons with a fawn-spotted Jersey calf. Named Tennyson by a poetry-loving researcher, the calf had lived 268 days with an artificial heart, dying only when he outgrew it.

Barney wanted to know how many animal implants DeVries had done. "One hundred, 150?" he asked. DeVries replied that the number had not been so large. "We'd know a lot more if the animals could talk," he said.

"Sounds to me like you've done all you can do, and now you are ready to put the heart in someone," Barney mused. "I think that would be a very rewarding thing to be involved in."

DeVries held up his hand. "We don't want anyone to undergo the surgery for that reason," he said. Mere curiosity or even pure altruism was not enough to make the potential benefit worth the risk. "We're not encouraging anyone," DeVries emphasized.

"Don't get me wrong," Barney responded. "I don't mean to indicate that I am completely philanthropic. Of course, I would hope to receive some benefit from the artificial heart."

DeVries persisted, "There are a lot of unknowns."

"I realize that. But still it would be a nice opportunity to do this for medical science," Barney said.

DeVries pressed on, determined to be as candid as possible. He explained that an evaluation committee would have to interview any potential candidate. The committee would have to certify that the artificial heart was the patient's sole alternative to death. The candidate would have to undergo a rigorous investigation to prove he and his family had the emotional resources to withstand the stresses the artificial heart would bring to their lives. He would have to live near the university. Significantly, unless the Food and Drug Administration approved a portable unit then under development, the patient would be tethered by two six-foot lines to a 375-pound cart that carried the compressed air mechanism to drive the heart. There was something else. No one could guarantee that the patient would ever come off the operating table alive. It was as realistic a portrait as DeVries could paint.

The Clarks were invited to visit the nearby animal lab in the old St. Mark's Hospital complex. They arrived just as a surgical team headed by Dr. Don Olsen, the veterinarian in charge of the research lab, had just completed implanting a pneumatically powered artificial heart in a calf. The animal had not yet been put in a recovery cage and was lying on the operating-room table—the worst time to see a surgical patient.

Olsen invited the Clarks in. He had known for some time that Barney was a potential recipient of the Utah-developed heart. The visitors watched as the calf was lifted into a recovery cage; then they visited the lab's manufacturing area, where they saw hearts in various stages of assembly. They continued to the animal holding area. Five calves with artificial hearts were standing eating hay or lying quietly in cages. "Calf sitters" had just placed one animal on a treadmill for exercise. The visitors were impressed.

The Clarks had some very pointed questions. Barney's Seattle cardiologist, Dr. Jeffrey Block, had accompanied them to Salt Lake City, and he joined in the lengthy discussions. Finally, with many thanks to Olsen and his colleagues, the group left the lab.

Earl Selby, in one of his extensive interviews with DeVries, asked the surgeon about his impressions of Barney Clark after the visit to the animal lab. "He [Barney] was very impressed," DeVries said. "He said, 'I hope I will not need this, but I think I will come to it sooner or later. It might be something I would be interested in doing. Why not? Doesn't hurt to investigate.' He realized that he was getting worse and going downhill fast."

Selby also asked DeVries's opinion of Una Loy. "Barney was the dominant one. He was just a tremendously happy, friendly, likable guy. But Una Loy felt that she could support him, and she was in it with him," DeVries said.

The seed had been planted, but the Clarks' decision was still in the future. "They didn't paint us any rose garden," Barney commented as the couple drove into Emigration Canyon east of Salt Lake City. The canyon was significant to these former Utahns. It was through this narrow defile in the Wasatch Mountains that thousands of Mormon pioneers had poured into the Salt Lake Valley in the mid-1800s, including their ancestors. They thought about those early pioneers and wondered if they might become modern-day successors.

Back in the Clarks' Seattle-area home, perched on a small bluff above Puget Sound, life started to go downhill. The grandfather clock chimed the hours as usual, but now it seemed to be ticking off the moments Barney had left. The cardiomyopathy was tightening its hold on him. When he ate, he vomited. His lungs, kidneys, and liver were acutely malnourished. He was constantly short of breath, and despite the thirty-plus pills he was required to take daily, he sometimes could barely raise an arm. "It's a fatigue you can't imagine," he told Una Loy.

His mental performance nosedived, a painful process to watch for Una Loy, who recalled how sharp he had been. Barney had been very business wise and could figure percentages and money easily in his head. Now he wrote numbers down and struggled with them. He used a calculator, which he had never done before. Despite his worsening condition, he taught Una Loy to look after the finances he had always managed.

The Clarks Jointly Decide

One day, when Barney had struggled to make his way to the couch in the den, Una Loy asked, "Honey, are you thinking about the artificial heart?"

"Well, yes. Are you?"

"I am," she said, leaning over to kiss him. The potential results of a move into unknown medical territory had become more concrete; now they were more personal. Barney was concerned that a decision to try the artificial heart would create a financial burden for them and their children. "If it is going to wipe out everything we have, I won't do it. I've worked too hard to leave you secure," he told Una Loy.

She put a practical face on it. "I don't think it would cost that much. And if it was a problem, I'd go to work like everybody else. I wouldn't be the first wife to do that," she said. She was less concerned about the financial effects than she was that some day she would walk into the den and find him dead. She watched in the evenings as he struggled to climb the eighteen steps of the circular staircase to the second floor. Exhausted, he flopped on their queen-size bed gasping for air. "Do you know what this feels like?" he panted. "Like a recently caught fish struggling in the bottom of a boat."

Determined to keep up with his golf buddies, Barney began using aerosol inhalers to enhance his breathing, not aware that the theophylline they delivered could possibly complicate his recovery after the epic surgery.

A dentist to the roots, he never failed to spend at least fifteen minutes each night cleaning his teeth. Some nights Una Loy said, "I'm just too pooped to clean mine." "Okay, you can sleep in the other room," Barney declared. "I'm not going to bed with a woman with dirty teeth." She brushed her teeth.

Every night they prayed—he on the bed, and Una Loy kneeling, holding his hand. Her plea was always the same: "Heavenly Father, please help us to make the right decision. To do the right thing. What would be best? Please help us know what to do."

Their children shared their burden and were willing to support any decision their parents made. "Dad's had enough medical training. He knows exactly where he's coming from physically," Stephen, a son who was himself a physician, told his wife. "He can diagnose his own feelings better than I can. He is nobody's fool."

By late November, the time had come to make a decision. Barney's heart was ready to quit, so the decision made itself. The Clarks contacted the heart team in Utah, who urged them to get Barney right to Salt Lake City. DeVries suggested they come by specially equipped air ambulance, but Barney would have none of that. He and Una Loy took a commercial flight south.

At Salt Lake International Airport, however, the media had already gathered. Barney and Una Loy were sneaked out of the airport and flown by helicopter east to the foothills, where the medical center snuggled into the Wasatch Mountains.

The Clarks had made their decision. Now a new set of decisions faced the little cluster of medical personnel gathered around the EKG monitor in the CICU. The conversation centered on one question—whether to wait until morning for the implant surgery or move more quickly lest the patient's heart quit on its own.

Fred Anderson already was there. DeVries, so tall he stood above his team members like a flagpole, stared at the V-tach printout, considered the fifty-four seconds it represented, and knew the duration was ominous. On the monitor, new—but shorter—bursts were visible. "We could lose him," DeVries said. There were drugs to jolt the heart out of irregular beating, but could Barney's heart stand the shock? If nothing was done, any one of those uncontrolled bursts of V-tach could trigger deadly ventricular fibrillation, and the heart would degenerate into such chaotic quivering that it would arrest.

Barney had been in the medical center for two days already. After his admission, DeVries had delayed surgery for sixty hours to warrant that the patient was a proper candidate and allow ample time for signing the requisite permissions. Also medical issues had to be sorted out. Barney's system had chemical imbalances, some of them related to heavy doses of anticoagulation drugs administered to keep his blood thin. They could cause uncontrolled bleeding during and after surgery.

The balance was agonizingly tricky. On the other hand, "We might lose him," DeVries repeated. It was a hard decision for this team that had prepared for surgery but not for these complications.

PART TWO

3

Willem Kolff's Story

Extreme remedies are most appropriate for extreme diseases.

—Hippocrates

A Pioneer in the Making

The road to workable artificial organs was long and rutted with potholes. Traversing it meant first of all altering long-held perceptions about the human body. Pioneers then faced unknown challenges that seemed destined to stymie introducing "foreign substances" into those bodies. Some scientists added a single strand to an unfolding tapestry; others wove large blocks into it.

One of these was Willem Johan Kolff, whose lifelong dedication to finding replacement parts for the human body justified his title of father of artificial organs. Whether as the primary researcher or the motivator for countless others, his efforts contributed to the ongoing design and development of artificial kidneys, hearts, lungs, eyes, ears, and arms. Kolff's contributions to the heart-lung bypass machine were also crucial to surgery on these organs.

Father and Son

Kolff's feet were set on the road to developing artificial organs when he was a boy in the Netherlands and listened to his physician father, Jacob Kolff, voice his frustrations when patients died despite his best efforts. The younger Kolff determined to follow in his father's footsteps and improve the odds of patients like these.

One frustrating case Jacob Kolff described to his son involved a young woman who was a patient in the Apeldoorn sanatorium where he worked. She suffered from tuberculosis. For four years, he had been treating her with drugs and bed rest, but everything had failed. Surgery was his last resort. Outfitting his automobile as a makeshift ambulance, he drove her to the hospital in nearby

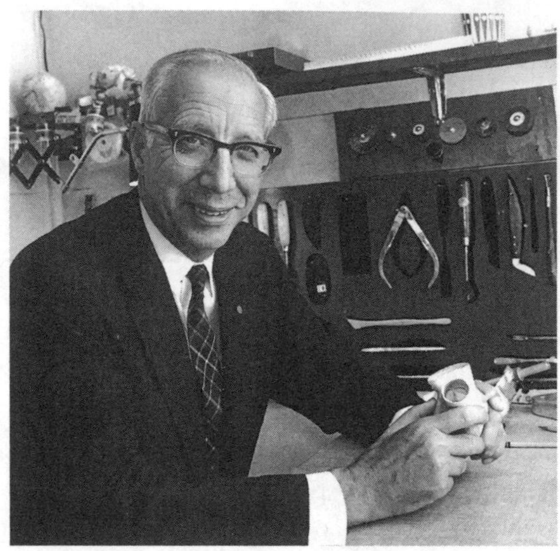

Dr. Willem J. Kolff was noted worldwide as the father of artificial organs.

Leiden and stayed with her in the operating room. That night he drove home disheartened, feeling again that he had failed his patient. Several days later, he went on a walk with nine-year-old Willem, known as Pim.

The two of them often walked through the woods near their comfortable home on the sanatorium grounds. Usually Kolff talked about the plants and trees, gratified that Pim knew every one by name. Sometimes, though, he talked about his patients.

On this particular afternoon, Dr. Kolff was anguished about the woman he had taken to Leiden. Pim saw the tears in his father's eyes. "Suffering, so much suffering," his father lamented. Pim had come to know how much the patients mattered to his father, and he understood that many of them died from their tuberculosis. That was the part of medicine Pim did not like. He could not, he decided, become a doctor; doctors were always too close to death.

That year—1920—Pim decided to become a zookeeper. He had been raising sheep and rabbits and kept caged crows, magpies, and parakeets. After two years, his father asked him, "Do you know how many zoos there are in Holland?" Pim did not. "Three," his father said. "If you studied biology to become a zookeeper, you probably would not become one. You would probably have to take a job teaching science in a high school. Is that what you want?"

A few days later, Pim told his father, "I don't like the dying, but I want to become a doctor like you." A commitment went with those words: becoming a doctor in his father's image meant really caring for patients.

At sixteen, Pim was in the gymnasium, the school for youngsters bound for advanced education. He was not an outstanding student, but he was good in science. Out of school, he was bright, handy, and ingenious. When earthenware fragments in a local field were upturned by plows, Pim helped pinpoint them as remnants of an ancient culture. His shard collection was accepted by a local museum. On Saturday afternoons, he worked with a carpenter because he wanted to learn the craft. Sawing, using the plane, hammering, and chiseling, Pim showed he had good hands.

Pim liked girls and was smitten with a young lady whose family had recently moved from Java. Restricted by the customs of small-town Holland in the 1920s, he could not just ask her for a date. He had to be formally introduced. The mechanics of arranging that were solved with the arrival of another family from Java, the Huidekopers, who had two daughters and a son. When he met the son, Pim immediately invited him to play tennis on the Kolff court, figuring he probably knew the girl Pim liked. The boy asked, "Can I bring my sister, Janke?"

"Of course," said Pim, not caring if he brought the Dutch army as long as he arranged the meeting Pim wanted. But once Pim met Janke, he was captivated and lost all desire to meet the other girl.

Janke

Janke Cornelia Huidekoper was long legged and had soft blonde hair and azure eyes. Her mother had died when she was six, and she had grown up in a fine house in Java, where her father was a trader in copra, rubber, and quinine. Janke (pronounced yawn-ka) laughed often, loved dancing, and played adult-level bridge. Learning to cook, clean a room, or make a bed was not for her. She thought it was much more important to have fun.

When Janke was thirteen, her father moved the family to his native Holland, intending to establish a large egg hatchery. Soon after Janke met Pim, she learned about his penchant for persistence. Though he was in the gymnasium, he came to her high school for chemistry and physics. Almost every day when she finished her classes, he was waiting to escort her home. Boys were not a high priority for Janke, and she made it plain she did not care if Pim was there or not. However, he waited every day; he had a hard time accepting the word "no."

For her part, Janke had to admit she liked Pim's looks. "Not that he is handsome," she explained to friends, but his narrow face and Roman nose made his features interesting to her. Eventually it just became natural for her to be with Pim.

Janke was shocked when she met Pim's family. In her home, people were lighthearted. They told jokes, played charades, and indulged in impish humor. The Kolffs were not at all like that; they were serious.

In addition to Pim and Dr. Kolff, there were four other sons and Mrs. Kolff, to whom the motherless Janke paid particular attention. Mrs. Kolff sat ramrod straight, head high, chin outthrust in what Janke thought was a queenly posture. Mrs. Kolff did not tolerate the word "no," a quality she had passed on to Pim. He worshipped her and would do anything to please her. She expected her sons to have high goals and work hard. There was no time for frivolity. New Year's Eve was an example. Everybody dressed up and then quietly sat in the living room reading books.

Janke could see why Pim adored his mother. She provided the children with the confidence of someone who always knew exactly what to say and do. Gradually Janke came to depend on her as well, doing what she asked and accepting what she said without question. "Janke," she said to herself, "Pim's mother is turning you into a Kolff."

On March 18, 1932, Pim and Janke became engaged. Both were students in Leiden, she to become a medical technician and Pim to attend the Leiden University medical school where his father had studied.

As soon as their studies were completed, the impatient Pim urged, "Let's get married."

"No," Janke said.

"Why not?"

"Not until I know we have a home. You will finish your schooling and go off for training in a hospital. You will have to live there, and I will never get to see you. That's not the way I want to live."

This time his persistence had met its match. Occasionally she went to his rooms, but she brought her textbooks with her. From experience she knew that Pim would be studying, too. He could sit for hours with the whole world blotted out as he concentrated on medicine.

In 1937 Janke took a sabbatical from Pim. She went to southern France, where she could learn patois French. Her landlady, an amateur graphologist, saw an envelope Pim had addressed. "What interesting handwriting," she commented. "This writer is someone who has the craziest, wildest ideas."

"Read my handwriting," Janke prompted.

The landlady studied a sample and concluded, "You are afraid to do something new. Yet, after you do, you always come out all right." There was some truth in that, Janke decided, and she returned to Leiden.

Late in the summer of 1937—during his seventh year of medical school—Pim learned that he could do his internal-medicine training at the University Medical Center Groningen. Calling Professor Polak Daniels, Groningen's head of medicine, Pim asked, "If I am accepted, would I have to live in the hospital?"

"Certainly not," replied the professor.

That night Pim told Janke, "All right now we can get serious." She agreed. In September they were married. While Pim finished his last months of medical school, their first home was on a nearby summer-resort beach. That fall and winter they had the beach to themselves. If Pim got too serious, she rumpled his hair, grabbed and wrestled with him, and tickled him and made him laugh. It was a lovely honeymoon.

Of Death and Birth

The ward in the University Medical Center Groningen was large and old-fashioned. Twenty or more beds lined its walls. Portable screens shielded the very sick, placed near the door. In October 1938, Pim, the youngest doctor in the ward, was assigned to four patients. One was behind a screen. At twenty-seven, the young doctor had a soldier's bearing; his head was erect and his flaxen hair cut short. His imposing image softened when he looked out from behind his horn-rimmed glasses and let his light blue eyes twinkle.

Pim made his daytime rounds, then came back to the ward in the early evening when it was peaceful. The sole island of light at the nurse's desk in the center of the room was a lamp with a dark green glass shade. Pim liked to sit there reading his patients' charts and thinking.

This particular night Pim was forcing himself to study the situation of the patient behind the screen, whose urine output was almost zero. He was vomiting and had staggeringly high blood pressure and shattering headaches. Blindness was rapidly closing in. This was all because the two bean-shaped kidneys in the back of his lower abdomen had virtually shut down and were no longer purging the blood of poisons such as urea and creatinine.

This was a compelling moment unlike any Pim had ever experienced. Instinctively he knew that his patient was going to die, and there was nothing that he—or indeed the whole body of medical knowledge—could do to save him. He was moved to tears when he realized that because his patient's body lacked the ability to drain its normal daily output of twenty grams of urea, he would die. Pim felt it was dreadfully unfair, mirroring his father's earlier frustrations.

The young man's mother came to the hospital. Pim's heart went out to her. Aware of what losing her only son meant, Pim told her the truth in the gentlest way he could. He felt helpless and wondered why he could not remove urea from the blood of this young patient and others like him.

Pim and Janke had a small house five minutes from the hospital. Because Janke was pregnant, Pim's mother visited them late that year to assure that the cradle, linens, and nursing arrangements were prepared. Janke was a nervous mother-to-be, and when she told her doctor she thought she was ready to deliver, he scolded her, "Your baby is due in two weeks, not today!"

That evening Pim and Janke went to the movies. Within hours the baby started coming. "You have got to help us," Pim told his mother.

She was dubious. "I might faint. I have never seen this before," she protested.

"Mother," Pim all but shouted, "you have to. Where are the scissors?" he asked Janke. She pointed to a drawer. He sterilized them over the kitchen stove's gas flame and asked for something to tie the umbilical cord. Janke said string and thread were in the sewing box. No anesthetic was available. They heated water and prepared cloths. That night Pim Kolff delivered his firstborn. He tied and cut the cord and wrapped his son to keep him warm. They named the baby Jacob after Pim's father. It was Janke's first glimpse of how organized and precise Pim was in a crisis.

The doctors at Groningen quickly perceived that young Kolff had a particular way of looking at disease. While in medical school, Pim had volunteered in the pathology lab. After doing postmortem examinations to determine the cause of death, he had snipped tissues from sick organs to examine under the microscope. The result was a road map to guide his diagnoses. "When I look at the sick," he told his Groningen peers, "I do not just think of a disease. I am concerned with anatomy. I see the sick organ as it is in the body: where it is, what it does, what happens when it does not function. I see the cells as I have seen them under the microscope. I put them all together, and then I know what I must do."

He had an image of the kidneys, the organs that pack up to sixty miles of little tubes connected to the glomeruli to filter blood impurities and discharge them in urine. He understood that no one could replicate everything the kidneys did, but why couldn't someone create a device to stop urea from killing people? He was thinking about that when the university's biochemistry professor, R. Brinkman, who had taken a liking to him, invited him to see something that had been imported from Germany. It was a sausage skin, but not just any sausage skin. It was made from cellophane! To Pim's astonishment, the professor demonstrated that the cellophane could filter out chemical particles.

Back in his own rooms, Pim knotted one end of a cellophane sausage skin, poured in blood, added urea powder, and knotted the other end. He tied the skin to a stick so he could immerse it in a saline solution and rocked it for thirty minutes. The blood was intact, but testing showed that the urea was gone! All of it had passed through the cellophane into the saline fluid, but the blood's molecules were too large to escape. Excited, Pim vowed that the young man in the Groningen ward had not died in vain. His death had opened the door to determining the way blood could be purified when the kidneys no longer worked.

Pim bought a generous supply of cellophane sausage skin, tantalized by the idea of creating a machine to do the work of the kidneys. Tackling such a task seemed impossible. Medical textbooks told despairing stories of researchers trying and failing to meet this challenge. Twenty-five years earlier, three Americans had invented an artificial kidney using dialysis to pass chemicals from one solution to another. They and those who followed could strain about two grams of urea from blood a day, only about a tenth of what would make their devices clinically useful.

Pim's solution was breathtakingly simple: build a machine that exposed enough blood for long enough to get rid of its poisons. He was aware that taking blood out of the body was courting danger. How could he be absolutely sure it would not clot? How could a machine keep the blood circulating while impurities were strained out? He addressed the blood-clotting problem by utilizing one of the serendipitous mistakes that mark medicine's landscape. In the United States, researchers at Johns Hopkins University had sought a drug to promote blood clotting to heal wounds. Instead, what they extracted from the lungs and livers of animals was a chemical that did exactly the opposite: heparin, the first true, laboratory-created anticoagulant. The researchers thought they had failed, but in reality they had stumbled onto one of the twentieth-century's greatest medical discoveries.

Pim was one of the first Europeans to request heparin from the United States to use in experiments. He realized that heparin was the magical ingredient to let him remove blood from the body, cleanse it, and return it with little fear of clotting. However, there was no artificial kidney machine anywhere in the world to purchase or replicate; he had to create one. His preliminary calculations of how long a cellophane tube he needed to strain twenty grams of urea out of the blood stunned Pim: almost a hundred feet! Where would he get the space? Did the tube have to be in a straight line? Could it be wrapped around a drum? He began to tinker with what he called his "apparatus."

Other doctors mocked him for wasting time on contraptions that were failures. Stubbornly, Pim ignored them. What drove him was the memory of that young man dying in the ward while he helplessly stood by. Pim did have one supporter—the only one that mattered, Professor Daniels, the medical chief who had told him he did not have to live in the hospital. Brushing aside staff criticism, Daniels said, "He has an idea. Who can know, now, if it is right or wrong? Let him continue." Pim said to Janke, "He does not make you think as he does. He lets you think for yourself. That is how research should be."

Pim used his small salary at the hospital to pay for his experiments, leaving the problem of providing food for their table and a roof over their heads to Janke, who contributed the dividends from quinine plantation stock she had inherited.

Invasion

As spring approached in 1940, the Nazis ramped up to conquer Europe. To mobilize its small army, the Dutch government called up thousands of men, including reserve-officer physicians, which left many small villages and towns without doctors. Pim was sent to another area as the internal-medicine physician. He arrived with strong ideas about the way medicine should be practiced. The director of the local hospital—a surgeon—had his own ideas. The ensuing clash of wills rattled enough windows that both were summoned before the hospital's board of directors. The showdown ended with the decision that Pim should return to Groningen.

After the meeting, however, the board's chairman sought out Pim. "I liked you in the meeting today. We are looking for an internist. Would you be interested?" he asked the young doctor.

"I don't know. I think I want to be in medicine with a university," Pim replied.

"Well, think about it," the bürgermeister said.

On May 9, 1940, the Kolffs left their young son in the care of a maid and took a train to The Hague for Janke's grandfather's funeral. The next day the Nazis invaded Holland. From the roof of the grandfather's house, Pim and Janke watched the German Luftwaffe dropping leaflets calling for surrender while the Dutch threw up flak against the airplanes. At one point, bullets spattered close to them.

Pim skipped the funeral and went to the local city hospital, where he knew some of the doctors. "With the invasion on, do you have a blood bank?" he asked. The officials said they did not. In fact, all of Europe had no blood bank. Undaunted, Pim told them, "With the war, there will be bombings. The injured will need blood. I have worked with blood. We will start a blood bank."

He made it seem so logical that the officials agreed. They gave him a car, a driver, and a soldier guard and authorized him to buy anything he needed at government expense. He returned with needles, rubber tubing, cotton, vials, and chemicals. Within four days, he had the blood bank in operation, stocked with more than eighty pints of blood.

That night the nearby city of Rotterdam was hit with incendiary bombs, and Pim's blood supply helped save lives. Although the Dutch government surrendered the next day, hospital officials were so impressed with the blood bank they decided to continue it. They did, however, ask Pim where he had learned how to start one since there were none in Europe. The answer indicated Pim's self-confidence. He had read of a blood bank at Chicago's Hospital of Cook County and decided that "if they can do it there, we can do it here."

Back in Groningen, the Kolffs found their young son safe but learned of a tragedy involving Pim's hospital ally, Professor Daniels. When the Nazi paratroopers had breached Holland's ancient Water-Line barrier, he and his wife had committed suicide. The Nazis appointed a Dutch sympathizer to replace Daniels, creating a moral dilemma for Pim. "I will not work under a National Socialist, ever," he declared to Janke, but he had months to go before completing his training at the hospital. Nights later he told Janke, "The good Lord has intervened. The National Socialist will not be coming for a while. He has tuberculosis." It took the Nazi sympathizer six months to convalesce, time for Pim to become certified in internal medicine. The day before the man reported for work, Pim resigned from University Medical Center Groningen.

Kampen

Pim, Janke, and their two children moved to Apeldoorn to stay with his parents. Pim told Janke he was "thankful to have a father who can afford to take in an unemployed son and his family." In early 1941, a letter arrived from the bürgermeister of Kampen. The Kampen Municipal Hospital was holding a competition for an internal-medicine director. Was Pim interested? He said yes but boldly announced he would take the position only with significant conditions: if he was in charge, if he had a staff, if he had a laboratory, if he had new X-ray diagnostic equipment, and if he could continue his research on his artificial kidney machine.

For an out-of-work doctor, this was very demanding, especially since he was the youngest of nine applicants. But Pim knew the city was competing with nearby, larger Zwolle and argued that "with this staff and equipment, Kampen can have internal medicine that is the equal of your neighbors in Zwolle." The bürgermeister and hospital officials gave him the job.

In some ways, Kampen—home to twenty-three thousand people—was an odd place for Pim to start his practice. With a town hall dating to 1278, its glories seemed to be in the past. In the late fifteenth century, it was Holland's largest city, but changing riverbeds eventually blocked access to the ocean. Now it was a little backwater community on the IJssel River, about fifty miles northeast of Amsterdam. Moreover, nineteenth-century writers had named it "the city of fools" based on a legend that the vanes of a large windmill hit people in the head and knocked them permanently silly.

Kampen exuded a quaint air. Its gates were stained with rust. On its narrow cobblestone streets, *klompen* (wooden shoes) could still be seen and heard. The town tower overshadowed its small buildings. The Germans essentially left Kampen alone. It was not strategic enough to merit a large occupation force.

On the surface, Pim was just a young doctor in town, pursuing his own experiments and causing no trouble for the Nazi occupiers. In fact, he was part of a group of resistance fighters who did whatever they could to harass the Germans. He later related that he was approached by an underground band that wanted to steal more than 125,000 ration cards from the Nazi distribution depot. "We're hiding Jewish families in homes all over," the underground leader said. "We need the ration cards to get food for them." The Dutch night guard at the depot was willing to cooperate but only if it looked as though he had been drugged and was unable to prevent the theft. Pim provided ether and showed the men how to use it. Soon after, the depot was "cracked," and the ration cards were stolen.

On other occasions, Pim gave injections to induce physical symptoms that prevented his countrymen from being deported to Germany to work in labor gangs. He secretly treated prisoners fleeing the Nazis and worked with a network of reliable doctors in other towns.

Frustrated in attempts to capture a patriot living near the Kolffs, the Nazis said they would strip the man's house of all its furniture and clothing if he did not surrender by the following noon. In the predawn hours, Janke and others hid the household goods in their homes, so, when the Nazis came, the house was empty. But Nazi spies exposed Janke and her friends. "If everything is not returned," the Nazis threatened, "we'll take all your furniture."

The group then went from door to door collecting old furniture to put in the patriot's home. The Nazis were fooled and called in trucks to haul off the junk, presumably to ship it to Germany. Janke told Pim with great satisfaction, "This has been our finest hour."

The Machine

In the nine-bed Kampen Municipal Hospital, Kolff lined up his staff, consisting of a medical assistant and some nurses and technicians, to do blood analyses around the clock and keep the equipment repaired. He also picked out a room for his thirteenth kidney experiment. Figuring he had enough odds against him without bucking superstition, he renumbered the experiment 12A. The room had a bed, a blackboard to jot notations, and space for a kidney machine and supplies. Pim had developed his plans for this machine, but where could he get it built with war casting a wide shadow?

Hendrik Th. J. Berk, principal director of the Kampen Enamel Works was, to put it mildly, astonished when the town's new doctor approached him, saying: "I'd like you to build me an artificial kidney."

Berk had never heard anything so outrageous. He asked, "What is an artificial kidney?" Pim told him it was a device that—if perfected—would help their countrymen live. He pointed out that everybody knew someone whose kidneys had failed. Pim said all he wanted was a "little help" in making a machine to do the kidney's work.

"How do you do that?" asked Berk.

Pim replied, "You take a barrel-like drum with about a hundred feet of cellophane casing spiraling around it. Put in an axle to rotate the drum. Then suspend it over a small, bathtub-sized tank of water with the bottom half of the drum submerged."

Berk found Pim persuasive. With materials shortages, his plant was hardly running full blast. "We'll do it," he told Pim. The Nazis did not discover the machine. Moreover, because Berk had orders to build nothing except for the German Wehrmacht, he kept the project off the books. It was the first of Pim's many contributions from industry.

When the machine was finally delivered in late 1942, Pim eagerly began experimenting, seeking the right chemicals to add to the water solution in the tank to filter out urea and other impurities without robbing the blood of vital salts and minerals. Blood was fed in at one end of the cellophane tubing wrapped around the machine's aluminum drum. The lower part of the drum and its tubing were submerged in water. As the drum rotated, blood moved to the cellophane tube's other end, pulled by gravity to the bottom of the rotating drum where the impurities passed into the water, leaving the blood pure.

In the early models, leaks developed where the cellophane tubing connected to rubber tubes that brought the blood in and out. Pim recalled that Henry Ford, the indomitable American auto designer, had perfected connections for his cars' water pumps. He visited the local Ford dealer to see how workers controlled dripping and borrowed the technique for his kidney machine. Pim then put blood doctored with urea and other chemicals into the cellophane tubing and let it run through the machine. Just as with the cellophane sausage skin that he had rocked by hand in water at Groningen, the urea was removed from the blood! The machine worked in the laboratory; would it function with live human beings?

The hospital, centerpiece of the Kolffs' lives, was a collection of low-slung old buildings. Sometimes Janke read a book while waiting for her husband to finish his work. Pim was building his practice and had to do his own X-rays and analyze the lab findings. It was absorbing work for the young doctor but not enough. At day's end, he headed for his unpaid job, the kidney machine.

One night he stopped at the bed of an aged patient in a coma who had, among other problems, a severe kidney ailment. Convinced the man was only hours from death, Pim had him moved to the special room. "He has nothing to lose," he told his nurse. "There is no harm in trying dialysis." Pim administered heparin to keep the patient's blood from clotting and then withdrew blood with a hypodermic syringe to run through his machine. He started the motor to get the aluminum drum rotating in the tank's water; suddenly, the motor stopped.

Since the blood was already in the machine, there was no time to investigate the problem. "Janke, you have to crank!" Pim ordered. Janke grabbed the hand crank on the drum and began turning it, trying to duplicate the motor's speed of twenty-six revolutions a minute. She continued cranking for almost twenty minutes. Finally, the blood was treated. Pim reinjected it into the patient.

There was no apparent change in the old man's condition. Did that mean the machine was a failure? Or had he simply purified too small an amount of blood to make a difference? There was no way of knowing, but at least he had demonstrated he could successfully remove blood, run it through his machine, and return it to the patient.

However, something unexpected occurred. When he removed the blood from the patient's veins, it was dirty blue, but when it came out of his machine, it had turned bright red, a dramatic change. That proved that he had found a way to perfuse blood with oxygen! Someday, he realized, this unplanned bonus might be useful.

A twenty-nine-year-old housemaid in Zwolle had dangerously high blood pressure of 245 over 150. Hemorrhages and edema in both eyes had stolen most of her sight. Blood oozed from her nose, and she vomited daily. Her breath smelled of urine, and her heart was enlarged with audible murmurs. The diagnosis was chronic nephritis with uremia: deadly kidney failure resulting in massive amounts of urea backing up into her body. Her doctor had heard of Pim's experiments with an artificial kidney. Satisfied she had nothing to lose and might enjoy a brief reprieve, the doctor got approval from her father to let Pim try dialysis.

"What is it you do?" the father, a farmer, asked Pim. In plain language, Pim explained the procedure.

"Will it help?"

"I do not know," replied Pim. Her father gave permission, providing the local minister could visit first.

On March 17, 1943, Pim added heparin to the girl's blood. She experienced chills, then a fever, but nothing else happened. There was no systemic shock from the heavy dose of injected anticoagulant. Her body had given him a signal to begin. Pim withdrew fifty milliliters of blood with his hypodermic syringe, let it flow through his machine, and replaced it. He continued until a half liter of blood was cleansed. When he finished, there was no change. The next day the patient's urea level increased. Pim tried another dialysis that night. No difference. The urea level rose again the following day. Was it possible he was wrong about dialysis? He refused to accept that possibility. He tried dialysis again, then two more times.

This time serious complications occurred. On the tenth day, the woman developed inflammation of the sac surrounding her heart. With her heparin-thinned blood, nosebleeds became so severe that she required repeated cauterizations. Tympanitis, an ear inflammation, spewed pus through her Eustachian tubes into her throat, causing more vomiting.

Other doctors and researchers might have retreated, unwilling to risk further complications, but how could Pim give up when he felt that he could give her a chance to live? He analyzed the few slender reasons to bolster hope. This housemaid had not been expected to survive more than a day or two, yet here she was, still alive in her second week in the hospital. After the fifth dialysis, the urea level had dropped minutely, but even that small gain was a possible indication he had arrested the poison's upward spiral.

He ordered a sixth dialysis and again noted only a tiny decrease in the urea level. Until then he had taken her blood syringe by syringe, but clearly that was not enough to produce a dramatic change. He decided to insert cannulas directly into the patient's veins and let blood flow continuously in and out. His biggest worry was that air bubbles might invade the bloodstream to form lethal emboli or blood clots. His defense was a glass "bubble catcher."

Pim arranged the tubing to direct the blood through his machine. Everyone in the room was tense. It was uncertain if the resulting trauma might kill the patient. Up to that point, Pim and his staff had purified no more than 5.5 liters of blood a day. With the new method, he was able to treat 12 liters! "Now we wait," he said.

The first blood tests showed a startling improvement. The urea level had plunged. The woman was able to read a newspaper! The palling patina that comes over uremia victims disappeared from her face. With the increased routing of the blood, Pim's machine worked!

Unfortunately, her kidneys did not. When she was off the machine for several days, the urea level again mounted. Pim had to bring her back for more dialyses. With the next four procedures, he basically maintained the urea at a stable level. Then he ran out of fresh veins to puncture to remove her blood. She died, but as a result of Pim's dialysis, she had lived forty-two additional days. That was six weeks longer than anyone could have predicted.

Isolated as he was in the Nazi net, Pim could not know what was being printed in the important medical journals of England and America. Still, he wanted to share his work, thinking other doctors could explore it to aid their patients. He had no study where he could write; his desk was in the living room in front of the window. However, he displayed the same concentration Janke had seen in medical school. The children could be underfoot, climbing his chair, shouting and laughing, but he was undisturbed.

In 1943 a Dutch journal published Pim's article about his dialysis machine. To get wider circulation, he sent it to the distinguished Swedish journal, *Acta Scandinavica.* The editors were probably puzzled by the lack of scientific credentials for the man identified as the paper's second author. Grateful for the help of the Kampen Enamel Works, Pim had shared authorship with Hendrik Th. J. Berk. It was the free world's first evidence that thirty-three-year-old Dr. W. J. Kolff had pioneered a way to perform the kidney's work outside of the body; he had created an artificial kidney!

Pim knew what his machine could do, but for his peers to accept it, he needed a patient who was alive because of dialysis. He contacted other doctors in the Kampen area. "Send me your chronic uremia patients," he urged. "Let me try my machine on them." Agreeing that Pim probably could not hurt their dying patients, the doctors shipped them to him in a slow procession. The patients almost always arrived in a coma and on stretchers. Pim's machine didn't save any of them.

On top of everything else, the machine began acting up. The motor shorted out or overheated. The bubble catcher exploded in a shower of glass. Wartime shortages barred fresh supplies of rubber tubing. In desperation Pim began using glass cannulas. Immediately the blood started clotting in the glass, forcing him to add heparin constantly, not always certain if the blood would become too thin. Leaks in the cellophane tubing released blood into the dialyzing water, generating a huge balloon of red foam that frothed over the tank sides onto the floor and out into the hall. The bloody foam was a grisly sight.

Nevertheless, Pim pushed on, tantalized by temporary recoveries. In one case, the patient came out of his coma and announced, "I want to write a new will." He did. He died the next day, however. After about ten cases, Pim invited the area's leading doctors and government officials to watch a dialysis treatment, hoping to gain their support. It was a disaster. Midway in the demonstration, the horrified Pim saw that the cellophane was leaking. He and his assistants made repairs but not before the audience was treated to the gut-curdling sight of the patient's blood foaming up and spilling onto the floor.

For days Pim was depressed. Then, from his schoolboy past, he remembered William, Prince of Orange, considered the father of the Netherlands, who had led his country's rebellion against Spain. Heartened by Prince William's statements, "Even without hope you shall undertake. And without success you shall persevere," Pim reassessed his experiments. He was dealing with the chronically ill. Even if his machine did provide some relief, the patients' kidneys were all ravaged by long-term disease. What he had to do was switch his emphasis from the chronically ill to patients with acute kidney failure. With dialysis, he theorized, he could give their temporarily stricken kidneys a chance to recover.

Theory did not become reality, however, because Pim could not find the right case. A fifty-two-year-old government worker lived after being dialyzed, but Pim acknowledged that the man probably would have survived without the machine. A woman with acute kidney disease was treated, but she died of pneumonia. A young woman brought in for dialysis succumbed from the effects of an illegal abortion. By the middle of July 1944, Pim had treated fifteen men and women but could claim no living success stories.

The escalating war eclipsed his experiments. With the Allies' D-Day invasion in France, the Nazis rounded up thousands of Dutchmen to send to Germany to build fortifications. Many came through Kampen where Pim, as the Red Cross medical director, examined them. The Red Cross organized an eight-hospital network with more than a thousand beds to care for the "ailing" Dutchmen whom Pim retrieved from the convoys. Without arousing Nazi suspicions, he also selected some not-so-sick men who had been leaders in the Dutch underground.

Holland's liberation in 1945 ended the emergency network, and Pim was able to return to his duties at the Kampen Municipal Hospital. He built new kidney machines, but disappointment was his constant companion. His sixteenth case also died. Then a sixty-seven-year-old woman in prison became deadly ill

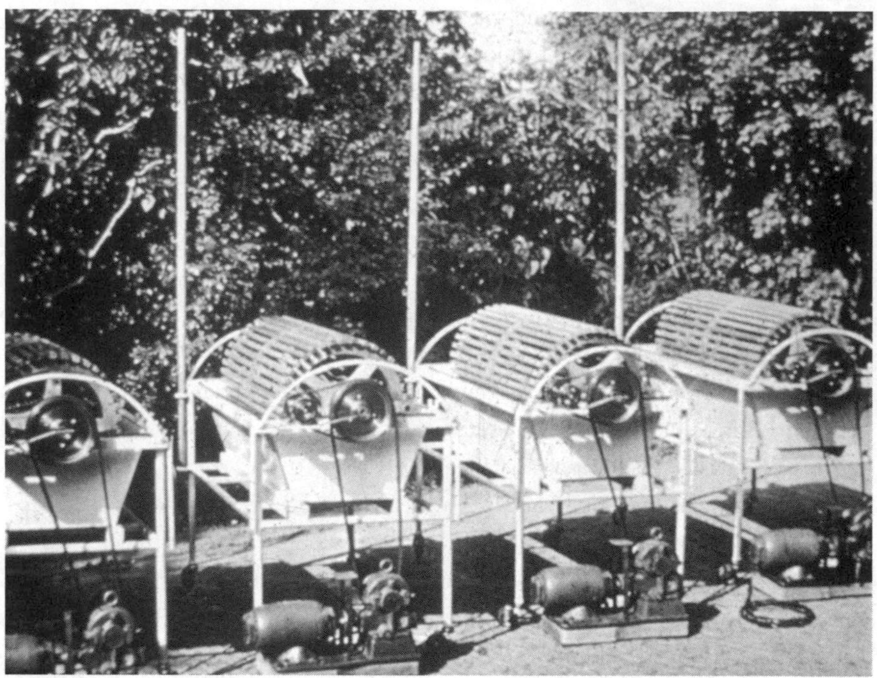

Artificial kidneys made secretly by Kolff and hidden during the World War II Nazi occupation.

of kidney problems. She was comatose, lying on her cot and snoring all day. Her jailers transferred her to the Kampen Municipal Hospital; some of them wanted her dead and hoped Pim would not treat her. A Nazi collaborator who had made many enemies during the war, she had been sentenced to a long prison term.

"I am a doctor. She is sick. What can I do? Of course I will treat her," Pim said. Standard therapies had accomplished nothing, so Pim put her on his machine. For eleven and a half hours, he kept blood flowing out of her body into the machine, then back into her veins, dialyzing eighty liters of blood. Sixty grams of urea—three times the amount normally created in the body daily—were removed. The woman woke up completely alert. She said, "Now I am going to divorce my husband," and she lived to do just that.

Rested and given time during dialysis to regenerate, her kidneys were once again normal. With her return to prison imminent, Pim was concerned that the guards would treat her cruelly. He appealed to an underground official he had befriended during the occupation: "I don't want this lady to die. She is the first person I have saved with the artificial kidney." The official made it possible for her to leave Kampen and live with a son hundreds of miles away, where she survived another six years before succumbing to a disease unrelated to her kidneys.

The Tourists

Pim was puzzled and disappointed. Doctors in the postwar world were paying no attention to his artificial kidney. Either they did not know about it, or they could not grasp its importance. This was intolerable. If the world would not come to him, he would go to the world by letting his kidney machines speak for him. He chose three prominent hospitals—London's Hammersmith, Montreal's Royal Victoria, and New York's Mt. Sinai—and donated a machine to each, suggesting they experiment with it. Eventually researchers at all three hospitals wrote scientific papers describing their work with dialysis. He told Janke, "They have proved that the kidney machine works in hands other than the Dutch."

With attention now beginning to focus on Pim, Dr. Isidore Snapper of New York's Mt. Sinai Hospital, a fellow Dutchman who had fled Holland before the Nazi invasion, wrote to say he could arrange a small lecture tour. When Pim and Janke arrived in New York, Snapper, as the tour's sponsor, said it was vital for Pim to make the best possible impression on the American doctors. He insisted Pim should go to his hotel room and write out his speech as a formal lecture. Pim later joked to Janke, "I know. He is worried because we are from Kampen, and he still believes that it is the city of fools."

The lecture went well, and in Boston Pim's words inspired doctors in Harvard's Peter Bent Brigham Hospital. Though he had no more kidney machines to give away, Pim carried blueprints, and Dr. Carl Walters built an artificial kidney. Pim felt that the Harvard doctors' testimony would be the best way to spread the word about the possibilities of his dialysis machine.

While Pim visited hospitals, Janke had her own tasks. Friends had given her lists and money to pay for an American shopping spree. Because there had been few new clothes during the war, the women needed dresses, coats, and undergarments. Janke spent her days in department-store bargain basements.

She and Pim never knew in advance how much he would receive for a lecture. Often when paying a hotel bill, she asked, "How much do we have?" The couple frequented restaurants where the entrees cost a dollar or less. They preferred places offering generous supplies of bread and butter. "We need quantity not quality," Janke explained. Hardly a meal went by without their asking for more bread, which she wrapped in paper napkins and slipped into her purse. The lean days of the war were firmly stamped into their memories.

In 1948 Pim returned to America to receive a prestigious award from the American Academy of Arts and Sciences. Janke worried their children might pay a price for Pim's growing fame. She was concerned he would be puffed up when he told the children about his big American award and the admiration of the American doctors. She said, "I cannot stand anyone who brags. Just behave naturally." Teasing, she added, "You are already silly enough."

Her mother-in-law told Janke, "You should speak with more respect."

Rather defiantly, Janke replied, "I have my own ideas. I am entitled to follow them." It was the first time she had ever contradicted Pim's mother. No one said any more, but Pim was restrained when he described his trip to America.

Blood, Bright Red

In America a Philadelphia doctor named John Gibbon was working in his Jefferson Medical College laboratory. Like Pim, he had been sidetracked into research by the haunting memory of his patients' deaths. The defining event for Gibbon had occurred at the Massachusetts General Hospital in 1931. Slowly and inexorably, a massive lung embolism was killing a patient. The only hope for successful surgery lay in being able to shut down the lungs and heart temporarily while the clot was excised, but there was no way to do that. Gibbon asked, "Why isn't there something that, for a short time, can carry a patient through this difficult period?"

He sketched out a design. Instead of blood from the veins returning to the heart, he wanted to divert it outside the body to a gas-exchange chamber—an oxygenator—where oxygen could flood the blood and strip it of poisonous carbon dioxide. The cleansed and nourished blood would then be fed into a mechanical pump to drive it back into the body and through the organs under pressure. The machine would perform the functions of the bypassed heart and lungs. On the surface, Gibbon's plan seemed no more difficult than an exercise in chemistry and physics. When Pim visited him in 1948, however, Gibbon was still struggling to develop a machine he could use on human beings.

Pim's reaction to Gibbon's work was direct: "There is a clinical need for the heart-lung machine, and it is not being met!" What attracted him was the enormous life-saving potential. He envisioned that a machine substituting temporarily for the heart and lungs would make it possible for surgeons to operate directly on the heart, something that currently was impossible. Pim decided he could create such a machine. He told his staff, "After all, who has more experience than we do in moving blood around outside the body?"

They began work with the mistaken notion that they had already met one challenge—creating the oxygenator. During his kidney experiments, Pim had repeatedly observed dark venous blood turn bright red, the consequence of oxygen passing through his cellophane tubing to revitalize the blood. However, when he did experiments to see how much oxygen actually flowed into the blood, he was disappointed to find it was not enough to match oxygen from the lungs. As an adequate oxygenator, his marvelous cellophane flunked.

He and a coworker, young physiologist C. P. Dubbleman, began to adapt a unit made in Sweden. As a youth, Pim had yearned to be a zookeeper. Now his work required him to use animals for experimentation, a somewhat discomforting prospect. "We will be humane," he assured his wife. His first adventures were with cows, chosen to test equipment able to handle at least five liters of blood a minute, the minimum supply for a human being. Gibbon and other experimenters had used two pumps in their machines: one to siphon blood out, the other to pump it back. Hoping to save money, Pim said, "I'll do it with just one."

In the Kampen slaughterhouse, he had a cow marched to a four-foot-high platform. With the animal strapped to a partition, technicians applied a local anesthetic and slit open the skin to insert cannulas into a vein and artery. The cow bellowed its unhappiness. With one galvanic shudder, it tore itself loose from its straps and jumped up, staring at Pim and the others with wild, rolling eyes. That was too much for the slaughterhouse's executioner. Drawing his gun, he shot the animal.

The research switched to calves and dogs, and the animals were anesthetized with sodium pentothal. One newly fed calf with a respirator on its tracheal tube could not belch, leaving it no way to expel the foul gas that fermentation was brewing in its rumen, the first of its four stomachs. The abdomen swelled gigantically. To keep it from exploding, the technicians punctured the rumen. People in the room immediately fled. "There's enough sour gas in there to light up the whole city of Rotterdam!" Pim laughed.

Pim and Dubbleman experimented with eighteen animals. They were successful with only one, a dog that recovered after the machine had done the work of its heart and lungs for forty-four minutes. Anxious to see if the dog's brain was intact, Pim offered it a cookie with his right hand. The dog spurned it. Then he remembered that in Holland, every well-trained dog learned to accept treats only from the left hand.

America Beckons

By late 1949, Pim's patients filled nearly every bed in the small Kampen Municipal Hospital. Amid grumblings among his coworkers that he was taking too much authority, Pim began to feel he had outgrown Kampen. To perfect the heart-lung machine, he needed a larger hospital with more resources and more skilled doctors, including cardiothoracic surgeons. He thought of going to the United States, even though Janke did not want to leave Holland. However, she was willing to go where her husband went.

In the United States, research hospitals were jammed with doctors trained on the military largesse of the G.I. Bill. An American friend suggested that Pim "write Page at the Cleveland Clinic. He may have some room." As it happened, Dr. Irving Page, the well-known head of the clinic's research staff, had recently received access to a building. There was space on the sixth floor that Pim could use if he chose to join the staff.

Pim accepted, but he told Janke, "I have to give up my independence to become a member of a team." To his old Groningen professor, Herr Brinkman, he wrote, "I will concentrate on developing the heart-lung machine, and I will leave the kidney to others."

Brinkman replied, "If you do not stay with the kidney machine, do not expect others to develop your invention." Pim thought that was good advice and packed all his dialysis data. Then he gathered up Janke and their five children and sailed to America.

4

Determination Gets Things Done

Kolff, if they just give you a chair, you'll make it.

—Dr. Isidore Snapper, Mt. Sinai Hospital

Interludes of the Heart[1]

No one knows when human beings first became aware of the heart. But twenty thousand or more years ago, an artist standing in Spain's El Pindal Cave drew what may be the first recorded suggestion of a heart.[2] Using fingers and an earthen paint, he or she sketched the outline of a giant mammoth. Below the left shoulder, the artist left a reddish splotch. It may be nothing more than the spot where the artist wiped paint from his finger. Perhaps it was intended to mark the target for a hunter's weapon. It is tempting to think of it as the earliest-known depiction of the heart.

Throughout history human beings have accepted one immutable law: when the heart beats, there is life; when it is still, there is death. Inevitably, a mystique grew around the heart. The oldest religions invoked it. Poets celebrated it. In their deepest psyches, humans thought of the heart as the font of love, courage, and compassion, the seat of the soul. Except for the most recent sliver of time, however, humanity has not known what the heart is or what it does.

In ancient China, medical men believed the heart was the seat of happiness and the beating they could feel at wrist and temple, the pulse, signified the balance of Yin, the female component standing for darkness, cold, and death, and Yang, the masculine source of life and heat.

To the earliest Egyptians, the heart was the wellspring of intelligence, a force so precious that of all the vital organs, it alone remained in place during mummification. The Greeks regarded the heart as the site of fiery emotions. The earliest attempts to understand the pump performance of the heart are probably lost in antiquity. The Egyptian Imhotep and his successors made observations of the pulse as early as 2980 BC.

Later, Greeks did more than poeticize the heart. They cut it out of animals, opened it, studied it, and took the first faltering steps to make scientific sense of its mechanism. Greek physicians who wrote under the collective name of Hippocrates (460 BC) said that the heart was an organ made of tissue that could expand and contract—in short, a muscle. They observed that it had valves, which were unbelievably durable flaps of tissue acting like folding doors that opened and shut, allowing blood to run in one direction only. Hippocrates also wrote treatises on the symptoms of heart disease, including dyspnea and peripheral edema.

In 400 BC, Plato described the way the heart works when he stated that it "pumps particles as from a fountain into channels of the veins, and makes the stream of the veins flow through the body as a conduit." From their dissections of dead animals, the Greeks were familiar with a network of blood-filled vessels that dead-ended in the heart, the *veins.* They also recognized that another network of vessels stemming from the heart had much less blood and seemed to channel air. These they named *arteries*: "a place that keeps air."

Aristotle (384–322 BC), the greatest mind in Greece's Golden Age, studied embryology using chicken eggs. He placed a clutch of eggs laid on the same day under a sitting hen, then opened one egg a day. On the fourth day, a tiny speck of red winked at him in the albumen, moving, he said, as if it had the force of life. On succeeding days, the spot grew until he realized it was the embryonic heart. From it fanned lines of red, the infantile veins and arteries.

Although Aristotle did not realize it, the whole miracle of circulation was spread before him. Blood flows in a continuous circle through the heart and arteries and veins. If he had nicked one of the red lines, the blood would have drained out and the heart stopped winking. He failed to understand that when the heart stops, no more blood goes into the arteries, and they collapse, supporting the illusion that they are tubes for air.

That myth survived for more than four hundred years until, in the second century after Christ, the ancient world's "prince of physicians," Galen of Pergamum (AD 129–216), doctor to Roman emperors, exposed an animal's artery while making a detailed study of the pulse. To prevent anything from entering or escaping, he tied two knots several inches apart and then sliced open the artery between them. Out gushed blood. After that no one thought the arteries were filled with air.

From his dissections, Galen knew that the heart had two chambers on each side. He discovered that blood came into the right side from the veins and flowed out into the aorta, the major vessel that exits from the heart. But how did blood get from the right to the left side? Galen fantasized that the blood passed through tiny pores in the heart's dividing wall, the septum. He recognized that vessels connected the heart to the lungs, but he regarded the lungs as just a source of air to cool hot blood. Galen noticed that the blood coming to the heart in the veins was dark, even appearing dirty. Yet when it came out of the heart and into the aorta, it was bright red. He imagined that the heart was a tiny furnace where the blood's sooty impurities were burned away.

For fourteen hundred years, Galen's blunders saddled medical minds. Partly this was a tribute to his towering stature as a scientist, but this was also the time when Europe's lights went out in the Dark Ages, stifling scientific inquiry, and the Church proclaimed "*ecclesia abboret sanguinis*," or "the church abhors blood." Priests who were surgeons abandoned surgery to barbers.

Not until 1553 was Galen challenged in a book that cost its Spanish author his life—he was burned at the stake. Michael Servetus, a physician with pronounced ideas on God and organized religion, denied there were any holes in the heart's septum. Emerging from his studies with a primitive, but correct, description of the circulatory system, he said that blood was expelled from the heart's right side into the lungs via a vessel called the pulmonary artery. The blood's color changed to "orangey yellow" in the lungs, not in the heart as Galen had written. Then it returned to the heart's left side through the pulmonary veins and went into the aorta.

Had Servetus confined himself to physiology he might have escaped his flaming end. His book also contained what both the Catholics and Protestant reformers deemed heresy. Not for a century did the three unconfiscated copies of his book emerge.

A feisty little Englishman named William Harvey (1578–1657) had no knowledge of Servetus's work when in the early 1600s he began to ask what the heart really did. At first he confessed his task seemed "so truly difficult" that he almost believed that "the motion of the heart was to be understood by God alone." Galen had said that the heart had two chambers on each of its sides. One was an atrium or "hall," and the other was a ventricle or "small belly." Patiently Harvey traced blood vessels. Blood coming to the heart through the veins flowed into the right atrium. A one-way valve let the blood drop through it into the right ventricle. From there it made its way through another one-way valve into the pulmonary artery and then to the lungs. He wondered what force propelled the blood.

Harvey examined the heart. When blood was coming in, the ventricle was soft and flexible. When the ventricle contracted and became hard, the blood was expelled. With each contraction or beat, the heart drove out blood, literally pumping. The number of beats per minute varied in response to the body's changing needs for blood (later defined as the "Starling effect").

Harvey saw why air-breathing vertebrates had a right atrium and ventricle. It was to project the blood through the lungs with enough force that the aerated blood was carried into the pulmonary veins and over to the heart's left atrium. There it encountered another one-way valve to steer it into the left ventricle. As the blood entered, the left ventricle filled like its right-side counterpart. It then contracted to pump blood through a fourth valve into the system of arteries. The pulse simply marked the contraction of the left ventricle.

Harvey demonstrated that the blood circulatory system was a one-way closed circuit pathway around the body and it was the heart that made its journey possible. He proclaimed, "The heart of animals is the foundation of their life, the sovereign of everything within them, the sum of their microcosm, that upon which all life depends, from which all power proceeds." In short, the heart was a pump, although a vital one.

Elementary as that seems, it had taken thousands of years to reach that understanding. It was up to others to prove that tiny capillaries were the bridges between the veins and arteries and that the lungs turned blood bright red. Nevertheless, what Harvey published in 1628 in *De Motu Cordis et Sanguinis* (*The Motion of the Heart and Blood*) helped to make it possible for Kolff and Dr. Tetsuzo Akutsu to stand together in their Cleveland lab some 329 years later wondering how they could fashion a mechanical substitute for the blood-pumping heart.

Getting Started

Dr. Irvine Page, the Cleveland Clinic's chief of research and Kolff's new boss, was short, curt, and crackling with live-wire energy. In his own words, he was "something of a martinet." His dream was one day to unlock the secrets of high blood pressure, and he zealously guarded his research funds to make sure that maximum dollars went to his pet project. He was anxious to hire Kolff, hoping to exploit his knowledge of the kidneys and, in particular, their role in hypertension. In turn Page impressed Kolff. He saw Page, ten years older, as a father figure who could shepherd him over rough shoals in his new environment. He wanted to please Page, even though he realized the new job was in clinical research and not in his special talent for creating new medical devices.

The clinic had no interest in that particular talent, either in its hospital or the research unit. When Kolff asked doctors to look at the heart-lung pumps and oxygenators he had brought from Holland and explained that they could open new horizons for heart surgery, his colleagues were politely indifferent. In the spring of 1950, heart surgeons were bewitched by another technique, the daring procedure of operating "in the blind," where they cut into the heart without acknowledging any need for Kolff's machine. For generations they had been taught that the heart was off limits to their scalpels. Then in the late 1940s, the heart was demystified.

Led by Philadelphia's Dr. Charles Bailey and Boston's Dr. Dwight Harken, surgeons found they could poke a tiny knife blade inside the heart through a small cut in the atrial wall. Although they could not see what they were doing, they could either cut open or manipulate stuck heart valve leaflets. This operation was the ultimate test of a heart surgeon's daring because the heart remained beating at the doctor's fingertips. The proof that the heart could be touched, even cut and sutured, encouraged many surgeons to explore more complex interventions. One approach was to quickly occlude the veins bringing blood into the heart, but this provided only four minutes to complete the surgery. The procedure could be repeated, however.

In 1952 Drs. Walter Lillehei and John Lewis used hypothermia to cool the body to eighty-one degrees Celsius, stopping circulation for ten minutes. It became apparent that an effective heart-lung machine could expand the field of cardiac surgery. In 1953 Dr. John Gibbon developed a heart-lung machine and successfully operated on an eight-year-old girl. His second patient died, however.

Donna, the twelve-year-old daughter of miner Lyman Glidden and his wife, Frances, died a miserable death with a ventricular septal defect (VSD), a hole between her right and left ventricles. To that date, only four children had undergone surgery to close a VSD, and all had died on the operating table. Frances had another child named Gregory on February 24, 1953. He was hospitalized at six weeks and again at eight weeks with symptoms of asthma and pneumonia very similar to those of his older sister. The Gliddens were very alarmed.

Initially Gregory was not diagnosed with a septal defect. X-rays, aided by a new technique developed at the Cleveland Clinic and used at the University of Minnesota called cardiac catheterization, revealed an enlarged heart. The tests confirmed that Gregory also had a VSD, and the Gliddens were devastated.

Lillehei and some colleagues were experimenting on dogs using an open-heart procedure called cross-circulation, where one dog's heart and lungs functioned for a second one undergoing open-heart surgery. They felt they were ready for the first human patient. "I think we can fix Gregory," Lillehei said.

However, Lillehei was criticized by the hospital staff, who said that cross-circulation was the first opportunity to have 200 percent mortality in one surgery. Lyman had the same blood type as his son, so he was chosen to be the donor. The connecting circuit between father and son was a beer hose and a milk pump to move an identical amount of blood between the two. The cross-circulation time was twelve minutes, and Gregory's heart was open for nearly ten minutes while surgeons closed the septal hole. This time period was well beyond hypothermia's accepted limit. Lillehei closed the incision through the right ventricular wall, and Gregory's heart took over fifteen minutes into the procedure. By nineteen minutes, the beer tubing and milk pump were removed, and Gregory was doing well.

As Lillehei's dogs had done, Gregory awoke promptly and showed no evidence of neurological damage. The team was elated with the success of the first VSD closure in a human patient. However, Gregory had difficulty breathing, went into cardiac arrest, and died eleven days after surgery. An autopsy revealed that the VSD had closed and begun healing; Gregory had died from severe pneumonia.

The second VSD patient to undergo surgery with cross-circulation, Pamela Schmidt, was successfully operated on with her father serving as the blood donor. A third success was logged before a press conference was held on April 30. Schmidt appeared and answered reporters' questions. Lillehei thought this was the first press conference ever held to announce such a marvelous breakthrough in surgery or medicine.

These surgeries and the advent of cardiac catheterization to identify heart pathology that might be corrected were evidence that open-heart surgery was feasible. Kolff was one of those who believed that a reliable heart-lung device providing temporary circulatory support for open-heart surgery could make these surgeries even more available.

However, he was disappointed at the lack of interest in his heart-lung machine and retired to the laboratory space that Page had provided. It was in a building adjoining the hospital, and when he finally got there, he shuddered. His facilities had been much better in Kampen.

The lab, which he shared with another researcher, was about fifty by thirty feet. At least he had the side closest to the windows. One piece of equipment was in the room—a gleaming artificial kidney that the commercial manufacturer had labeled a "Kolff-type." Included was a manual telling him how to operate the device he had invented! Page had obtained the machine for Kolff to use in dog experiments.

The practical Kolff saw no reason why the machine should not also be used to help human patients with acute kidney disease. There was a catch, however. Kolff could not move the machine to the bedsides of hospital patients. That meant that before a patient could be treated, all the experiment dogs had to be stored elsewhere and the floor scrubbed. Because of corridor steps and a double turn, patients could not be wheeled to the room. Beds had to be taken apart, carted to the lab, and reassembled before orderlies hand-carried the patients in. After dialysis the process was reversed. "I really need additional space for the dialysis," Kolff told clinic officials.

"We all need more space. Make do," was the answer. Kolff did.

Wandering by Kolff's lab one day, a new, up-and-coming clinic surgeon, Dr. Stanley Hoerr, was astounded to see the kidney machine at work on a patient. "That Kolff is something," Hoerr said to other clinic doctors. "He's been here only a couple of weeks, and already he's got a dialysis program going."

On one thing, Kolff was adamant. "I will not be just a technician using a dialyzer," he said to the medical staff. "I want full responsibility for patients on dialysis. If a person is sick enough to need the artificial kidney, then my service is in charge until the patient returns to the referring service." He was not the nine-to-five type of attending doctor. The night staff grew accustomed to having him drop in at 10:00 PM, midnight, or predawn to check on his patients.

High blood pressure is a malady in which—for causes not fully understood—blood exerts strong force on the walls of blood vessels, creating extra work for the heart and vascular system and the possibility of heart failure and stroke. Some doctors thought its source lay in the kidneys, but a Texas researcher reported that dogs could get the illness with or without kidneys. Page wanted Kolff to duplicate the Texas experiments to see if they were correct. Kolff validated the findings, then did work that indicated the kidneys put out a substance to ease high blood pressure. The scientific reports he wrote with Page were accepted for publication but caused little stir.

Nevertheless, Kolff made the most of his assignment. He anticipated that at some time in the future, kidney transplants in humans would be possible and taught himself enough surgery to transplant kidneys from one dog to another. However, Kolff grew restless. Page became less of a father figure as he and Kolff, both strong-minded individuals, began to disagree.

Kolff had nostalgic recollections of Kampen, where he did research he found interesting and had a staff to assist him. At Cleveland he did not have even one secretary. Forced to scurry around asking other doctors' secretaries to type his letters and reports, Kolff determined to unravel the typewriter's mysteries. He took a machine on a family vacation and for an hour each morning hunted and pecked among the keys. The ineluctable truth was that the man who had given the world its first artificial kidney could not learn to type.

More seriously, Page would not give Kolff an assistant. He had to do all his professional tasks himself. Walking through another part of the clinic one day, he saw a young doctor huddled behind a lab table. He looked so unhappy that Kolff introduced himself. The man was W. G. Tu, a twenty-five-year-old Taiwanese. "My wife was born in Indonesia," Kolff told him. "I am sure she would like to have you to dinner tonight." Overwhelmed, Tu accepted.

On the drive to Kolff's spacious three-level home in Cleveland Heights, Tu explained why he was so unhappy: "I hoped when I came to the clinic to be assigned to research the chemistry of the kidney. Instead, all I do all day is work on dogs' nervous systems for Dr. Page. I am afraid I will not be able to do what he wants, but even if I can, I do not want to do it."

At dinner Janke told the family not to talk medicine. She wanted dinner to be a family affair with their daughter and four sons participating. By barring medicine from the table, she let the children learn about the world from their visitors and made sure that Kolff was in close daily touch with his children. But after dinner, Kolff and Tu discussed Tu's future at the clinic. "I will work it out so that you can come to my laboratory," Kolff told Tu.

Page did not easily agree. Finally, he said that Tu could work with Kolff on kidney chemistry but only if he first prepared the dogs and other animals for various Page research projects. From a life insurance group, Kolff got the funds to pay Tu, who was his first medical assistant. Tu found that Kolff asked nothing of him that he did not require of himself. When the two stayed late to finish experiments on animals, they cleaned up after themselves. Tu thought it an honor to work side-by-side with a world-class scientist, even if he had to swab up dog droppings.

Kolff initiated Tu into the code of a researcher: to be original, persistent, and honest. "You cannot get reliable long-term results," Kolff said, "with just short-term experiments." So day after day, they took kidneys out of animals, induced high blood pressure, and noted that the pressure readings went down when they put new kidneys in. When Tu left fourteen months later, he broke into tears as he said thanks and good-bye to his mentor and friend.

Kidney in a Can

After nearly five years being a Page laboratory specialist, Kolff figured he had paid his dues. "There are other things I want to do," he told Page. "I have an idea for a better artificial kidney. I want three weeks to work on it." Kolff was

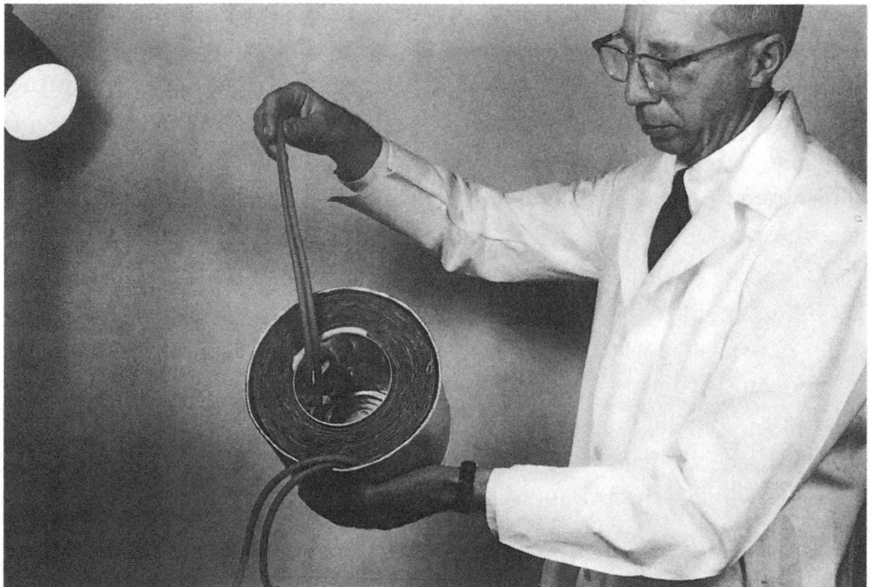

Kolff with his coil kidney.

aware his kidney had not had the general acceptance he believed it deserved. By his estimate, perhaps only one of every four machines purchased by hospitals was in regular use. The devices were too big, too complicated, and too expensive. In Philadelphia two youthful researchers had devised a small artificial kidney housed in a simple pressure-cooker pan. Discovering they had done nothing further, Kolff concluded it was too good an idea to abandon.

In his basement workshop, he set out to improvise his own simple kidney. He used his old standby—cellophane sausage casing—and combined it with tin cans, ordinary plastic window screening, and a connector for garden hoses. Two twenty-foot sections of casing were threaded between the openings and coiled around a family-sized juice can, which could be immersed in a dialyzing fluid in a larger can to remove the urea and impurities from the blood circulating through the cellophane. He then soldered on the hose connector to bring the fluid from a tank. His device, technically a twin-coil artificial kidney, was portable, efficient, and easy to operate. It was also typically American: the inner can was cheap enough to be thrown away after dialysis.

The tinkering was textbook Kolff, adapting everyday items to create a scientific device that could save lives. The result was that doctors from both developed and Third World countries came to work with him and learn his techniques. Page's research budget could not afford fellowships for these doctors;

they had to get stipends from their home countries. Because many came from nations with different hygiene, Kolff prepared a two-page list of what he expected. To combat body odor, he handed someone a bar of soap with instructions on the art of bathing. Occasionally he paid for haircuts. He marched some people to thrift stores with a pointed suggestion on what to wear. People at the clinic joked that foreigners tutored by Kolff spoke English with a strong Dutch accent.

Kolff's staff met each weekday precisely at 8:00 AM to prompt everybody to get to work on time; Kolff berated latecomers. Each day one staff member gave a short report on a work-related topic of his choice. Kolff cut off windy speakers and translated jargony talk, training his people to communicate briefly and clearly.

Kolff's laboratory had been quiet and deserted when he arrived in 1950. Now it bustled with new investigations. Concerned that his staff would spill over, the clinic ruled that he could have no more than eight fellows in his lab at one time. On the other hand, his dialysis program, which by then had a room in the hospital, brought in thirty thousand dollars a year to support his entire lab.

The clinic assigned a maid to clean up. Aslean Cooper was a seventeen-year-old high-school dropout from an inner-city ghetto. Kolff believed she was bright. Hearing she wanted to go to night school for her diploma but lacked funds for books and fees, he asked if she was serious. "I am; I am," she said.

"I will give you the money," he replied, and several months later, she brought him a paper from school. "What's this?" he asked.

"My report card. I wanted you to see that I am serious about my education," she explained.

Breakthrough Oxygenator

The Cleveland Clinic's chief cardiovascular surgeon was Dr. Donald B. Effler, a tall, gregarious thirty-nine-year-old. In Kolff's dialysis room, he noticed that blood coming out of a patient was dark and unhealthy looking but abruptly changed to vivid red in the artificial kidney. "Why is that blood changing color?" he asked. Kolff was so familiar with this phenomenon that he merely said that the blood was taking on oxygen. Effler burst out, "If you can do that for kidney patients, why can't you do it for heart patients? Hell, you've got an oxygenator for a heart-lung pump!"

Effler had desperately been looking for a device to take over for the heart and lungs during surgery. Operating in the blind had very limited possibilities. Most surgeons recognized that to attack serious defects they needed to be able to open the heart and see what they were doing. That required an effective heart-lung bypass device, but Philadelphia's Dr. Gibbon had given up on his machine. It had been successful in the operation on Gregory, but the next two patients had died. The anguished Gibbon had walked out of his lab.

That baffled Kolff, who had seen fifteen deaths before he had proved that his artificial kidney worked. "He should continue," Kolff said. Others felt the same way. At the Mayo Clinic and the University of Minnesota, surgeons were doing animal experiments with heart-lung machines. Effler's words spurred Kolff to renewed action.

In Holland Kolff had learned that cellophane was a disaster in heart-lung machines because it failed to pass enough oxygen into the blood. He was not aware that the amount of oxygen in his kidney-rinse solution was very low. If he had used cellophane in oxygen-rich air, he very likely would have been successful. Other scientists had since discovered that oxygen permeated a plastic called polyethylene more efficiently.

Modifying his twin-coil kidney, Kolff wrapped polyethylene tubing around a fruit-juice can with openings for blood to flow in and out. Instead of immersing the device in dialyzing fluid, he put it into an ordinary plastic bag. With the bag partially closed, he funneled in pure oxygen while the blood coursed through the coils. Deep purplish blood entered the tubing and came out red. To dramatize that he had created what ultimately became a membrane oxygenator, Kolff sealed both ends of a four-foot strip of polyethylene and hung it horizontally on a wall of his lab. The tube was filled with water, and a small goldfish swam around in it. Had the fish been in a sealed glass jar, it would have died for lack of air, but oxygen permeated the plastic to keep it alive.

The question was, could Kolff's membrane work in a heart-lung machine? After some consultations at the University of Minnesota, he anesthetized dogs back in Cleveland for surgery to test his membrane oxygenator. The first ones died. When examination showed an acid buildup, he treated the next series of dogs with bicarbonate of soda, a remedy for heartburn. The dogs still died. Kolff was stumped. Then he and Effler determined the cause of the deaths: during the heart-lung bypass, Kolff's machine was not perfusing the dogs' blood with enough oxygen. Adding more oxygen corrected the problem, and the next dogs survived.

Effler and his team moved into Kolff's lab, practicing the way to tap the heart-lung machine into the vessels of anesthetized dogs. A surgeon opened the dog's chest, then spread the ribs to get access to the pericardium (the sac where the heart nestles) to reach the aorta, the major artery from the heart. One of the aorta's branches carries blood to the brain and upper torso while another branch loops down to bring blood to the rest of the body. The surgeon implanted a cannula into this branch near the heart. He put two more cannulas into the inferior and superior venae cavae, the two main veins directing blood back to the heart. By tying off these blood vessels, he redirected the entire blood flow away from the dog's heart and lungs through the cannulas into Kolff's machine. After the blood was oxygenated, a pump drove it back into the body at the desired pressure. Bypassed and temporarily not needed to maintain life, the heart and lungs could be operated on.

What no one knew was how long a dog could tolerate having its heart bypassed and its circulation dependent on Kolff's machine. Effler's first experiments were simple: get the dog on bypass, open the heart, make a hole in the inner wall, patch it, sew up the heart, then restore the natural circulation and close the chest. In the beginning, Effler and his team did their work in less than fifteen minutes. The results were very encouraging: thirteen of the first sixteen dogs survived.

Cautiously Effler and his team ventured into more complex surgery. The time on the machine went to twenty and then twenty-five minutes. An unending worry was that a lethal air bubble, an embolism, would enter the circulation system. The longer the blood went through Kolff's machine, the greater the danger that vital red cells would be chewed up in a process called hemolysis.

Nonetheless, Effler and Kolff pushed on. The number of experiments reached seventy-five. At this point, they were daring to keep the dog on the machine for thirty to thirty-five minutes. They had to cope with postsurgery problems such as infection and hemorrhage, but the surgeons were undeterred.

Throughout the series of dog surgeries, Effler was confronted with what amounted to a moving target. Even though bypassed by the heart-lung pump, the heart continued contracting because its natural pacemaker was still sending out electrical impulses. Effler was playing catch-as-catch-can with the beating heart. Moreover, his vision was sometimes obscured. Although most of the dog's blood was shunted to the heart-lung machine, two small trickles still got to the heart. Before oxygenated blood in the aorta went anywhere else, some of it was siphoned off for the coronary arteries, which lie atop the heart like a crown of thorns to ensure the heart tissue is nourished. This blood, plus another tiny supply to feed the lung's trachea and bronchi, returned to the heart, where it occasionally pooled, blocking Effler's view.

How much better it would be, Kolff thought, if there was some way to give surgeons a perfectly still heart and a dry field. He remembered that in

Minnesota he had seen a researcher attempting to verify work reported by a British scientist, Dr. Donald Melrose. Melrose thought that clamping off the normal blood flow to the lungs and the coronary arteries could deliberately slow the heart. Additionally an injection of potassium citrate would paralyze the heart. Other doctors had known this for decades but did not know how to restart the heart. Melrose's contribution was merely restoring the normal blood flow to the coronary arteries to flush out the potassium, and the heart spontaneously resumed beating. However, Melrose experimented with cardiac arrest on animal hearts, not on human patients.

The audacity of treating the heart as if it had a stop/start switch fascinated Kolff. When Effler and his team were not working in the lab, Kolff anesthetized a dog, opened its chest, and put it on bypass with the heart-lung pump. After clamping the aorta near the coronary arteries to prevent blood from entering, he injected potassium. The heart stopped. He allowed it to be still for several minutes before restoring blood flow to the arteries. The heart started, so Kolff injected more potassium. The heart stopped. With blood back in the arteries, it started. Then he called in Effler and Dr. F. Mason Sones, a heart-disease specialist in his thirties. "I've got something you should see," he said. He repeated the potassium demonstration.

Effler was incredulous. Then he stopped a dog's heart, started it, stopped it, started it, stopped it, and started it again. Sones reached over the inert dog to shake Kolff's hand. "This is it," he declared.

Sones had a particular reason for wanting a heart-lung machine with potassium arrest. Like cardiologists throughout the world, he had watched helplessly as babies died of congenital septal defects like the case with Gregory. Because doctors could not get inside the heart, they could not make repairs. As a result, many babies with septal defects became progressively weaker due to inadequate blood flow, and most of them died.

Sones had a list of patients with these congenital defects. He hoped that Kolff's heart-lung apparatus would enable surgeons to correct them. Kolff said, "Before we use it on babies, we will try it on puppies to be sure our techniques work on tiny creatures." After 139 successful experiments, Kolff said, "We are ready."

On Monday, March 13, 1956, Sones admitted a seventeen-month-old boy with a large hole in his inner heart wall into the clinic hospital. Four days later, Effler operated, Kolff ran the heart-lung machine, and Sones monitored the beating of the heart with an electrocardiogram. With a long incision, Effler opened his gateway to the heart, where he and his assistant quickly inserted the cannulas to bypass the blood from the heart into Kolff's machine. The surgeon let the heart pump a few more times to empty as much of the blood in it as possible and then applied blood-vessel clamps. "We are on the run," Kolff said. His machine now controlled the child's circulation.

Effler stuck a syringe with twenty cubic centimeters of blood and potassium citrate into the aorta below the clamp and pushed in the plunger. The drug inched through the coronary arteries. The heart shuddered and then halted. Effler cut through the heart's flaccid outer wall with his scalpel. When his assistant had suctioned out the remaining blood, the surgeon had a dry, passive surgical field. Effler remained motionless for a few seconds, examining the hole high in the inner septum. He then made four stitches to close the opening and checked to make sure they were secure.

Now came the moment of life or death. Effler withdrew the clamp to allow blood from the aorta to enter the coronary arteries and rinse out the potassium. According to numerous laboratory experiments on dogs, the baby's heart should start. None of the people in the room could be sure it would work with a human patient; perhaps the potassium had caused some irreversible damage to the heart.

The group waited. Five painful seconds went by, but the heart remained lifeless. More seconds passed; there was still no motion. Effler stifled the almost irresistible urge to reach in, massage the heart, and somehow get it going. And then the heart moved after twenty-five seconds, shaking itself back into motion. Its color changed from a dull crimson to a vigorous red. Effler stitched up the outer wall's incision, separating the heart from Kolff's machine, and closed the chest. Fifteen days later, a healthy baby was discharged from the hospital. It was history's first successful use of a heart-lung machine combined with cardiac arrest to repair a human heart!

Within several weeks, the Effler/Kolff/Sones team operated on a four-year-old. The surgery went off flawlessly. Again there was the time of peril: would the heart restart? This time thirty-seven agonizing seconds went by before the beat resumed. The child regained color, his reflexes normal. However, ten hours after the operation, the child was sitting up in bed and fainted. By the time doctors got to him, he was dead. There was no evidence that anything had gone wrong in the surgery, and an autopsy revealed no reason for the abrupt death. This was starting out like Gibbon's experience: one success, then a disappointing death. Clearly there were mysteries the Cleveland team had not fathomed.

Two days later, a third child—a three-year-old—was operated on for a septal hole. The following day bleeding broke out around the chest incision. Physicians moved fast to control it with pressure dressings, and the bleeding stopped. On the fourteenth day after surgery, the child was discharged, completely recovered.

Of the first thirty-seven patients operated on, thirteen died. The team, treading into the medical unknown, frankly acknowledged that ten of them could be considered surgical failures, often because the doctors ran into unanticipated problems far greater than a septal hole. Diagnostic techniques to identify cardiac defects before surgery were still not very well developed. Nevertheless, they held out hope that with further experience, most of the problems could be overcome.[3]

Kolff was in the operating room for the first hundred surgeries. His polyethylene oxygenator worked with septal-defect patients weighing less than fifty pounds, but as the surgeons operated on older and larger patients suffering from other heart diseases, he switched to different types, including one known as "the bubble." Due to the units that he and others were perfecting and surgeons who had the courage to persevere, operations to repair the heart became commonplace.

To Be So Brash

In Japan twenty-five-year-old Dr. Tetsuzo Akutsu was anxious to learn about surgery with the heart-lung machine and wrote Kolff asking if there was room in the laboratory. When Akutsu arrived, Kolff took him to the 1957 meeting of an organization that became the launching pad for the "bionic man." It was the American Society for Artificial Internal Organs (ASAIO). A cosmopolitan German doctor, Peter Salisbury, along with Kolff and four other investigators, had founded it two years earlier.

Trained in biochemistry at England's Cambridge University and a graduate of an Italian medical school with a PhD in physiology from the University of Minnesota, Salisbury had also developed an artificial kidney in the early 1950s. When he exhibited it at the 1954 American Medical Association convention, the response convinced Salisbury that a growing number of doctors were interested in the burgeoning field of artificial organs. "We ought to start our own organization," Salisbury said. It took him a winter's work, but in the spring of 1955, the ASAIO held its first meeting. The fifty-five scientists present chose Kolff as president.

When Salisbury became president in 1957, he had tough words for his fellow members. He asked why ASAIO members were so fixated on artificial kidneys, heart-lung pumps, and other out-of-body machines. Why weren't they thinking about developing artificial organs that could function inside the body?

Specifically, why not an artificial heart that could be implanted to do the work of a failed natural heart? Was it unethical to think of replacing the heart, the most hallowed organ? Absolutely not, Salisbury declared. Was it possible to build an artificial heart? The answer was "of course." Already he had theoretical plans with ideas borrowed from a Swedish scientist, who in turn had taken his heart design from a milking machine.

Salisbury was not alone. Also at the ASAIO was Dr. Selwyn McCabe, a New Zealand researcher who had worked for the National Institutes of Health (NIH) in Washington, DC and actually built a model of a plastic artificial heart.

Kolff sat spellbound. Never had he been so brash as to suggest that a man-made device could replace the natural heart. The grandeur of that vision stunned Kolff. He saw that an artificial heart could mean new life to thousands of people with irreversible heart disease. What a goal to strive for! "I can do that; I can build a heart," Kolff vowed with the certainty that had driven him to create the artificial kidney and the heart-lung bypass machine. He determined not only to fashion an artificial heart but have it for the next ASAIO meeting: one year to develop a replacement for an organ that humanity had struggled for millennia to understand.

Heart of Plastic

Kolff realized that outside of the ASAIO, the mere suggestion of building an artificial heart to replace a worn-out one would be considered too bizarre for valid scientific experimentation.[4] Therefore, he did not tell Dr. Page what he intended to do. He revealed his plans to only a few clinic doctors he trusted.

The project was truly staggering. The human heart weighs only about eleven ounces in a man, nine in a woman, and is about five inches long, three inches wide, and less than three inches deep. Electric impulses that travel through a small column of special cells known as the bundle of His drive it. On an average day, the heart pumps nearly two thousand gallons of blood through approximately sixty thousand miles of arteries, capillaries, and veins. In a year, it beats forty million times. Over an average lifetime, this remarkable muscle generates two-and-a-quarter-billion pulses.

The challenge of duplicating that action was formidable. What material would be flexible and durable but also blood compatible so clots would not form? How would the heart connect to the body? What would power it to pump the way the natural heart does? How could he regulate the device's beating to approximate natural rhythm and flow?

His group began by considering size. The heart had to be large enough to handle the necessary volume of blood yet small enough to fit in the chest without compressing anything else. Akutsu cut out the heart of a dead dog and made plaster-of-Paris casts to give them some idea of the overall size. They modeled their heart on the one that McCabe had displayed at the ASAIO. It was made of polyvinyl chloride, a plastic that could be easily molded. Replicating the human heart's function required four chambers. McCabe had used an electroplating process to form his artificial heart's chambers. Neither Kolff nor Akutsu had the dimmest idea how to electroplate. Fortunately the clinic's machine-shop chief had a book, and Akutsu followed the directions to create metal molds to fabricate the atria and ventricles with the plastic.

At that point, Kolff heard he was about to lose his job. Seven years earlier, Dr. Hoerr had been impressed with Kolff's speed in setting up a dialysis program. He was now chair of the surgery division and had heard that Dr. Page was becoming increasingly disenchanted with Kolff, feeling he was working too much with surgeons and not doing enough kidney research. The intensity of the Page-Kolff disputes had escalated.

"You are in trouble with Page," a grim-faced Hoerr told Kolff, "but I know how important your work is with Effler and the other surgeons. We do not want you to be separated from the clinic. Although you are technically not a surgeon, we're offering you an appointment in our division."

Kolff said he certainly would accept Hoerr's offer, but he did not intend to resign from Page's division. "If I leave research, I will lose my laboratory foothold in this building. Page will surely want it back," he told Hoerr. "You cannot offer me the equivalent, and once I am out of research, I will have to endure the tedious procedures of the Research Projects Committee for everything I need. No, I must have appointments in both divisions."

Amazingly, Kolff got his way. The clinic created the new Division of Artificial Organs with Kolff as its boss, responsible to both Hoerr and Page. Kolff maneuvered so deftly through the bureaucratic minefield that not only did he keep his laboratory but for the first time he finally got a secretary.

Replicating the Heart

The human heart vaguely resembles the artwork on valentine cards. It has a rounded apex at the bottom as if a make-believe heart were upside down. There are six openings for vessels ferrying blood in and out: the superior and inferior venae cavae, aorta, pulmonary artery, and pulmonary veins. The left and right sides, separated by a septum, wrap around each other with the right ventricle and atrium in front.

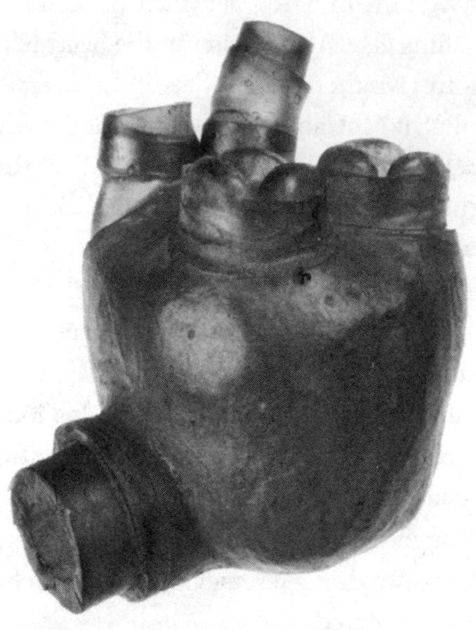

Kolff's first artificial heart model sustained life in a dog.

The first artificial heart Akutsu's adroit fingers created didn't look like that. It was a rigid plastic can with a cluster of tubes that were designed to connect to the body's blood vessels. Sealed inside were the four chambers, the flexible atria and ventricles with plastic valves mimicking those in the natural heart.

To replicate the muscle power that drives blood out of the natural heart, Akutsu used pulsed compressed air. A hose pushed bursts of air into the can, squeezing the ventricles and blasting out their blood. When the air shut off, the empty chambers expanded and refilled with blood. Regulating the number of airbursts per minute gave the heart a steady pulse rate.

Kolff and Akutsu rigged up a mock circulation system to verify that the heart could actually move blood from one side to the other. "Now we try it in a dead animal," said Kolff. He felt driven to get the work done before December 21, 1957, the ASAIO's deadline for reporting projects to be discussed at the next meeting.

Akutsu replaced a dead dog's heart with the artificial model, testing the fit. Blood left over from other animal experiments was injected, and air mechanically blown into the lungs. Akutsu turned on a pump so that compressed air could drive the mechanical heart. Although the dog had been dead ten hours, its circulatory system became active. The dog even had blood pressure, measuring when the ventricles were emptying (systolic phase) and when they were filling (diastolic phase). Kolff was certain he would be able to inform the ASAIO he had met his personal deadline.

Aslean Cooper, the high-school dropout who had cleaned Kolff's lab, had finished night school with his help. Now he noticed that she had an important quality—good hands. Moreover, she was always willing to pitch in to help Akutsu and the lab technicians. "We will promote you," Kolff informed her. "You will be an apprentice technician for the operations."

At 8:30 AM on December 12, 1957, Akutsu and Kolff moved to the operating table. With Aslean serving as his scrub nurse, Akutsu anesthetized a dog the size of a fairly large cocker spaniel. After giving heparin to keep the blood from clotting, Akutsu opened the chest and inserted cannulas to attach the animal to the heart-lung machine. He deftly scissored out the natural heart and then connected the veins and arteries to the tubes coming out of the artificial one so that blood would flow to the atria and then into the ventricles. Akutsu threaded a single cannula through the chest wall to bring in the compressed air bursts to power the heart. The question was what would happen when circulation was transferred to the artificial heart.

Slowly Kolff started pulsing the compressed air. A leak suddenly spouted blood from the pulmonary artery, and Akutsu promptly sutured it. "Are you ready to go off the pump?" Kolff asked. Akutsu nodded. The heart-lung machine slowly shut down. Now the artificial heart dictated whether the dog lived or died. Kolff and Akutsu could hear the compressed air unit wheezing and whoozing. They set it to pulse a hundred times a minute. Akutsu touched the cornea in an eye, and the dog blinked. He stuck a pin in a tendon, and its leg moved. Akutsu and Kolff were satisfied the dog had its normal reflexes so they closed the chest.

The dog lay on the table, kept unconscious with intermittent anesthesia. Steadily the lungs filled and emptied. The heart kept pumping. Solid blood-pressure readings proved the blood was circulating. For ninety minutes, the dog lived on its artificial heart. Kolff decided that was long enough and turned off the compressed air to stop the heart. The dog died.

Kolff and Akutsu drank no toast to their achievement. No press release was issued. No television cameras were invited. Neither man had any intention of rushing his news into any scientific journal. Kolff's rationale was that if they said what they had done, "people will think we are nuts." Not until they were among friendly ears at the ASAIO spring meeting did they announce their ninety-minute success. The era of the artificial heart had been born!

Notes

1. The phrase comes from "The Stopped Heart Operation: New Era in Surgery?" *Reader's Digest,* August 1956. The title was prophetic. Today with some modifications, potassium heart arrest is standard procedure in many of the more than 100,000 heart surgeries done each year.
2. The El Pindal Cave in the Asturias area of northern Spain contains remarkably preserved Paleolithic cave art.
3. Donald B. Effler, Laurence K. Groves, F. Mason Sones, and Willem J. Kolff, "Elective Cardiac Arrest in Open-Heart Surgery," *Cleveland Clinic Quarterly* 23 (1956):105–14; Willem J. Kolff, Donald B. Effler, Laurence K. Groves, and Patrick P. Moraca, *Journal of the American Medical Association* 164 (August 10, 1957): 1653–60.
4. Kolff was unaware of it, but a Russian researcher claimed that he had kept a dog alive for some hours with an artificial heart powered by a rotating drive shaft through its chest in 1938. He said he reported it the following year to a youth conference but did not write a scientific paper until 1949.

5

Sputnik Affects the Artificial Heart

Men must be taught as if you taught them not.
And things unknown proposed as things forgot.

—Alexander Pope

The era of the artificial heart had arrived, but its survival was fraught with uncertainties. A growing number of eager scientists joined the chase to a horizon that seemed ever to recede. The years from 1957 to 1960, when Sputnik led the world into the Space Age, were exciting for the members of ASAIO. They also were on the threshold of scientific breakthroughs, hopefully leading into an era when human minds and hands could create replacement organs for the human body. No one was sure what they might accomplish. There were no guidelines; they invented their own procedures. They measured triumphs in hours, sometimes minutes. They knew they would stumble, be misled, or commit errors. They had no assurance they could ever reach their goals. That only drove them harder.

Inevitably, controversies arose about the way the new science should focus its energies. The rivalry over the artificial heart quickly took shape. Willem Kolff was on one side, and on the other was almost everybody else. He believed in creating a mechanical pump to replace the natural heart. His critics worried that cutting out a patient's natural heart was too radical. With the heart gone, there would be no way to preserve life if the artificial heart broke. It would be better to keep the heart in place—even if it was dying—and support it with pumping. They envisioned an assist device, something that could piggyback on the natural heart and add mechanical thrust to keep the blood flowing.

"You miss the point," Kolff said. "With his sick heart still in his chest, the patient continues to have angina [chest pain]. His palpitations do not stop. The mere idea that he has a dying heart can lead to cardiac neurosis. How wonderful it would be to spare him the pain and other symptoms. That is what we look forward to with the total artificial heart."

Neither side budged. It was soon clear that it was Kolff against all the others. "We'll set up a race," he said, "and we'll see what comes out." Those who supported the idea of an assist device started out as the hares in this race. Kolff and Tetsuzo Akutsu told the doctors at ASAIO's 1958 meeting about their ninety-minute dog, but Yale University's Dr. Bert K. Kusserow had news that topped theirs. He reported developing a small electrically powered assist device that was implanted in a dog to pump along with the natural heart. It had worked for ten hours, he said. The ASAIO commentators gave their praise to Kusserow, not Kolff.

Kolff was unperturbed. He had plans for newer and better total artificial hearts. As he had in Holland, he sought help from private industry. While Akutsu had been fashioning the first heart model, Kolff had gone to Thompson Products, a Cleveland-based manufacturer that later became TRW Inc.

He was already a polished persuader. He told Thompson executives that diseases of the heart and blood vessels kill a million persons a year. What better public service could they do than focusing some of their engineering talent on designing an artificial heart? Thompson happened to have a creative engineer, S. Harry Norton, who could help Kolff. Norton was retired but still acted as a consultant and wanted the assignment, but he told his Thompson bosses, "I am an automotive engineer. What do I know about a heart?"

They replied, "A heart is a pump. Can you make a pump?"

"Sure, I can make a pump."

"Then make a heart."

Kolff advised Norton not to be overwhelmed: "Do not think you can create something that will do everything the natural heart does. Figure just what you must have and be satisfied."

In addition to the obvious need for pumping, Norton realized it would be best if the beat rate could vary like the pulse of the human heart.

Norton built a heart the Tin Woodman of *The Wizard of Oz* would have loved. It was metal, shaped like a hexagonal box. Because Kolff and Akutsu believed polyurethane was more compatible with blood than polyvinyl chloride, two polyurethane sacs were immersed in hydraulic fluid in the box. Electrically activated magnets moved a piston back and forth to exert pressure on the fluid, which in turn compressed the sacs and drove blood through small tubes. By controlling how many times a minute the current activated the magnets, Norton could change the pumping rate.

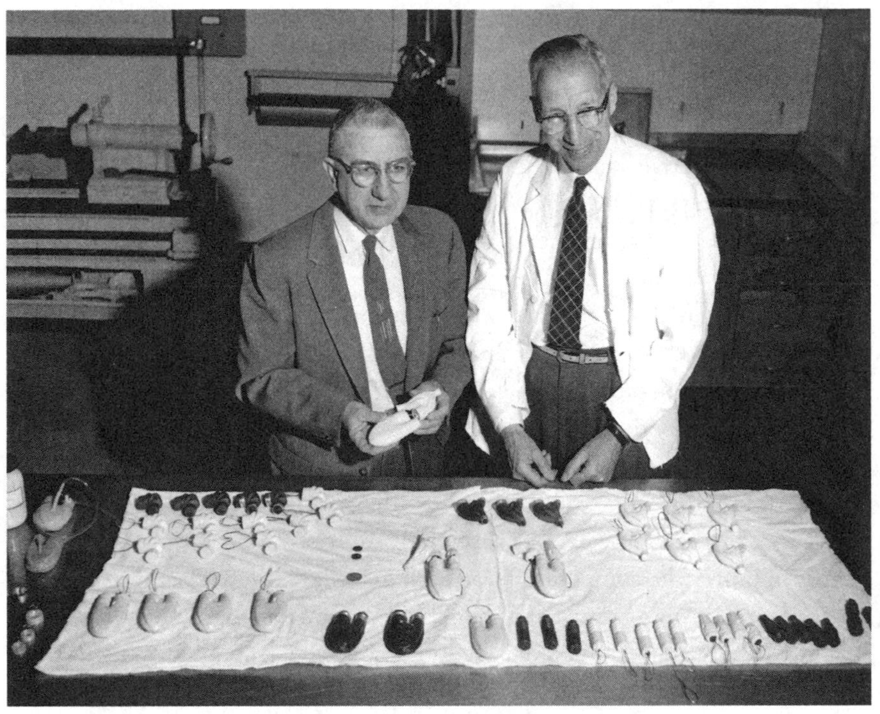

Dr. Harry Norton (left), pictured with Kolff, was a NASA engineer.

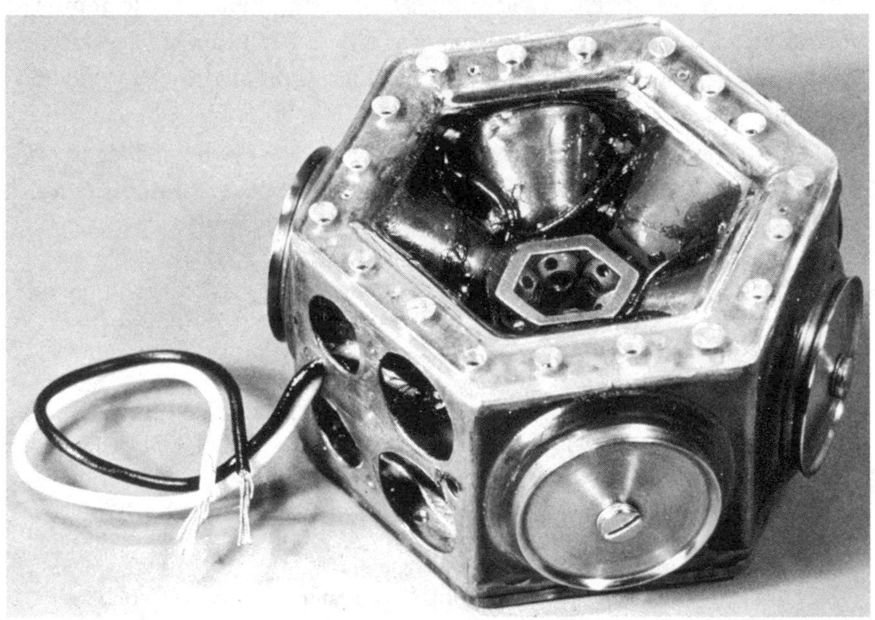

Electrohydraulic heart designed by Norton.

Norton's design was tested in January 1959 in Kolff's lab. A dog's heart was excised while it was on the heart-lung machine. Its major blood vessels were connected to the mechanical heart. Two thin wires from the mechanical heart were brought out through the abdominal wall to supply current for the magnet. Kolff injected contrast material into the dog's blood and then weaned the animal off the heart-lung machine. The lab was silent as he signaled to turn on the heart. Everyone in the room stared at an X-ray image, watching the dye-stained blood course through the dog's veins and arteries.

The blood dropped into a sac on the mechanical heart's right side and was propelled into the pulmonary artery to the lungs. It travelled through the pulmonary veins to the sac on the mechanical heart's left side and was ejected into the aorta and around the animal's network of arteries and veins. Norton had built a workable heart.

Several months later, Kolff returned to the ASAIO and reported that Norton's electrohydraulic heart had sustained life in a dog for three hours and twenty minutes. The competition was back as well. Kusserow had improved his assist device. The new version kept pumping in a dog for twelve hours.

But Kusserow had a problem. The longer his device pumped, the more red blood cells were destroyed. His pump was not gentle enough. Hemolysis, the destruction of red blood cells, preceded death. He told the gathering he would have to modify his designs. Kolff could sympathize. While the Norton heart worked, it, too, had critical shortcomings. It was too heavy, too awkwardly shaped, and got too hot. Like Kusserow, Norton was headed back to the drawing board.

Neither Kolff and Kusserow nor anyone else was anywhere close to winning this race. McCabe, whose heart had inspired the first Kolff-Akutsu model, proclaimed,

> We are aiming at the sky in hopes that our struggling efforts will go higher than if we set our sights on the top of the trees. The era we live in is shocked by some systems of society that claim we can do anything. But I believe it is time for us to look into the archives of our own civilization and wipe off the complacent cobwebs of our cozy thoughts. There we will find that there lies in our Hebrew-Christian heritage a more fantastic concept. It is this—and I need to use the symbol word "god"—in the god of absolute truth, of great patience and of tender persistence, in the god willing to make sacrifices and who bonds by trust and love, man can do anything.
>
> It is my belief that that kind of god lies latent within every one of us. If it is true that we want to, if we have faith to do it, man can make

> a suitable replacement for the heart. We may then not only draw from our efforts a clinical satisfaction but also the reward of having helped broaden man's philosophy by increasing his understanding of his own boundlessness and the remarkable humility of his creator.

Back in Cleveland, Kolff asked Akutsu, "What can we do for another design?" Akutsu developed a heart packed inside a circular container, a pendulum suspended between two blood sacs and driven by a small electric motor. When it swung back and forth, it compressed the sacs to propel blood. Called the pendulum heart, it increased the dog-survival time to six and a half hours. Unfortunately, the small motor's lifespan was too short to be practical.

Kolff continued to be attracted to the notion of hearts driven by electricity. He went to engineers in the Cleveland lab of the National Aeronautics and Space Administration (NASA). They advised Kolff, "You are trying to do too much within the chest. You should have one unit inside the body to do the pumping: no motors, no magnets, just pumping. Your power for driving the pump should come from outside."

"But what would the power source be?" Kolff asked.

"Compressed air" was the reply.

Kolff was skeptical.

The NASA scientists were blunt: "Look, you haven't yet solved the problems of heat, weight, and sufficient electric power. That means you don't know if an artificial heart is feasible. Compressed gas is easy to work with. It's reliable. With it you can test your heart and then worry about developing some other energy force." The engineers said they would use technology spin-offs from the space program to build Kolff a driving mechanism for his heart.

After a particularly wearying encounter, Dr. Donald Effler, the clinic's chief of surgery, told his wife, "Kolff has only one speed—top speed. He has only one direction—straight ahead."

But Kolff was struggling with problems aside from his artificial-heart research. His Division of Artificial Organs was undergoing growing pains. By 1960 he had three subdepartments: dialysis, heart/lung, and experimentation with artificial organs. He divided his expanding staff between "my kidney boys" and "my heart boys."

The science of dialysis was growing, and Kolff had to keep up. He needed space for his expanding patient load because a Washington researcher, Dr. Belding Scribner, had developed a shunt that made it possible to use artificial kidneys on chronic as well as acute kidney patients. Although some prestigious institutions scoffed at the shunt, Kolff immediately accepted it as a life-saving innovation.

Shunt patients began coming to the Cleveland Clinic. In 1961 his staff gave 491 treatments. Kolff pleaded with clinic officials for more space than the one room he had for dialysis. He set his sights on one of the clinic's older and less attractive buildings and hired an architect to draw up plans, but finance officers flatly informed him, "The building will be torn down." Kolff thought that was a most "convincing way" to deny his request.

Kolff had to scramble chronically for money to keep his lab going. He got funding from a variety of places: the Public Health Service, the Cleveland chapter of the American Heart Association, local industries, and the Rotary Club. A legend about Kolff grew up at the clinic. It was said he always asked for twice as much money as he needed to be assured of minimum funds. If the research was successful, he began asking for four times as much, figuring he was sure to get at least a quarter of it. One day he went to a clinic finance official to say, "I know where I can get $120,000 from a foundation for patient care. Can I ask for this much?"

"Absolutely not," replied the official. "We've never done anything like this before."

"We've never had a situation like this before," Kolff replied.

"If you had only asked for $25,000, I would not have objected."

Kolff looked the officer straight in the eye, "I'll settle for $60,000," he declared. They agreed on $50,000.

Just a Balloon

In running his lab, Kolff remembered his old Dutch friend, Professor Daniel, who believed that young scientists should be encouraged. It was always understood that anyone with an idea would get a hearing. In 1961 an unlikely combination of men in their twenties—a voluble American engineer and a trim and reserved Greek cardiologist—were in Kolff's lab to break new ground. The American was Stephen Topaz, an engineer who had read about Kolff in *Time* magazine and thought he would like to work for him. Topaz's sole qualifications for a job were an undergraduate degree from Purdue University and a summer making and repairing orthopedic devices at a crippled-children's camp.

Kolff teamed him with Greek cardiology fellow Dr. Spyridon Moulopoulos, whose interest lay in aiding a stressed heart before surgery was needed. Moulopoulos had seen heart-attack patients go into shock following an infarction (death of heart tissue from blood clots) and knew the reason was that the weakened heart could not supply enough blood to the coronary arteries. "But suppose we could mechanically pump blood to the coronaries," Moulopoulos proposed.

Brainstorming, he and Topaz figured out the way to do this. Moulopoulos was familiar with inserting catheters into veins and arteries. He and Topaz realized that tying a plastic balloon around the end of a tube would turn it into a pump. The tube could be inserted into the aorta near the mouth of the vessel that sends blood to the coronary arteries. Gas injected into the tube would inflate the balloon. Any blood in front of the gas would then be forced into the coronaries. They quickly constructed a working model.

Moulopoulos and Topaz were at their lab table when Kolff saw the contraption they had rigged. "What is that?" he asked.

Topaz cheekily answered, "That is a *great idea!*"

Kolff smiled. "Good," he said and walked away.

By the next day, the two young experimenters had connected the balloon-tipped cannula into a mock circulation system. Sure enough, when the balloon expanded, it pushed the fluid in its path. When the gas was sucked out, the balloon collapsed. But how to know when to activate the balloon in the cardiac cycle of filling and pumping? That turned out to have an easy answer. All they had to do was hook up an electrocardiogram. Its recording of the heart's electrical impulses would tell when to inflate and deflate the balloon.

Now it was time to show their device to Kolff. Grasping its possibilities for treating shock due to circulatory failure, Kolff said, "We'll try it on dogs. If that is successful, I will get you a cadaver." With the balloon catheter in the dog's aorta, Moulopoulos signaled for the jury-rigged pump to start inflating the balloon with gas. They installed an image amplifier over the dog's chest to monitor the flow of dye-stained blood. The balloon began expanding and collapsing. As it inflated, it drove blood to the heart's arteries.

"Son of a bitch" exclaimed a startled cardiologist in the lab. "Look at that blood fill the coronaries!"

Kolff helped with some small modifications, but his primary contribution was that he had not killed the experiment in its infancy. Tried in a cadaver, the device created by the two young scientists—and now called an intra-aortic balloon pump—worked in the human circulation system.

After this invention was announced at the ASAIO meeting, an enthusiastic Kolff sent out bulletins to the clinic staff letting them know the pump was available as a tremendous tool to tide patients over cardiogenic shock. Only one doctor showed any interest. The physicians' response saddened Kolff, but he was sure that the day would come when the pump, or one like it, would save thousands of lives.

Calves in the Clinic

The NASA machine intended to power an artificial heart with jets of compressed air was overwhelming. It stood more than five feet high and had a large array of electronics stacked in a rack. Technicians could manipulate its twenty-four dials to drive a heart at any tempo. An electrical impulse controlled the air driving the artificial heart. As it turned out, hearts worked best when there was a sudden spike of air pressure followed by a drop to a plateau and then complete collapse.

The driver was attached to a new heart that Norton created and built. The heart was almost as complicated as the NASA machine with bellows, sacs for blood, and four sets of mechanical pistons. Like his ill-fated, magnet-driven heart, it circulated blood in dogs but was too cumbersome. Kolff shelved it.

Akutsu also came up with a new heart model—two chambered sacs that were the ventricles. Each sac was sealed inside a canlike container with tubes to connect into the aorta and the pulmonary vessels. Compressed air was pumped in to squeeze the sacs, which then expelled blood. Since the two ventricles had separate drivelines, the left one could be driven at the necessary higher pressure. Suction restored the sacs to their original shape for filling.

The heart had two six-foot hoses that tethered the animal to the air compressor. Akutsu remarked, "It is not a solution that a healthy man would look forward to, but for the patient in desperate heart failure, the alternative of death probably would not be popular, either."

Kolff's team had grown to include surgeons, cardiologists, biologists, engineers, and technicians. They started off on a high. The first dog implanted with Akutsu's new heart survived twenty hours, a lab record, giving rise to jubilant hope that perhaps they had found the secret. In fact, they were off on a toboggan ride of wild ups and downs. Most dogs did not live more than nine hours. Some even died on the operating table.

Some of the deaths were due to technical difficulties with the bewildering NASA machinery. Surveying its maze of controls, Kolff said, "It's beautiful, but to operate it, you have to be a licensed airplane pilot." Even its size was intimidating. He told an American Medical Association writer, "Our ultimate goal is not a patient with an air-driven heart accompanied by a tower of electronic equipment."

Though he was concerned that most of the dogs died so quickly, Kolff took hope from the three that survived twenty hours or more. They sat up, their reflexes were intact, and they barked and swallowed water; when Kolff reached to pet them, they licked his hand. The downside was that they all followed the same pattern. They were first lively and then abruptly turned listless. When reflex tests showed their central nervous systems were failing, Kolff turned off their artificial hearts. That was more humane than letting them live with dead brains while the hearts kept beating.

Why did the dogs' nervous systems fail? Autopsies provided the first unmistakable evidence that the complication Kolff feared most was taking place. As the dogs' lives extended, their artificial hearts became breeding grounds for thrombi—deadly blood clots. The heart valves were sheathed with them. Eventually some of the material broke free in the circulatory system and clogged a blood vessel.

One of Kolff's early acts in the heart program was setting up a long-range study of thrombosis (clotting). It was already well known that when blood contacts a foreign substance, it lays down a layer of protein, making the surface seem more compatible. But the added layer can also attract blood cells (platelets) that sometimes congeal. The rough surface creates barriers where cells can take root. From the beginning, therefore, the heart researchers had chosen smooth materials that offered no catch holds for blood.

Akutsu had followed that guideline. Kolff was especially puzzled because thrombi formed in less than a day. That was odd because valve replacements for humans were made from the same material his lab used in artificial hearts. After months those human valve replacements were clear of all clotting. The suspicion grew that dog blood was especially vulnerable to thrombi formation.

"We will start using calves," Kolff said. The researchers also decided to change from polyurethane to Silastic, a rubberlike compound. Calves had drawbacks, too, however. A hospital was associated with the research clinic, and many doctors said that having the place people visited for medical treatment also admit cows did not project a good public image. The solution was to build a box big enough to enclose a calf so it could be placed inside and shielded from public view.

Once in Kolff's cramped lab—the same fifty-by-thirty-foot room he had originally had—a calf was penned only feet from a secretary's desk. Puzzled telephone callers sometimes heard more moo than voice. One patient in a sixth-floor hospital room told a technician that she was delirious all night: "I kept hearing a cow, and I know that on 93rd Street in Cleveland, there aren't any cows."

The calves also turned Kolff into an insomniac. In their first ten experiments, he and his team could not get a single calf to live more than five hours with an artificial heart. Everything in the surgery, starting with the time on the heart-lung machine, proceeded without trouble. However, the calves soon died. The autopsies were startling. Ordinarily blood coming from the lungs into the left atrium is bright red since it is 95 percent saturated with oxygen, but in the calves, it was black and had an oxygen level of only 34 percent.

Was the fault in the heart-lung machine, the artificial heart, or the surgical technique? The team members reviewed their entire procedure, hunting for some obscure error but found none. Akutsu told the assembled ASAIO, "We welcome your suggestions." Nobody had any so Kolff suspended further calf implants.

Competition

In the hill-country coal town of Harlan, Kentucky, Dr. Frank Hastings, a surgeon in the Miners Memorial Hospital, was sitting in his basement watching an anesthetized dog lying on an operating table. Its chest was open, and multiple tubes ran to a small pump. Hastings was caught up in the fever of making an artificial heart and—with several associates at the hospital—was experimenting. He outfitted a lab in his basement for nights and weekends.

By his own definition, Hastings was a humanist. A Quaker, he had attended Swarthmore College and was a conscientious objector. After getting his training as a thoracic surgeon, Hastings declared he wanted to practice in small rural areas where he could "really help people." He was a thoughtful man with a taste for research. His natural interest was sparked when he read of Kolff's artificial-heart experimentation.

Initially he and his associates envisioned a heart that would drive exactly the same amount of blood into the lungs and arterial circuits with each beat. However, veins do not always deliver identical amounts of blood to the heart. For instance, the flow is less during sleep than when exercising. Half a century earlier, an Englishman, Ernest Henry Starling, had discovered that a heart can only pump out the volume of blood it receives. An artificial heart would need to have flexible output depending on the changing amount of blood sent to it.

Therefore, the Harlan group built a new heart run by hydraulic power. They implanted the device in a large mongrel dog. Hastings intended to close the chest, but surgical complications caused a blood leak that could not be repaired. Hour after hour the dog lay unconscious while the artificial heart kept going, and Hastings siphoned out the loose blood. The dog lived for thirty-two hours—the longest survival period yet.

In Argentina another doctor, Domingo Liotta, had also experimented with hydraulic power in an artificial heart. He and Hastings came to an ASAIO meeting on the same day in 1961 to report on their work. After they spoke, the program chair said their projects showed that, "whether you're in Cordoba, Argentina, or Hazard, Kentucky, if you want to do it badly enough, you do it." The chair was Kolff, and no one corrected him to say it was Harlan, not Hazard.

Liotta wrote Kolff, and he got funds from the Rotary Club so that Liotta could come to the United States. For five months, Liotta worked with Kolff. Then he got an offer he could not turn down. Houston's Michael DeBakey, one of the world's leading cardiovascular surgeons, invited him to join his lab at Baylor University's College of Medicine. DeBakey recognized Kolff as a fellow pioneer. He felt that he and Kolff were bucking the tide by maintaining that the artificial heart was both feasible and desirable. He hoped that Liotta could work with his staff to create a made-in-Texas heart.

The goal was more easily stated than achieved. DeBakey's team soon encountered problems it could not solve. The focus quickly switched to a cardiac booster pump, an assist device to supplement the work of the heart's left ventricle.

The Baylor team, which included one of DeBakey's prize protégées, the ambitious Dr. Denton A. Cooley, designed a device that mirrored the pneumatic principle of the Kolff sac heart. It was a tube within a tube. The inner tube ran blood from the natural heart's left atrium directly to the aorta, bypassing the left ventricle. The outer tube, sealed at both ends, had a space where injected air could compress the blood-filled tube, emptying its contents into the aorta and augmenting what the left ventricle was pumping. A single cannula injected the air.

Liotta returned to the ASAIO in 1962 to describe the double tube's success. He said it had functioned in dogs up to forty-four hours, far beyond anything Kolff had achieved. A report—signed by Liotta, Cooley, and others—said their pump, because it was light and small and didn't generate heat, was ideal.

The following year a forty-two-year-old man made history with the Texas device without ever knowing it. He suffered from congestive heart failure and was operated on to replace a clogged heart valve. Eighteen hours later, his heart stopped. Surgeons speedily opened his chest and hand-massaged the heart in hopes it would resume beating. However, the patient went into a coma; the arrested heart had damaged his brain. His kidneys were failing, and his lungs were filling with fluid.

The doctors decided his situation was hopeless so he appeared to be an ideal candidate to test the assist device. On the night of July 19, 1963, DeBakey directed the pump designed for a dog to be put into the man's chest, the first time an artificial ventricle had ever been implanted in a human patient. The man's lungs began to clear; his breathing deepened, and neurological sensitivity improved. After forty-eight hours, clots began to form. Urine output was zero, and dialysis was started. On the third day after the implant, the patient developed bronchopneumonia, and death followed.

The autopsy showed an enlarged heart and liver, clot-induced tissue death in all four quarters of the brain, and long-standing damage in the liver, lungs, and kidneys. Nevertheless, the DeBakey team was encouraged enough to put the device in two more patients whose hearts stopped during open-heart surgery. In neither case could the pump restore cardiac function. The team did no more human experiments.

Kolff's research continued to have problems, but the team would not give up seeking an explanation for the black blood coming out of the calves' lungs. They eliminated potential causes one by one. Finally, there was only one possibility—the force and amount of blood being pumped out of the artificial right ventricle were excessive. When Akutsu drove the blood with high force into a calf's lungs, it came out black. After he slowed the pump to ease the flow, it came out red. Starting the artificial heart at full driving power flooded the lungs' tiny arteries, the researchers realized. These capillaries constricted, and blood rushed by without being oxygenated. "From now on, we start the artificial heart very slowly," Kolff directed. Its rate would be allowed to increase only after tests showed that the blood was satisfactorily saturated with oxygen.

Eagerly Kolff and his staff resumed their calf work. The first animal lived less than three hours, and the next two also died quickly. The deaths were from mechanical failures, however, not physiological or biological ones. Persisting, the researchers logged a calf survival time of twenty hours in 1964. The animal stood up and drank water. That was a world record, prompting Kolff to state, "There is no doubt that in the near future, the symbol of life, the site of life, and the habitat of the soul—the human heart—will be replaced by a mechanical pump."

The Great Society

In Houston the redoubtable DeBakey was proving just as stubborn as Kolff in refusing to give up the idea of a total artificial heart. DeBakey already had a young surgeon as the scientific director for his artificial-heart program. Dr. C. William Hall had been at the University of Kansas experimenting with man-made heart valves when DeBakey lured him to Houston. From nearby Rice

University, DeBakey also brought in engineers, chemists, and physicists to work with Hall, Liotta, and others on solving the artificial heart's enigmas.

Even these expanded efforts were not enough for DeBakey. He thought the work was so important that it merited a national crash program like the one for a U.S. moon shot. That kind of financial input was necessary. In Washington one man, who had survived a heart attack, listened. The new president, Texan Lyndon B. Johnson, admired DeBakey and thought a solution to heart disease should be part of his vision of the Great Society. Johnson said he would support heart research on a scale never before dreamed.

With White House approval, DeBakey sent Hall to Washington to lay the groundwork for this program. Johnson appointed a national commission to study the problem, choosing DeBakey as its chair. The National Heart Institute was started under the umbrella of the NIH to foster artificial-heart research. That probably would not have happened without DeBakey's special influence in the White House. The program's first director was Hastings, the former coal-country surgeon.

The first grant went to DeBakey's multiyear $4.5 million program, which ultimately failed to produce a successful artificial heart and was dropped. Hall returned to Houston, where DeBakey had him write the proposal for a new program. Hall was proud of the plan that he drafted, especially because he was sure the work could be done for $25,000. DeBakey heatedly told him, "This is not what I want, not at all." Hall rewrote the program to reflect DeBakey's ideas, and Washington loved it.

However, after several years, DeBakey's research lost its momentum. The secrets of the artificial heart had eluded the acclaimed DeBakey.

Kolff's Peril

Kolff never could avoid run-ins with the Cleveland Clinic's bureaucracy. When he announced plans to seek a seven-million-dollar NIH grant to fund all his heart and kidney work for seven years, others in the clinic said they would resign if he submitted the proposal. They said that with such a budget, the tail would be wagging the dog. The clinic's board of governors decided it would be best to abolish his Division of Artificial Organs and put him back under Page in kidney research. Kolff pleaded with the board, promising he would not submit the grant proposal if his department was allowed to continue.

The board agreed, but there were more clouds. Objections were made to Kolff's research animals being in a building so close to the hospital, and his lab workers were accused of taking home meat from calves terminated after experiments and eating it. Fearful that the charges could mean the demise of his program, Kolff appealed to the board chair. A meeting was arranged, but when Kolff arrived, he suddenly felt very ill. He recognized the symptoms as psychosomatic, stemming from the realization that his life's work was in jeopardy, but the pain was very real.

The dreaded meeting proved to be quite pleasant. Kolff pointed out that it was common practice to eat experimental animals because it was inexcusable to waste good meat. Moreover, newspaper photographs had publicized the fact that calves were used in his work without public objection. Finally, he reminded the board that both the clinic's research committee and the board itself had approved the calf experiments. The objections were dismissed, and Kolff went back to work on the artificial heart.

He was still confronted with personnel shortages. A Swiss lab had hired away one of his biomedical engineers. His chief heart designer and surgeon, Akutsu, left to work in a much larger Brooklyn lab. "I am glad for Dr. Akutsu," Kolff told the doctor's new boss, Dr. Adrian Kantrowitz, head of cardiovascular surgery at Maimonides Medical Center. "But this leaves me without a surgeon."

Kantrowitz, a bluff and imposing man, had known Kolff for years through the ASAIO. He was an advocate of the heart-assist device and had regularly disputed with Kolff about removing the natural heart. Still, he could understand Kolff's point. The two agreed that Kolff could ask another young surgeon working with Kantrowitz if he would like to transfer to the Cleveland staff. He was Yukihiko Nosé (pronounced "no zay"). Nosé was not sure he wanted to go to Cleveland. In fact, he was not even sure he wanted to stay in America. In Japan he had worked on artificial kidneys. His experience with Kantrowitz had prepared him to go back to Japan to develop an artificial-heart program.

After a preliminary visit, Nosé returned to Kolff's lab, assured he would be its surgeon, heart designer, and chief of staff. During his first surgery on a calf, Kolff stood nearby, saying, "We do this stitch this way," and, "We insert the cannula here."

"You are a surgeon?" Nosé asked.

"No."

"I am a surgeon. Do not tell me my work. Would you please leave?"

No one had ever kicked Kolff out of his own lab before, but he left.

After the surgery, Nosé explained what he had done and answered Kolff's questions. Subsequently the two became close friends. Nosé, a bachelor with a quick sense of humor, was often invited to the Kolffs' home and farm. At the farm, Nosé, like all other guests, was assigned to various fix-up projects. One day he was sandpapering a picnic table with another guest, Bonnie MacDonald, a clinic technician. "Do you like to do this sandpapering?" Nosé asked her. When she said no, he smiled. "Then why do we do it?"

"Let's just take a walk and talk," she replied. Courtship followed, then marriage. When their first child, a daughter, was born, Kolff claimed the right to name her. He chose Wilhelmina for the former Dutch queen. It did not occur to him that Wilhelmina's father would have trouble pronouncing all those "l's."

Kantrowitz, meanwhile, was studying some distressing statistics. Of all heart attack victims suffering acute heart muscle infarctions, 20 percent went into cardiogenic shock. Almost all of them failed to respond to any therapy. Kantrowitz decided to do something about these figures. Reviving the idea of the intra-aortic balloon pump devised in Kolff's lab by Moulopoulos and Topaz four years earlier, Kantrowitz made changes possible with new materials, then tried it on dogs. Satisfied it worked, he waited for the right human patient to test it.

That turned out to be a forty-five-year-old woman who came to Maimonides with chest pains, shortness of breath, and marked weakness. Her skin was ashen, cold, and clammy, and her lips and nails were bluish. The diagnosis was acute heart-muscle infarction with early congestive heart failure and cardiogenic shock. Five hours after admission, she was still in shock despite medication. When all seemed hopeless, Kantrowitz called for the intra-aortic balloon pump. He kept the balloon in her aorta for seven hours, turning it on and off. When it went off for the ninth time, her skin was dry and warm, the blue color was gone, and she was out of shock. Shortly thereafter she was discharged from the hospital.

More successes and some failures followed, but it was clear that the balloon pump had proved its worth in combating cardiogenic shock.[1] As of 2011, nearly every hospital had the balloon pump available for emergency situations. An estimated 100,000 balloons were being used in the U.S. each year.

In New York City, a third-year medical student, Theodore Stanley, went to the funeral of a young man only thirty-five who had not recovered from surgery to replace a defective heart valve. Although Stanley had known the man only during his stay in Presbyterian Hospital, he admired the patient's fight against his disease. "His death was needless," Stanley said to one of his professors. "People like him are okay in everything, except they have a pump that is failing. Why can't we replace it? Would that be so tough?"

"There's a man in Cleveland who's trying," his professor said, "Name's Kolff." The accounts of Kolff's early struggles to make an artificial heart inspired Stanley. "I'm going to build a heart," he vowed. His professor suggested he visit the company that made Silastic, the material Kolff was using to make artificial hearts.

"Give us your design for a heart," the company said. "We'll make it for you." Within several months, the firm sent him prototypes of his heart, ready for implant. Impressed, Stanley's professor persuaded staff members to help the young physician by implanting his device. However, the heart failed. It failed in dogs, a calf, and a sheep. Later, while interning at the University of Michigan's hospital, Stanley wrote to both Kolff and DeBakey, saying he wanted to visit their labs. Both said he was welcome.

DeBakey's lab was impressive, covering an entire hospital floor with an array of expensive, modern equipment. It was very professional and subdued. "Dull, dull, dull," Stanley thought. DeBakey was too busy to see him.

Cleveland was something else. Kolff personally introduced Stanley at a morning conference and asked him to describe his heart design. When he finished, Kolff had sharp, but constructive, criticism. It was animal-experiment day, and Kolff suggested Stanley help Nosé implant an artificial heart. For an intern, this was heady business. Much of the lab's equipment was old, often patched together. Under the operating table were open pails to catch blood. Yet Stanley sensed that the men around Kolff believed in the artificial heart. Kolff had instilled the feeling that they were on the cutting edge of history.

With his latest heart design, Nosé had kept a calf alive for thirty-three hours and fifteen minutes, a new record. At day's end, Kolff invited Stanley into his tiny office. "We have much to do," he said, "many technical problems to overcome. Yet there is progress." Then he stunned Stanley. "Why don't you do a fellowship with us? I think you would like it. We would like to have you." Kolff took him home to dinner with Janke and the children. Stanley went back to his internship, looking forward to joining Kolff's team as soon as possible.

By the end of 1966, Kolff's unit had performed 12,000 dialyses and 126 kidney transplants. With yet-another new heart design, Nosé kept a calf alive for forty-eight hours. More than ever, Kolff felt he needed greater clinic support, which meant more staff, space, and money. One official asked him, "Why should you get it? We're all strapped."

Kolff felt he had no future at the clinic. That winter he called William Hall, DeBakey's chief of staff, and asked, "Is there room for me in your program?"

"Pim," said Hall, "both of us are strong people. There isn't a program in the world big enough to hold us, not to mention DeBakey. It would never work."

"What I would like is a place in a regional university where I could set up an institute of artificial organs," a rebuffed Kolff explained.

The University of Utah: Kolff's New Home

At about the same time, Dr. James C. Fletcher, president of the University of Utah (1964–1971), who later became the head of NASA, contacted Hall in Houston. Fletcher asked Hall if he was interested in moving to the University of Utah to form an Institute for Biomedical Engineering. Hall informed Fletcher that a doctor at the Cleveland Clinic was very good and looking for a move.

At Utah Dr. Keith Reemtsma, chief of surgery, wanted to expand into kidney transplants and was spearheading a drive for a new artificial-organs program. Hall had been just about to turn down the offer to direct Reemtsma's project when Kolff called. "Stay where you are," Hall told Kolff. "I'll call you back." Hall then telephoned the Utah officials who were recruiting him. "I can't accept," Hall said, but how would you like to have Pim Kolff as your director?"

"Kolff? Are you sure? Would he come? Can we get him?"

"Here's Kolff's number. Wait fifteen minutes and then call him." Hall then telephoned Kolff. "The University of Utah is thinking of starting a program in artificial organs," he said.

"Do I have a chance there?" asked Kolff.

"They'll be calling you in fifteen minutes. Ask them yourself," Hall replied.

Fletcher contacted Kolff, and after much conversation and Fletcher making two visits to Cleveland, Kolff agreed to move to Salt Lake City. He planned to bring two men from Cleveland: a surgeon, Dr. Clifford Kwan-Gett, and Tom Kessler, a dental technician trained in the navy who built artificial hearts. Some adjustments had to be made. Fletcher wanted the name to be Institute for Biomedical Engineering (IBE), and Kolff wanted Artificial Organs in the title. In the end, the Division of Artificial Organs became the major component of the IBE.

As the plane carrying Pim and Janke Kolff came into the valley of the Great Salt Lake, Janke, who had grown up amid mountains in Java, felt a rush of emotion as she saw the ranges cradling the valley—the Wasatch to the east, the Oquirrh to the west. Snow-garlanded peaks stabbed ten thousand feet into the sky. "It is all so beautiful," Janke enthused.

Kolff's mind wasn't on mountains. He was sketching the artificial-organs institute he wanted to found. He would have a dialysis program, a heart program, and an open door to anyone wanting an adventure in research involving replacements for almost every part of the body.

When they got off the plane, Reemtsma was there along with the university's vice president for research, the dean of the College of Medicine, and other officials. "My husband is very honored that you would have him here," Janke said to one of the greeters.

"We were honored the minute he stepped off the plane onto Utah soil," was the reply.

They took the Kolffs to Fletcher's office. He had a bold plan to elevate the university's stature with new programs in science. "We are glad you are here, and we hope you will stay. And if there are opportunities for you to start companies furthering your work, count on us for help," he told Kolff.

In a mountainside restaurant with a magnificent view of the valley, the Utah delegation laid out what they could offer. Kolff would have an appointment as professor in the Department of Surgery. The university could not pay him what he had made in Cleveland, but he would have autonomy in his program and be responsible only to the vice president for research. He could take over the dialysis unit for University Hospital, and his work could include research on all artificial organs.

It was all acceptable to Kolff. Talking privately to Dr. Kenneth Castleton, medical-school dean, Kolff said, "To make all this work, I will need money. I am sure you know many rich people here in the valley. In time you must introduce me to them." Kolff told Janke that the opportunity in Utah was like liberation.

Nosé, who had been visiting in Japan, returned to Cleveland to find that Kolff was going to Utah. "And I want you with me," Kolff told him. At first Nosé was tempted. Then he thought of the sixteen lab workers who might be out of work.

"I am Japanese," Nosé told friends. "I could not leave them with no jobs." The clinic said that if Nosé stayed, he could have Kolff's position. He accepted and managed to keep most of the staff. The personnel office called Theodore Stanley, who was planning to start at the clinic within a month or two. "You're welcome to come, but Dr. Kolff will not be here. He is going to Utah," he was told.

That was the first Stanley had heard of the move. "What is going on?" he asked Kolff when he finally got him on the phone.

"I think I have a place for you in Utah," Kolff replied. Actually the Utah move was great news for Stanley; it led to a wedding. Earlier the woman he wanted to marry had refused because she thought they would be living in Cleveland. When she heard the destination was Salt Lake City, she said that was quite a different story.

The University Struggling to Become a Harvard or Johns Hopkins

The dust was hardly off the first pioneer wagons in the mid-1800s when the Mormons, holding to a fundamental belief that salvation could never be attained in ignorance, set up the first university west of the Mississippi. After the Pilgrims came to Plymouth Rock, it took twenty-six years before Harvard College opened. The University of Deseret (later Utah) was launched in 1850, three years after the vanguard group of settlers had arrived in the valley. At times it shut down for lack of money, but it always reopened and expanded, moving into three buildings at the start of the twentieth century on land set aside on Salt Lake's east bench, a plateau nestled against the Wasatch Mountains.

The University of Utah was fifty-four years old before it opened a two-year medical school. The delay was perhaps a reflection of Brigham Young's view that he would rather die a natural death than "be helped out of the world by a doctor," no matter how fancy his medical pedigree. He thought a doctor's main jobs were to treat fevers (of which there were few) and deliver babies (of which there were many), although he later conceded a bonesetter could be useful.

The creation of the University of Utah Medical Center proceeded by small, but visionary, steps, guided by the determination of people who had the same grit as the earlier settlers. Another thirty-seven years passed before the school expanded to a four-year program. A recruiter lined up a staff of brilliant young doctors by comparing the school to Johns Hopkins.

As soon as he came to Salt Lake, Dr. Maxwell M. Wintrobe knew that the claim was false. Wintrobe was from the real Johns Hopkins. He was appalled to find the school's only clinical facility was a dismal county hospital, run by politicians "whose only difference from the Tammany Hall crowd was that, being Mormons, they didn't smoke cigars." Wintrobe asked the president of Johns Hopkins, "Should I stay?"

"Of course," he was told. "Utah is the center of about a third of the country. From Canada to Mexico, Denver to the Pacific, it has the only medical school. Take the job! It's the last frontier in American medicine."

Wintrobe did, and so did a cadre of other Young Turks who infused the infant program with standards of excellence. Wintrobe became world recognized in hematology. The school eventually achieved national praise for its research in pharmacology and other fields. Ironically, *Newsweek* later described the University of Utah School of Medicine as "the Johns Hopkins of the West."

Salt Lake City was a setting to soothe the soul of a pioneer's son. As far as the eye could see were mountains, jagged rock spines soaring above the timberline. On the valley floor sat the Mormon Temple, topped with the gold-plated figure of the Angel Moroni blowing his trumpet; the State Capitol, patterned after the U.S. Capitol; and the Great Salt Lake, the eighty-mile-long remnant of a vast prehistoric sea four times saltier than any ocean.

That was what awaited Pim and Janke in 1967 when they arrived to start over in the land the Mormons called "Zion, home of the pure in heart."

Note

1. In 1983 Kolff said the pump was used 110,000 times a year on heart-attack victims in the U.S. alone. "I shall forever be grateful that Dr. Kantrowitz had the courage and the wisdom to use it," he said.

6

Come to the Mountains of the Pioneers

Why is there so much work on the artificial heart in Utah?
Because I am here.
—Dr. Willem J. Kolff

Theodore Stanley and his bride, Mary Ann, arrived in Salt Lake City on July 23, 1967, following a cross-country honeymoon. When they telephoned Kolff, he arranged to have his assistant take them to dinner. Ten minutes later, a man with a decidedly British-Australian accent called. "I am Dr. Clifford Kwan-Gett," he said. "Dr. Kolff has told me of you. If you will be outside your motel at eight this evening, I would be most happy to have you and your wife as my guests at dinner."

At 8:00 PM the Stanleys were waiting. Standing nearby was a lean Chinese man, fairly tall with a sharp, intense feeling about him. He started to walk toward them but stopped when they turned away. Five minutes later, the three of them were still waiting. "Do you suppose . . . ?" Mary Ann asked.

"No, I don't think he's our man," said Stanley. Finally, the Chinese man walked up to the Stanleys. Tentatively he asked, "Dr. Stanley?" Noting the incredulity on Stanley's face, he added, "I am Clifford Kwan-Gett."

"But I was looking for an Englishman," Stanley replied. Over dinner Kwan-Gett explained that his parents had emigrated from Canton, China, to Australia before he was born. After receiving a University of Sydney degree in mechanical engineering, he realized that was "not the right spot," so he went back to school to become a medical doctor. Following a two-year residency, Kwan-Gett took stock of his prospects. Australian physicians mostly got their degrees, launched their practices, and stayed put. To his wife, Joo Een, a lithe and beautiful émigré from Singapore, he said, "They're all tied to their practices, so before we are locked into that, let's get travel out of our systems. Let's see the United States."

Kwan-Gett had read scientific articles about the artificial heart. "I want to do that," he said. "I am an engineer, and I am a doctor. I can combine my training in that work." He asked a professor in Australia, "Who's the best in the field?"

"There are two" was the answer: "Kolff and DeBakey." Kwan-Gett wrote to Kolff, saying he had a fellowship that would pay some of his expenses if the scientist could find a place for him.

Kolff answered, "Yes. I can use you, but do not come as a student. You are then at the mercy of the immigration people about how long you can stay." Kwan-Gett gave up his fellowship, bought airline tickets, and applied for a visa.

"Sorry" was an American official's response. "The immigration quota from Australia is filled." Kwan-Gett was frantic. Then the official took another look at the couple's papers. "Wait a minute. Your wife is from Singapore, and the quota from there is open. If she applies, you can go with her as her husband."

By that thin strand of circumstances, the Kwan-Getts entered the United States in 1966. Cleveland was a time of learning for Kwan-Gett because Kolff let him experiment with both the artificial kidney and heart. When Yukihiko Nosé declined to move to Salt Lake City, Kwan-Gett eagerly accepted Kolff's offer to be chief of the new Utah lab.

Fiefdom on a Hill

Building 512 stood on a small rise at the foot of the Wasatch Mountains near the University of Utah's hospital/medical school complex. It was a dingy, one-story wooden affair with age-stained paint and dirt-encrusted windows. During World War II, it had been a barracks for soldiers at nearby Fort Douglas. Donated to the university, it was first a lab for entomologists. Long after they moved out, the residue of their research lingered: bugs littered the floors and walls.

This inauspicious structure was the first home of the Division of Artificial Organs. The promise was that the university would later organize a new IBE, a synergistic blending of Kolff's work with engineering and biology. Until then he was stuck with the old barracks building. Later, he expanded across the street into Building 518—grandly named the Hercick Building after a benefactor—to house his office and dialysis group.

Building 512's initial mangyness did not bother Kolff. It had what he needed for his fiefdom—space for an operating room (OR), offices, a machine shop, laboratory for fabricating hearts, and stalls for research animals. There was also

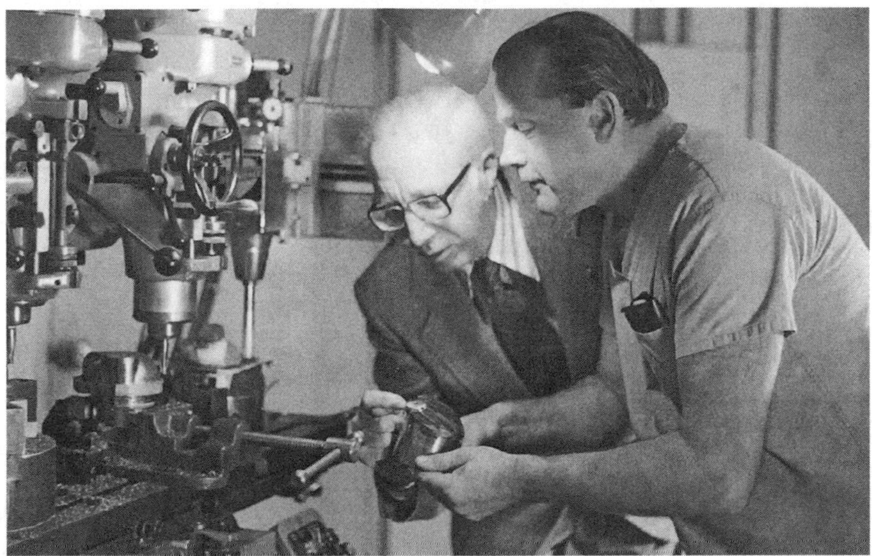

Dr. Kolff (*left*) with Walter Rohloff, one of many machinists.

a room where he and his staff—small as it was—could meet every morning at 8:00 AM for his famous morning conference.

Paint took care of the surface appearance. Cement floors were sealed with plastic to make them impervious to blood stains in the surgery rooms and animal stalls. Finances did not cover office rugs, but the father of a staff member contributed one. Kolff hung some pictures, and others brought vases of flowers. "With the little touches," Kolff said, "we make this our home."

The OR equipment was pitiful. Stanley scrounged a table that was being discarded at the nearby Veterans Administration Hospital. The old heart-lung-machine oxygenators Kolff salvaged from Cleveland were so inefficient they periodically turned blood into a froth that could not be defoamed. The respirator to aerate the lungs of anesthetized animals was an antique made in Sweden. There were some air pumps to drive the artificial hearts, but much of the critical equipment was missing or defunct, including blood-chemistry test kits.

Kolff could count the personnel for his first Utah team on two hands. Kwan-Gett and Stanley would do the surgery. Kolff had brought Tom Kessler, a solemn, ascetic looking man, from Cleveland to make hearts. The chief technician to start the kidney-dialysis program was another Cleveland export, Dietz Van Dura. In Salt Lake, Kolff hired Peggy Miller, a chic and cheerful clinical social worker, to counsel dialysis patients. Several OR and lab technicians, two secretaries, and a few student volunteers rounded out the staff.

Kolff told them he was wide open to proposals for replacing human organs with mechanical substitutes. At a staff brainstorming session, however, reproductive organs were quickly eliminated as possibilities. The group came up with another interesting idea, however. During lunch one day, Stanley and another lab worker were sprawled on the grass when a coed in a very tight skirt walked by. "Wow," said the friend, eying her backside, "it's great to make artificial hearts, but you could never hope for anything as cute as that."

"That's it," said Stanley, suddenly animated.

"What's it?"

"Do you know how many people have colostomies?" asked Stanley, referring to the devices that empty the colon into a rubber sac after surgery. "Why not an artificial anus?"

Kolff liked the idea. With the help of Kessler, now supervisor of the prosthetics laboratory, Stanley designed a miniature signal device for opening and closing the colon. To test the units, Stanley wore old boots into the animal area every morning to give enemas to sheep rigged with the new device. The boots became legendary. Eventually one of Stanley's boots mysteriously disappeared; it was bronzed and returned to him as a symbol of his prowess at pathfinding research. Scientific publications printed three reports on his experiment, but in the end it was clear that the scientists who could build artificial hearts could not come up with a satisfactory artificial anus.

Otherwise, a bionic man began taking shape on the drawing board with a variety of internal organs and artificial eyes, arms, and ears that responded to neural stimuli.

In his younger years, Kolff was primarily a hands-on scientist. Now he believed his role was to inspire, prod, and nursemaid others. Kwan-Gett learned this early. He scheduled a calf for an artificial-heart implant in the first surgery at 512, but when he arrived in the OR, there was no animal. "Surgery's cancelled," he was informed. "Kolff said something about working with sheep."

Kwan-Gett, annoyed because he was supposed to run the lab, raced into Kolff's office to protest. "In Cleveland you tried sheep. It was a disaster. You said you never wanted to see another sheep."

"Here, I want them," Kolff responded. Calves cost $150 apiece, but a mature ewe could be bought for $5 and a ram for $15. In addition, an inexperienced veterinarian had convinced him that Salt Lake's altitude of four thousand–plus feet made young calves vulnerable to lung problems. It was advice, unfortunately, that simply was not true. But for the practical Kolff, there was one more persuasive point: sheep droppings were far easier to clean up.

Kwan-Gett still objected. "Try the sheep," Kolff coldly replied. His tone of voice told Kwan-Gett the decision was final.

The lab staff called the particular heart they were working with the green heart. It consisted of two separate blood sacs (ventricles) inside canisters covered with Teflon tinted the color of grass. Designed in Cleveland by Nosé, it was the model used in the calf that lived a record-setting forty-eight hours. Nosé was seeking to demystify making a heart. Instead of having technicians work days or weeks to handcraft each one, he believed the hearts could be mass produced. He bought sacs from a factory that specialized in Silastic rubber and added commercially available valves and tubes to connect to the body and air power. Enclosing them in separate containers, he could assemble a heart in a matter of hours.

Kolff designated the green heart for his Utah team's first series of implants. It was not a grand opening for the lab, however, because the heart was designed for calves. Neither Kwan-Gett nor Stanley was a trained cardiac surgeon, so they had trouble implanting it in the sheep without impinging on the lungs and great veins. Additionally the sheep's tissue tore easily, so suturing was difficult. The sheep died on the table. Animals that lived experienced frightful hemolysis and uncontrollable hemorrhaging. Kwan-Gett pleaded with Kolff to switch to calves.

Kolff again refused. "I have done the autopsies. I know the problems. They are not insoluble," he stubbornly insisted.

The Burden

In academic research there are two kinds of money: hard and soft. Hard is better because it is a steady, reliable source of funds, such as a perpetual endowment that provides salaries for a professorial chair. Those who work with soft money are like Willie Loman in Arthur Miller's modern tragedy, *The Death of a Salesman.* Willie ventured forth with a smile and a shoeshine, hoping for the best, and failed miserably. In Utah—as he had done in Cleveland—Kolff hustled for soft dollars because federal grants were unreliable. From the University of Utah, he received thirty thousand dollars for salaries—two-thirds of what he had received in Cleveland. The burden of raising money to support his division was up to him. "We live on the brink of bankruptcy," he wryly commented.

He started with a $100,000 federal grant to further the artificial-heart work in Utah. The first time he sought renewal, the National Heart Institute refused. The indefatigable Kolff wrote a flotilla of letters to corporations, saying he knew that they would not want his life-saving work to end. Back came a piddling drizzle totaling $35,000 to keep the division going.

Kolff planted seeds among the federal agencies that had big dollars for research. From the U.S. Public Health Service, he got a contract to do cost analysis on kidney-dialysis programs. Though he had to fight to renew it, it was ultimately worth $1,277,000. He returned to the National Heart Institute with a different proposal and netted a $110,106 contract for the artificial-heart lab.

At last he had the money to hire part-time physicists, chemists, a biologist, medical researchers, and engineers to round out his team. He could even add an administrator to track office finances. He felt secure enough to set up the Division of Artificial Organs Development Fund, a high-sounding name for petty cash to cover expenses federal grants didn't meet, such as meals for workers at nighttime meetings. Somewhat nervously, John Warner, the new administrator, asked, "Where is the money coming from?" The answer was out of Kolff's pocket.

In his usual high-handed way, Kolff also obtained an administrative assistant, Mary Johnson. When her husband's job took them to Salt Lake City, Johnson, a five-foot, two-inch ash blonde, sought work at the Veterans Administration (VA) Hospital. The hospital had a hiring freeze, but just across Foothill Boulevard was the University of Utah. A personnel worker suggested she "go see John Warner in the Division of Artificial Organs. There is an opening in his office."

Making artificial hearts and kidneys sounded weird. "I'll think about it," Johnson told Warner. She finally accepted the job, although it did not pay much. She kept the lab books in the mornings and did secretarial chores on the dialysis program in the afternoons.

One day a white-haired man with a strong accent introduced himself: "Hello, I'm Dr. Kolff." Without her knowing, he had been watching her. He liked her forthright manner, the way she spoke up and attacked her work. He thought she would make an excellent administrative assistant to bring order to the mountain of paper work and correspondence engulfing his desk.

Before he could talk to her, one of her friends at the VA Hospital learned the hiring freeze had ended and called Kolff for a recommendation for Johnson.

Kolff bawled him out. "You do not steal secretaries. I will not allow you to take her."

The friend repeated the incident to Johnson: "Dr. Kolff will not release you." Enraged, she marched into Kolff's office and declared, "You can't stop me. The VA Hospital pays more than you do."

Kolff stared at her. "We'll see about this," he replied. He contacted the university's personnel office. "She has a much higher-paying job offer at the VA Hospital. I don't want to lose her. I want approval to pay her more than it can." Cowed by his ramrod insistence, the office agreed. Then he informed Johnson, "I have all this arranged for you. Wouldn't you like to stay?" She could think of nothing to say but yes.

Before Mary Johnson took the job as Kolff's private secretary, she was warned that she was about to be consumed in a workaholic's unending grind of letter writing, speeches, grant applications, financial worksheets, and assorted other headaches. The Cassandras who voiced the warnings underestimated; working for Kolff was even worse.

Night after night Johnson was in the office trying to match his pace. Finally, she could stand it no more. "Dr. Kolff, this work is wonderfully exciting, but I can't go on like this. My husband is complaining."

"Oh," Kolff replied. "We can't have that. From now on, you must leave every day at 4:30." Regularly as that time approached, he admonished her, "It's time. Keep your husband happy."

To office staff and scientists alike, Kolff was an odd blend of curtness and courtliness. When people talked longer than he wanted to listen, he shut them off. When he took his staff out for dinner meetings, he lectured them on what to order. Yet when a receptionist's grandson died in Ohio, Kolff paid her round-trip airfare to the funeral. The staff collected Kolffisms. Noticing that three-hole punches scattered small white paper circles on the floor, he instructed the secretaries, "Each girl will pick up seven holes." After a particularly heavy storm piled snow on the walks outside 512, he announced, "Every man will shovel for seven minutes." He refused to use the American slang of "doohickeys" for the valves, molds, and other objects in the lab. To him they were always "hickeydoos."

Kolff liked to tell his people to "take time to smell the roses." One morning while on the telephone with a researcher in Rome, he excused himself, explaining that he wanted to look at an interesting bird perched outside his window. He planted so many flower bulbs the staff called him "the tulip king." Visitors from Europe, Africa, and Asia trooped to his door. They usually received written invitations to cocktails at his home. In the lower left corner were the words, "Tricks by the dog." Diane, the family dog, entertained visitors with her routines. Many of the visitors spoke limited English, but everyone could understand Diane.

Barnard's Miracle

In 1967 the American College of Surgeons was rife with reports that the world was about to enter the era of human heart transplants. After years of research, Stanford University's Dr. Norman Shumway was close to doing the operation. In Virginia Dr. Richard Lower, who had worked with Shumway, put a dog's heart into the chest of another and showed fellow surgeons a movie of the recipient dog jumping and playing. In Brooklyn Dr. Adrian Kantrowitz was also planning cardiac transplants, and great strides were being made in understanding the greatest bugaboo—immunologic tissue rejection.

None of these surgeons did the first human transplant, however. In South Africa, Dr. Christiaan Barnard, who had done a residency with both Lower and Shumway, used techniques developed by Shumway to put a donor heart into a patient named Louis Washkansky. Although Washkansky only lived seventeen days, the operation enthralled the world; the press called it the "Miracle of Cape Town." Kantrowitz was next with a transplant in a baby. Shumway and his team then performed the surgery on an adult. Barnard did a second transplant. In Houston Michael DeBakey and Denton Cooley added transplants to their surgical repertories. Other doctors in many parts of the world followed.

In Salt Lake City, Kolff heard the news with unruffled equanimity, unconcerned with conjecture that transplants might end the need for an artificial heart. Noting a government report that tens of thousands of heart patients were sick enough to qualify for transplants, Kolff prophetically said, "There will never be enough donors to meet the demand." Moreover, he told his staff that regardless of the number of potential donors, the actual number would be fewer because of "sensitive questions surrounding the timing of death and the taking and using of a heart." Kolff definitely felt that "the world will still need the artificial heart."

To the uninitiated, scientists often seem to inhabit a world governed by blind alleys, phantom theories, and unbelievable missteps. Kolff thought it was better to risk error than avoid experimentation for fear of committing mistakes. Clearly, however, he had to do something about the high mortality in his sheep experiments. He began investigating a new heart design, what he called the "soft-shell mushroom heart," possibly the oddest design to emerge from his lab.

As envisioned in his sketches, the heart had two units, each with a hollow stem and cap that resembled a mushroom, anchored inside a flexible bag. With the mushroom deflated, blood could come into the bag. When the stem and cap were inflated with compressed air, they filled the bag and drove out the blood. While inflated, the cap covered the inflow ports, acting as a valve to stop blood from backing up.

Kolff filed formal notice that he considered this a patentable invention. He would develop it with funds from his U.S. heart contract, but he needed malleable material. The manager of a plant using liquid latex, a natural rubber, to manufacture gloves invited him to visit his factory. Kolff saw at once beyond thumbs

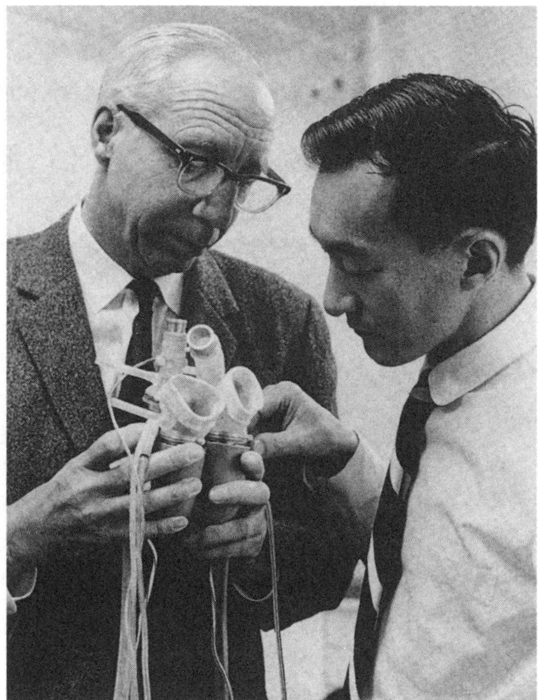

Dr. Kolff (*left*) with Dr. Clifford Kwan-Gett.

and fingers of gloves to hearts of latex. Latex could take almost any shape merely by dipping a mold in it; the thickness was controlled by how many times the mold was submerged.

For Kolff the tinkerer, latex was like a new toy. He filled an entire room at the lab with vats, racks, sinks, latex drums, and other dipping equipment. Instead of paying five thousand dollars for a mechanical arm to rotate the mold during dipping, he rigged a cheap counterpart from a child's erector set. To create his mushroom heart, he persuaded a glass blower in another university department to make a mold. The effort failed. At first Kolff reported delays to federal program reviewers, but eventually he had to abandon the design.

Kwan-Gett also was designing a heart. Instead of one canister as in the green heart, it had two, each with its own blood sac. Kwan-Gett hoped that these could be maneuvered to conform more accurately to a sheep's chest cavity. Kolff believed that latex should be used for the sac heart, but Kwan-Gett was not sure about its durability.

Kessler fretted because he could not produce identical latex sacs every time. The factory manager who volunteered to be Kolff's consultant explained why

Kessler was having problems. The liquid latex had to be kept moving in the vat. Kolff turned to California physicist Gerald Foote, whom he had recently hired to improve the instrumentation in artificial kidneys. Foote told them to put a small pump in the latex to agitate it constantly.

New problems surfaced. To achieve blood compatibility, the latex had to be purged of certain chemicals, but without them, the rubber appeared weaker. Moreover, it was all but impossible to bond one piece to another. A university specialist was called in and concluded that latex was not the best material for the lab to use. Kolff reversed himself and directed Kwan-Gett to use Silastic for his sac models.

Enter a Veterinarian

Despite the changes, the animals continued to suffer from severe hemolysis. The team managed to get one animal to survive for fifty hours, a mere two-hour advance in four years. Kolff was not dismayed; he said, "Look, if what we are doing were easy, it would have been done long before us." In 1967 Kwan-Gett attended a meeting where a veterinarian from the University of Nevada, Reno, Dr. Don B. Olsen, presented a paper on using sheep in cardiovascular research. Olsen was energetic, quick moving, and enthusiastic.

Thinking Olsen's expertise might be just what Kolff's staff needed, Kwan-Gett traced him to the Desert Research Institute. The institute had hired him after he had spent seven years in a private large-animal practice. Kwan-Gett urged him to become a consultant in Kolff's lab. Olsen agreed to visit Salt Lake City, but he was not sure who Kolff was. He had to look him up in the library to discover he was being asked to advise a world-ranking scientist.

Olsen was self-effacing with twinkling brown eyes that reflected his gentle sense of humor. As a Utah native, he liked to tramp the wilderness and was a crack shot. In the lab, his fellow researchers respected his meticulous skills. On his visit to Kolff's lab, he was impressed with the doctor's warmth and charm. He expected that Kolff would know a little about veterinary science without being terribly deep. Instead, Kolff raised questions about animals that pushed Olsen's knowledge. He told his wife, "I found myself in awe of him."

In his role as a consultant, Olsen was supposed to attend implants to monitor the animal's condition. Though he knew nothing about surgery with a heart-lung pump, he assumed he could use standard techniques to measure vital signs.

On his first try, Olsen inserted a probe to monitor the animal's temperature. Receptors to record the heart's electrical impulses with an electrocardiogram (EKG) were attached. He asked the surgeons to thread in an arterial cannula for tracking blood pressure. What happened next humiliated the veterinarian. The heart-lung machine had a cooling chamber to chill the blood and reduce the animal's need for oxygen. That left Olsen's thermometer meaningless. On bypass blood pressure doesn't pulsate, so his blood-pressure line told him nothing. Once the natural heart was excised, the EKG didn't function.

"What's the status of our sheep?" Kwan-Gett asked Olsen.

"According to what I'm monitoring, the sheep is dead," Olsen answered.

He had a lot to learn about cardiopulmonary bypass and implants. Nevertheless, Kolff thought he was bright and would make an excellent addition to his heart team. Olsen, however, was not ready to make a full commitment to the Utah program. He hoped to accept a postdoctoral fellowship from the NIH to earn his PhD. He asked Kolff if he could work as a consultant for four years.

Olsen visited the Artificial Heart Research Laboratory several times in 1967 and again in early 1968. He recommended switching from sheep to calves as the artificial-heart test animal. This made some points with Kwan-Gett. Kolff offered Olsen full-time employment, but he had received the four-year NIH postdoctoral fellowship to attend the University of Colorado School of Medicine. The alternate opportunity in Salt Lake City intrigued his scientific curiosity, but in the end, Olsen indicated he would consider working for Kolff after he completed his four years at the University of Colorado.

Kolff said, "We are keenly interested in your future."

In 1970 Olsen was briefly in Salt Lake City to visit his wife's relatives. Kolff invited him to give a lecture at the lab. He saw Olsen staring at the shabby plywood floor in the shower. Kolff said, "I assure you, Don, that if you'll come with us, I'll put new tile on the floor." Olsen had never heard bathroom tile used as a recruiting tactic.

Hoopla in Houston

In 1969 a forty-seven-year-old Skokie, Illinois, printing estimator named Haskell Karp became the catalyst for a series of events that launched the artificial heart into a media event. Cardiac trouble ran in Karp's family. A heart attack killed his father, and when Karp was fifteen, he contracted rheumatic fever, a disease that nearly always damages heart valves. Between his thirty-seventh and forty-seventh birthdays, Karp had five heart attacks. He once suffered complete cardiac block, requiring a pacemaker to keep his heart pumping at all. The heart was enlarged. Two coronary arteries were shut off and a third compromised. Angina stabbed him upon any exertion. Karp was on the borderline of the most severe class of heart disease. In addition, he had emphysema.

In early March 1969, Karp entered St. Luke's Episcopal Hospital in Houston, an affiliate of the Baylor College of Medicine headed by DeBakey. Karp was there to see whether DeBakey's one-time protégé, heart surgeon Denton Cooley, could help him. Cooley was now a full professor at Baylor and leader of his own competing Texas Heart Institute. Having read newspaper stories about heart surgery, Karp knew what he did and did not want. He thought himself a candidate for ventriculoplasty—surgery to cut out some of the dilated heart's dead tissue—repair of an aneurysm, and some other patchwork. What he assuredly did not want was a heart transplant.

In the fifteen months since Barnard's first transplant, physicians had grown both hot and cold about the procedure. On the plus side, Barnard's second patient lived more than five hundred days. On the downside, the high death rate from rejection of transplanted hearts was alarming. The Montreal Heart Institute declared a moratorium on further transplants. Of 170 cardiac-transplant patients in 1971, 146 had died of infection or rejection. Surgeons stopped the flood of transplants except for Shumway at Stanford. Ultimately, the tissue rejection problem was solved with a drug called cyclosporine.

Fourteen of Cooley's first seventeen transplant patients died, but he still found the surgery promising. However, he told Karp he would not do one on him if he opposed it. When an intensive medical regimen failed, Cooley scheduled Karp for ventriculoplasty on Good Friday, April 4, 1969. Cooley talked one more time with Karp, who said he would agree to a transplant if there was no alternative. Karp's wife later said her husband had told her he wanted to "live like a man, not lie like a vegetable."

Cooley did not have a donor heart for Karp, but he did have an artificial heart. The fact he would even consider an artificial heart was surprising. Only the previous August, he had told a California meeting that the device "borders on science fiction and wishful thinking." He thought it would not be feasible for another three to five years. Nevertheless, as Cooley reported, when Karp's heart failed to restart after surgery, an artificial heart was brought to the OR. Cooley cut out Karp's heart and stitched in the mechanical device.

The electrifying news that—for the first time—a man-made heart was beating in a human chest swept the world. Tabloid newspapers saluted Cooley as a "cardiowhiz." The *New York Times* ran the story on page 1. Television hailed Cooley as a national hero, ranking his achievement alongside Barnard's transplant. Kolff was on a camping trip. Informed of Cooley's operation, he telephoned congratulations to the Texas surgeon for a "fantastic accomplishment."

Cooley had never intended the mechanical heart to be other than a stopgap to buy time to find a heart donor. Almost from the beginning, Karp's kidneys were failing. He passed no urine, and at least one person who saw him described him as "semicomatose." With radio and newspapers relaying her every word, Karp's distraught wife made a unique anguished appeal: "Someone, somewhere, please hear my plea, a plea for a heart for my husband. I see him lying there, breathing, and knowing that there is within his chest a man-made implement where there should only be a God-given heart."

Her words touched the family of a thirty-nine-year-old Connecticut woman who had been in a coma for three weeks with irreversible brain damage. The family agreed to have her flown in a chartered air ambulance to St. Luke's so that if she died, Karp could get her heart. Less than two hours after she reached St. Luke's, doctors with no stake in the Karp case certified she was dead. After sixty-four hours on the artificial heart, Karp underwent transplant surgery. Cooley cut out the man-made heart and replaced it with the woman's. The artificial heart had been used for the first time as a bridge to cardiac transplant.

Mrs. Karp's plea for a heart for her husband was answered, but her broader prayer—that it nurture life in him—was not. Thirty-two hours after receiving the donor heart, Karp died. Cooley said death was due to pneumonia and kidney problems.

No one was more stunned by the Karp implant than DeBakey, who heard the news while attending a Washington conference—ironically one on the artificial heart. DeBakey and Cooley had an edgy, complex relationship. To the media, they were the Texas Titans, two of the world's great heart surgeons—but they were rivals who did not really like each other. As Baylor's medical-center president, DeBakey was Cooley's boss. The tantalizing question was whether Cooley's daring implant revealed ambition to outstrip DeBakey. The implant erupted into a lawsuit by Karp's family and a lengthy series of confrontations among those involved.

The news accounts of Karp's surgery mentioned Cooley's lead associate, Dr. Domingo Liotta, the Argentinean heart researcher who had left Kolff's Cleveland lab to work for DeBakey. In DeBakey's program, Liotta had concentrated on heart-assist devices. When Barnard launched transplants, emphasis had returned to a total artificial heart that could be implanted to maintain life while patients waited for donor hearts. The majority of patients hoping for a transplant died while they waited. A workable artificial heart could bridge the gap.

DeBakey later recalled that such a heart was being developed in his lab at that time. According to him, Liotta had worked on the device and pressed for human implantation. DeBakey stated, "He was very strong about it. I said, 'That is perfectly absurd. You can't put this in a human being.' His [Liotta's] idea was that if we did, we would develop publicity and get support for the program. That is what he was trying to do. He thought it was very important. I said, 'That is not our objective. Our objective is to do good scientific work.'"[1]

After returning to Houston from Washington, DeBakey got another jolt. The program for the upcoming ASAIO meeting listed him as one of the coauthors of the abstract of a paper describing calf-implant tests of his lab's total artificial heart. He was unaware of the abstract and paper. Furthermore, he was positive that no animal implants had been done in his lab recently. He was baffled as to how the paper could report that ten calves had been given the heart and had lived twenty-four to forty-four hours. Liotta was the abstract's lead author.

DeBakey reported that he told Liotta, "I haven't seen anything like the results described in this abstract. Where is the data?" According to DeBakey, Liotta said the experiments would be done before the ASAIO meeting. Assuming this meant the experiments had not been done when the abstract was written, DeBakey recalled saying, "You can't do that. It is not honest." Incensed, DeBakey asked the ASAIO to withdraw the Liotta paper.

He then asked for accounts of all animal implants with the artificial heart in his program for publication in the *Cardiovascular Research Center Bulletin*. There were seven. Four of the seven had died on the operating table. Two others had lived eight and twelve hours, although both had kidney failure. An artificial heart was kept pumping in the seventh for forty-four hours, but the animal had no reflexes.

DeBakey did not think these results justified human implantation. He also wanted to know how Liotta, an employee in his lab, had cooperated with Cooley. Where had Cooley, once so opposed to an artificial heart, gotten one to implant in Karp? After his talk with Liotta, DeBakey said, "We knew that the heart was ours because Liotta admitted he took it out of our lab and brought it to Cooley. Liotta was not really moonlighting or working with Dr. Cooley. He was conspiring with Dr. Cooley to put it in a human being."[2]

Liotta and Cooley had conferred several months before the Karp implant, but DeBakey had not been told of Liotta's arrangement to work nights and weekends with Cooley. Meanwhile, because Liotta was associated with DeBakey, the government wanted to know whether any of the millions in research funding it had given Baylor for heart research had gone into developing the heart implanted in Karp. The NIH said Baylor had guaranteed that the artificial heart would not be implanted in a human without prior approval by a college committee overseeing human experimentation. These committees, called institutional review boards (IRBs), are required for all institutions using federal money in research. They require informed consent by the patient to experimental procedures.

Baylor acknowledged that Liotta was paid from NIH funds but indicated that no IRB had approved the Karp implant because permission had not been asked. To the *New York Daily News*, Cooley stated, "I have done more heart surgery than anyone else in the world. Based on this experience, I believe I am qualified to judge what is right and proper for my patients. The permission I receive to do what I do, I receive from my patients. It is not required from a government agency or one of my seniors."

Cooley had received no NIH funds, so the agency had no power over him. After an investigation, Baylor discharged Liotta, who was promptly hired by Cooley. Since the school received millions of NIH dollars for cardiovascular research, Baylor also announced new rules stipulating that a condition for current and future appointments to the professional staff was a written agreement to abide by U.S. regulations. This satisfied the NIH.

Cooley was not ready to sign this agreement and asked Baylor's IRB to approve his protocol for future implants of the artificial heart. DeBakey told the committee he had no evidence that the heart would be helpful as a pretransplantation device and might be harmful, so Cooley's request was denied. Cooley resigned from Baylor, the only one of 1,350 staff members who refused to sign the agreement.

Not all these details had been disclosed when the ASAIO convened its 1969 meeting after the Karp implant, but the NIH had publicly raised its questions. The chair of the program on which Liotta was going to appear was anxious to hear details of the Karp procedure. He praised both Liotta's "persistence" and Cooley's "vision and surgical ability." Then he asked Cooley to speak. Cooley was ready with a five-thousand-word paper. The chair then called on Liotta, who thanked him for his generosity in allowing both men to talk. He said, "The chairman has been my teacher all these years, the force behind my work." The chair called for a standing ovation for Liotta. The chair was W. J. Kolff.

The Sac Heart

Despite the furor in Houston, the Utah researchers continued their plodding progress toward a workable artificial heart. Kwan-Gett was puzzled by the persistent destruction of red cells in the lab animals' blood. The red cells carry a precious cargo of hemoglobin, the body's vehicle for ferrying oxygen to the tissues. If the cells are destroyed, the hemoglobin is released into the plasma, the blood's liquid element. It can then neither oxygenate nor buffer acidosis, a potentially fatal acid buildup. It is also very toxic and causes renal shutdown.

Kwan-Gett wondered if hemolysis resulted from the design of the sac heart and its air driver. He reviewed the pumping cycle and blew into the air hose of a sac heart. The sides rammed into each other. He stopped and thought about that. In such a collision, blood would be squashed, crushing red cells. He had no doubt: the sac heart design was a spawning ground for hemolysis.

Moreover, when he sucked air out of the heart's hose, it took all his might. Puzzled, he examined the tube. Its diameter was only an eighth of an inch. Elementary physics told him that the smaller the hose, the greater the force needed to draw air through it. That meant the heart driver required a strong vacuum. Later studies demonstrated that the walls of the sac heart nearest to the outflow valves were the first to touch. This created a narrow slit for the blood to pass through, causing even more hemolysis.

Kwan-Gett reasoned that the vacuum—while prying the sac apart—generated a force that pulled at the anastomoses—the junctures where materials joined the heart tissue. He reasoned that this created tiny holes around the suture lines, a gateway for air bubbles. With the help of another researcher, he built a new heart driver equipped with bigger air hoses. Though not requiring such powerful suction, it unfortunately did not reduce the rate of hemolysis. What the lab had to have, he decided, was a different-style heart. By day Kwan-Gett continued doing what Kolff wanted—making and implanting sac hearts. At night in his home, Kwan-Gett started to design a heart better than any the lab and world had ever known.

Young William C. DeVries, the gangly medical student who approached Kolff for a summer job in 1969, attended a medical Grand Rounds lecture at the University Hospital. The subject was blood coagulation. Inspired by the discussion, he investigated why so many sheep were dying with the artificial heart.

The way the body mobilizes coagulation to fight blood loss is one of nature's marvelous dramas, as exciting as watching waves of firemen respond to multiple alarms. The first alarm sounds when a cut or other trauma lets blood escape. Instantly the walls of the punctured vessel contract around the wound, seeking to diminish the blood loss. The contractions set off a second alert, attracting hordes of microscopic protein discs known as platelets. Within seconds the platelets expand, sending out tentacles at the site of the cut, becoming sticky, and clinging together to coalesce into a plug to seal the wound.

If that does not staunch the flow, the body turns in more alarms that summon chemicals that engender minute threads of fibrin—little strips of protein that form a mesh with the platelets at the break in the vessel and net blood cells from the passing flow. Somehow at the right second, the body transmits a signal for this mass to contract, squeezing out its liquid and leaving a clot that usually patches the rupture. One portion of this clot actually becomes part of the vessel wall. Other chemicals then dissolve the excess clot.

Impressive as this mechanism is, it is not foolproof. It can be tricked by false alarms. Under certain circumstances, the body believes it has been besieged by blood leaks. Even though there are none, the coagulation agents swing into action, sprouting clots throughout the vascular network. These can produce a state of shock by jamming veins or arteries and stopping blood from nurturing tissue. When the clotting is rampant, physicians diagnose it as disseminated intravascular coagulopathy or DIC. Ironically, while the body is in the grip of DIC, it can also hemorrhage. The DIC consumes so many of the platelets and other coagulation factors that not enough are left to stem blood loss if there is a genuine wound.

In the late 1960s, DIC was something of a fad in medicine, a catchall to explain otherwise-inexplicable conditions. Before leaving Kolff's lab for his residency in New York's Presbyterian Hospital, Stanley had done some preliminary exploration of DIC in animals. DeVries wanted to build on that by mounting a case-by-case study to see if DIC was indeed the sheep's "final, fatal environment."

With Kolff's support, DeVries examined the records on the lab's twenty-four sheep implants between February and August of 1969, when the average survival with an artificial heart was slightly more than twelve hours. Everywhere DeVries looked he found what investigators said were among the thirty-six presumptive causes of DIC. Not one of the animals could breathe without a respirator, indicative of lung problems. Of the thirteen that lasted longer than eight hours, each had a rising tide of destroyed red cells. The platelet counts were low, indirect proof of excessive coagulation. Falling blood pressures evidenced circulation failure. All the animals died in shock with autopsies revealing hemorrhagic disorders or pernicious bleeding.

The question for DeVries was whether this syndrome identified DIC as the sheep killer. Given the state of blood analyses in 1969, DeVries could not be positive, but he postulated that this was the case. That was important for Kolff. It gave him a medically trendy explanation for his lab's poor survival rates. Coupled with the news that he had recruited a prominent hematologist to investigate further, the rationale offered Kolff a credible stratagem for continued government funding.

The final experiment covered in DeVries's study occurred on August 14, 1969, with an implant in a 125-pound ewe. It was a disaster. The artificial heart's left blood sac blew a hole, and the animal died from a massive air embolism. Kolff declared a moratorium on further surgery. He and the staff needed time to regroup and break through their agonizing defeats.

Starling-Like Response of the Artificial Heart

Among the questions that plagued artificial-heart researchers was, how can the (mechanical) heart increase and/or decrease the blood flow to meet the changing needs of the patient? Kwan-Gett studied this issue and published the answer for pneumatically powered hearts, an approach that did not require changing the heart rate. He adjusted the heart-driver pressure so the ventricles emptied completely at every beat. The heart rate was set so the heart did not fully fill at each beat. When the recipient required increased blood flow, the venous return increased; thus, the ventricle had a greater volume of blood for each beat. This effect was demonstrated in calves with artificial hearts placed on treadmills for exercise. Kwan-Gett's discovery, published in 1970, has been used with the pneumatically powered SynCardia artificial heart well into the 2000s.

The moment was ripe for Kwan-Gett to unveil the heart he was developing at home. He called it the hemispherical heart. It looked as if he had severed a three-inch ball, giving him two equal half domes of Silastic. He bonded the open ends to bases made from aluminum shaped like saucers. The two units formed the pumping chambers, the equivalent of the natural heart's left and right ventricles. Inside each he placed a second dome to serve as a diaphragm, a wall separating the blood from the pulsing air. Through a one-way valve, blood entered from the top (atria) to rest on the supple diaphragm, causing it to sag. When air was pumped against the diaphragm's underside, it rebounded, ejecting the blood through another one-way valve, much the way the natural heart pumps. The diaphragm was the key. It had to be flexible enough to collapse with the incoming blood but not so stretchable that it bumped into the outer dome when inflated.

Kwan-Gett found the system reduced hemolysis. In his design, high levels of suction were not needed to fill the heart since blood just dropped in. Kolff and others had talked of this principle, but Kwan-Gett argued his heart was first to use it successfully. He and Kessler further refined the prototype in Kolff's lab. After testing in a mock circulation system, the heart and a new air driver designed and built by engineer Hank Wong and Kwan-Gett were ready for implant trials when Kolff lifted his moratorium on animal experimentation in January 1970.

In the first surgery, the two artificial ventricles were fitted into a sheep's chest with the metal bases abutting each other the way the septum separates the two sides of the natural heart. Although the heart pumped blood, the animal never breathed on its own and died in twenty hours. The next six experiments with the hemispherical heart were scarcely more encouraging.

Kolff called another halt. For more than two years, he had mandated using sheep. Perhaps he should rethink this, discard the reasons to choose sheep over calves. Olsen, the consulting veterinarian, had advised calves as much more resilient. Three months later, the implants resumed—with calves. The heart was put in a two-hundred-pound animal. It breathed spontaneously, drank water, and survived thirty-one hours and fifteen minutes. Two experiments later, another calf survived sixty-six hours and forty-five minutes—a new world's record for life with an artificial heart.

Kwan-Gett had been with Kolff for four years, and they had had disputes. Still, Kwan-Gett admired Kolff for "staying the course and damn the disappointments." Now it was time for Kwan-Gett to move on. He believed he had done what he set out to do—create the best artificial heart system, pump, and driver yet for the lab. In July 1970, he resigned to begin residencies to become a clinical cardiovascular surgeon. He told Kolff, "I'll still be around to do whatever else I can."

In the fall of 1970, Kolff faced another departure. Hans Zwart, the tall, bespectacled doctor who was in Kolff's Division of Artificial Organs for two years, was a fellow Dutchman. While in the Netherlands, he had written his PhD thesis on an extracorporeal pump to aid weak hearts without major surgery. Interested, Kolff had invited him to Utah to work on the idea. A Dutch government grant allowed Zwart to accept.

Technology was not sufficiently advanced to provide the materials Zwart's system had to have. After writing a flock of scientific papers on what he had learned, Zwart was about to close up shop when Kolff suggested, "Why don't you join the heart work? Take some time, look at everything. Perhaps you can find ways to improve what we do." Zwart agreed to stay.

He was not overly impressed by the implant program and its protocols. He sensed that the philosophy was "put the heart in and see what happens." With the Kwan-Gett heart, the lab had kept one calf alive for ninety-two hours. Hemolysis remained a major complication, but as so often happened with the artificial heart, easing one problem invited another. The dome design seemingly spurred thrombi. Clots formed when blood pooled and coagulated at the V-shaped diaphragm-housing (D-H) junction of the diaphragm and the outer dome. The

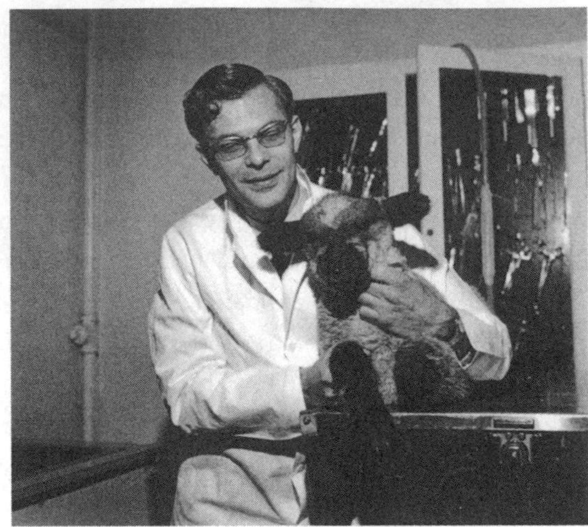

Dr. Hans Zwart with a wooly patient.

longer the animals lived, the greater the peril of these clots breaking up and showering the circulation system with emboli.

There was some hope, however. Troubled by thrombi in a heart-assist device, two Boston researchers had found a way to combat them. They coated the interior of their unit with glue and then dusted on hundreds of thousands of infinitely small fibrils of plastic Dacron. This actually invited thrombus formation, but because the fibrils were anchored, they locked the clots in place, reducing the danger.

"I like the idea," Zwart said. Kolff sent him to Boston to learn the technique. Returning to Salt Lake with Dacron fibrils, Zwart spent weeks with Kessler until they felt confident they knew how to layer them over the heart's blood-contacting surfaces, including the D-H junction. Zwart also had some revolutionary ideas about postsurgery care, which had been haphazard. "We should treat each animal as if it were a human patient recovering from a very serious open-heart operation," Zwart said.

In early April 1971, a black-and-white Holstein calf was selected to receive a fibril-coated Kwan-Gett heart. Though she was female, the staff named her Latino. She had a good disposition and liked to be petted. Zwart put Latino on bypass, then cut out and replaced her heart. The operation took almost five hours. An hour later, Latino awoke from the anesthesia. Treating the calf as though she were in the medical center's surgical intensive-care unit, Zwart instituted constant monitoring: blood pressure, cardiac output, urinalysis, and no fewer than twenty-eight continuous blood-chemistry tests.

The only possible concern was a higher-than-normal reading of blood pressure on the heart's right atria. Zwart guessed that this indicated the heart was not quite a perfect fit and was squeezing veins. The day after surgery, Latino was helped to a standing position. With the respirator removed, she recovered her voice and repeatedly mooed. To guard against infection, Zwart administered antibiotics.

On Sunday signs turned bad: Latino's urine was dark red. That was a clue to what blood tests confirmed—hemolysis. In a heart specifically designed to eliminate hemolysis, this was a shocker. Then Zwart remembered that when running his finger over the Dacron fibrils, he had felt little stabs. Were the fibrils' stiletto ends puncturing the blood cells? If they were, there was nothing he could do about it.

As the hours went by, the urine noticeably cleared. When Latino mysteriously hyperventilated, then equally mysteriously calmed, the occasion called for champagne. Even doctors and staff from the university's medical school and hospital came to celebrate as Latino broke the previous survival record of 102 hours and lived for another 72 hours. When she had no reflex responses, Zwart terminated her.

An autopsy confirmed Zwart's guess about the heart restricting venous flow. Blood had backed up and fatally damaged the liver, a symptom of what doctors call right-heart failure. The hemolysis had also taken its toll; the kidneys were starved for oxygen. These were problems for future corrections, but Latino was reason for hope. The heifer was the world's first animal to live an entire week with an artificial heart!

DeVries was in North Carolina when he got Kolff's letter describing the success with Latino. First in his class at medical school, DeVries was accepted to do his internship and surgical residency at Duke University Medical Center. Kolff applauded DeVries and knew that Duke's senior cardiovascular surgeon, Dr. David C. Sabiston Jr., was among the country's leading medical educators. Kolff had long-range plans for DeVries; he thought DeVries might one day be the first person to implant a permanent artificial heart in a human.

Aftermath

Continuing their work in the maelstrom that surrounded the Texas Karp case, Kessler was focused on stopping the sharp Dacron fibrils from puncturing red blood cells in what jokesters were calling the "hairy heart." As he thought, he rubbed his chin. He needed a shave. Of course! So did the fibrils! Getting out a Norelco razor (a good Dutch company, Kolff noted), Kessler barbered the prickles until he could trim them evenly and still leave enough Dacron to hold the thrombi. A well-groomed heart was tried in a calf. The results were inconclusive because nine hours into the experiment, a compressed-air regulator failed, and the heart exploded like a balloon.

The lab had a new recruit, Dr. Jun Kawai, an experienced Japanese cardiac surgeon. He persuaded Kolff to approve a novel surgery to implant a heart without a heart-lung machine. The secret was deep hypothermia. The body was chilled until it no longer had any metabolism and temporarily did not need oxygen.

On May 11, 1971, Kawai anesthetized a calf named Taro. The animal was put into a tub of ice for ninety minutes before surgery. Packing him in ice dropped his blood temperature to sixty-eight degrees. Because the time tissue can exist without metabolism is limited, Kawai had to work fast. In two hours, he implanted one of the shaved diaphragm hearts. Taro ate, drank, and mooed until felled by an infection that Kawai traced to organisms that had taken root in the fibrils. Nevertheless, Taro lived an unprecedented 260 hours—almost eleven days.

Five days before Taro died, Kolff wrote to Lowell T. Harmison, acting chief of the Medical Devices Application program in the National Heart and Lung Institute (NHLI), the new name of the National Heart Institute. The government's program had lost much of the vigor DeBakey had generated under his friend Lyndon Johnson. Alarmed by the Cooley-Karp furor, federal officials were shying away from total-heart implants and focusing on much-less-radical assist devices. Kolff had already asked the federal program to reassess its priorities; he wanted more frequent implants to learn as much as possible as soon as possible.

"Our recent results have been most encouraging," Kolff informed Harmison. "After we adopted the technique of coating the inside of the heart with fibrils, the thromboembolism that killed our animals has been reduced to where we obtained a survival of more than a week and the clinical condition of our recent animals seems to have been greatly improved." Then he got to the point—money. The experiments were getting expensive. The cost of surgeons, OR personnel, around-the-clock calf sitters, technicians, feed, drugs, laboratory tests, and overhead expenses was five thousand dollars to implant a heart and keep one animal alive for a week. Illustrating his thriftiness, Kolff itemized the surgeon's hourly fee at $9.68.

Noting that his lab only had a $60,000 contract, Kolff continued, "It would be of great importance to us, if instead of allocating the funds over an entire year, we be allowed to spend most of it in a ten-week period." Harmison said that he saw no point in speeding up the "activity of implanting the same device repeatedly in animal after animal without very careful and time-consuming consideration of the results of the previous trials."

As Kolff's staff administrator, John Warner, tried to spread out the government money, Kolff was hitting other sources for funds. From another unit of the NHLI, he received a grant worth nearly $300,000 a year. The Atomic Energy Commission (AEC) awarded him $60,000 annually to work on a nuclear-powered heart. Adroitly, Kolff found the money to shift his program into high gear.

Kolff's crow of victory over clotting was short lived, however. The first calf to receive an implant after his letter died in twenty-six hours. The autopsy showed multiple clots. In a second calf, thromboembolism invaded the kidneys, and in a third, the artery funneling blood from the heart to the lungs was blocked. Hoping for better results, the lab tried using ponies. The first came off the table with possible brain damage. "Went loco," a technician explained. Within eight hours, the animal was dead. Another succumbed in surgery. One pony lasted only five hours. The pony trials were abandoned. The researchers incorrectly conjectured that the ponies could not tolerate the hypothermia procedure.

It was not, in fact, the hypothermia. Routinely large-animal surgery recovery rooms have floors and walls padded with foam rubber. While under sedation, horses are gently placed on the floor and left to recover very quietly, monitored via video. For an animal implanted with an artificial heart that had drivelines through the chest wall, this was not possible.

The researchers returned to calves and the vexing quandaries of thromboembolism and infection. The problem of fit that had killed Latino continued to be a stumbling block.

Notes

1. Based on news and videotapes of interviews of Dr. Michael DeBakey speaking about the lawsuit filed by Haskell Karp's widow (see chapter 7).
2. Ibid.

7

New Materials, New Designs, More Success

Nature begins with the reason and ends with experience, but researchers must follow the opposite path—from experimentation we must understand the reason. Why did nature not arrange things such that one animal could live from the death of another?

—Leonardo DaVinci

John Warner was surprised to see Robert Jarvik reporting for work as a research assistant. "What can a young kid like that possibly contribute?" he asked.

But Kolff treated Jarvik as an experienced professional and personal friend in what amounted to a father-son relationship. "There is something I want you to do," Kolff said. "We have been having trouble with too-high venous pressures. I'd like you to build a heart that avoids that problem." He did not say what Jarvik would have to work with or what his relationship was to other researchers; Kolff did make it clear Jarvik would be on his own, doing whatever he thought necessary. After asking why an artificial heart should not be shaped like a natural one, Jarvik settled in to learn the craft of artificial-heart designing.

Tom Kessler was pleasant when Jarvik asked him to explain the technique of fabricating a heart. Kessler showed him but added, "I've got schedules I've got to meet, a lot of stuff to build for the actual implants."

Sensing that Kessler would not have time to fashion a heart from his design, Jarvik replied, "What you mean is that I do it myself." Kessler nodded.

Wrestling with the problem of a better-fitting heart, Kolff asked Jarvik, "What would you think of a heart with each ventricle shaped like a pancake?" Two flat pouches for holding blood could be placed against the sides of the rib cage. Presumably this would avoid any interference with the lungs, great veins, and arteries. Jarvik said he would try it.

When Kolff saw the silicone-rubber pouches, he thought they looked strange. It was as though a heart had become a set of water wings. An implanted calf maintained normal venous pressure, evidence that the pouches were not jamming any of the great veins. However, they could not pump a high enough volume of blood to sustain life. To increase the flow, Jarvik developed a design that looked like a Valentine's Day heart. It was too big to fit inside the chest. The numerous setbacks did not depress him. Confident that he would find some solution, Jarvik told his wife, Elaine, "It's no more than an exercise in geometry and anatomy."

Jarvik had applied to the University of Utah's School of Medicine earlier and been turned down; now he reapplied as a state resident. Cardiologist Dr. Fred Anderson, chair of the Admissions Committee, said, "I have been pressured by legislators, wealthy individuals, and a few governors as to why their students or relatives were not accepted into the medical school, but I have never been under as much pressure as Kolff applied for two years to get Jarvik accepted. We finally accepted him to remove the pressure."

Jarvik was waiting for an answer when he and Elaine went to the Kolff home for a small reception honoring Dr. A. G. Guyton, a celebrated physiologist consulting for the Utah artificial-heart program. During the party, Kolff clapped his hands to get the attention of the fifteen or twenty guests for a champagne toast. "This toast," he said, "is for—" he paused. Jarvik assumed the name would be Guyton. "Robert Jarvik. I have just been told he is accepted to medical school." Jarvik paled. Being finally accepted shocked him. The fact that he was second from last to be chosen, as he learned later, did not matter at all.

The Veterinarian Says Yes

Coincidentally that afternoon in the spring of 1972, the veterinarian who had earlier consulted with Kolff's lab decided it was time to face some hard realities. For almost four years, Don Olsen, now forty-two, had been in Colorado working for his PhD in molecular biology. Now he had to choose between supporting his family and writing the thesis for his degree. Seeing no real choice, he telephoned Kolff, who had once offered him a job. "I'm close to finishing my work here," he told Kolff. "I'm disappointed at not finishing the PhD, but it's quite obvious that I will not have enough money to continue."

Kolff said, "That's the best news I've heard in months. Not having the PhD doesn't matter. I'll see you at the Hotel Utah in Salt Lake City at 8:30 tomorrow morning."

There was a flight out of Denver that night. Calling his wife, Joyce, Olsen requested, "Pack me a bag. I'm going to see Dr. Kolff." It reminded her of the first time he had gone to Salt Lake City to see Kolff in 1967.

When Olsen arrived in Salt Lake City, he found that Kolff had arranged for both a room and a basket of fruit to welcome him to the Hotel Utah. The next morning Kolff chauffeured him to the lab. Though they had not talked salary, Kolff acted as if all the arrangements had been completed. "Dr. Olsen will be joining us this summer full time," Kolff announced to the staff at the morning conference.

Theodore Stanley, who had returned to the lab after completing his residency, said, "Great. It has been the pits. Not one calf survived or got off the table when I first arrived." Always impatient, Stanley was concerned about the snail's-pace progress during his first years in Utah and relieved that another skilled professional would hopefully speed up the progress.

The time was ripe for a veterinarian with infinite patience to join Kolff's lab. The lab was experiencing a sea of troubles. After Taro the survival record of calves had advanced by only three days to fourteen. Thirty-one of the thirty-six animals operated on in the eight months before Olsen's arrival had failed to live even fifty hours. Six had died on the operating table. Some developed fatal thromboses, and others died in convulsions or surgical hemorrhaging. The plastic hearts occasionally ruptured.

The lab staff believed the cause of some deaths was inadequate blood flow. They worked to overcome this with a smaller version of Kwan-Gett's design and speeded up the pumping rate to 165 beats a minute. Because that was like having a machine gun in the chest, the technicians had to slow the heart rate. To line the hearts, they switched from Dacron to rayon and back to Dacron. No matter what changes they made, the same problems continued.

Zwart had moved on and left behind a heritage of treating the animals as if they were open-heart surgery patients, a practice accepted by most of the staff. Kolff felt it was not practical to do that for every experiment. He hired Olsen because he needed someone to treat the calves as animals—a knowledgeable veterinarian. Olsen immediately validated Kolff's thinking. "You're not giving the calves enough liquid to meet their needs for mastication," he said. "They're like kids. They need fluids. I'll grind five hundred grams of alfalfa in a homogenizer with four liters of water."

"There's no way a calf's stomach can hold four liters," the staff objected.

Olsen knew that calves have four stomachs to aid regurgitation—chewing the cud. Taking a stomach from the next autopsy, he cleaned and then inflated it like a giant balloon. Showing up with the inflated stomach at morning conference, Olsen said, "Does anyone doubt I can get four liters of water in this?"

Olsen then ground up his slurry and put in a tablespoon of bicarbonate of soda. "Bicarb?" someone asked in surprise.

"Calves have lots of acidity," Olsen answered. "They need help in neutralizing it." He drove the gruel into a contented calf with a pump.

Kolff gave Olsen an assignment to solve. Frequently animals with implanted hearts had lung problems, including severe swelling and edema, which jeopardized their internal organs. Having done work on lungs in his PhD studies, Olsen took a week to draw up a sophisticated experiment. Kolff examined Olsen's protocol and shook his head: "This is not what I had in mind. This would take you a year to do. I don't have that kind of time. Just look at the operations; see what they're doing. We don't have all the fancy tools you had in Colorado anyway. Use your own eyes. Run some autopsies. Then make the changes."

The lab's set routine was driving the right side of the artificial heart at four pounds per square inch, while the left side was set at six pounds because that side has to push blood through the entire body. Olsen recalled the published observation of a Boston scientist who was testing ventricular-assist devices. He said that lungs often swelled with fluid (edema) when he drove blood into the right ventricle at high pressure. However, there was no pulmonary edema if he dissipated the driving force.

Olsen informed the Kolff researchers they were pumping both sides of the heart at too much pressure. For the next implant, he ordered almost half the pressure. The serum stayed in the blood vascular system, and no edema puffed up the lungs. A major complication was averted.

Kolff asked Olsen about his goals and objectives. Olsen had thought carefully about what he wanted to do. He replied, "I want to know more about a calf with an artificial heart than anyone in the world." After a short pause, Kolff asked how he intended to do that since Yukihiko Nosé, Dr. William Pierce, and the Texas group had all implanted hearts in calves for many years and were excellent surgeons.

Olsen responded that they were medical doctors and had many other responsibilities. Nosé headed a large group of investigators working on artificial kidneys, artificial lungs, and plasmapheresis devices. Pierce at Hershey had a very demanding cardiothoracic surgery practice that limited his time in the laboratory. The Texas group also had many other interests. Olsen was trained as a veterinarian; he knew the complexities of the ruminant digestive system and understood the anatomy, physiology, and pharmacology of animals, which differed greatly from humans. And he was working full time on the artificial heart. Based on Olsen's contributions, almost all of the artificial-heart research teams in the world included a veterinarian within the next four years.

Olsen's move to Utah on June 19, 1972, coincided with the trial of the ongoing court case of Karp versus Cooley. Haskell Karp's widow sued Denton Cooley,

Domingo Liotta, St. Luke's Hospital, and Sam Calvin, a Baylor electronics engineer, over her husband's implant surgery. Mrs. Karp said the heart was not adequately tested and that her husband was not told that experimental animals had died soon after their implants, so he could not give informed consent. The case was eventually closed and settled without fines.

The Karp lawyers intended to use Michael DeBakey to buttress their charge that the Liotta artificial heart was not ready for a human implant. However, the judge barred him from testifying. At that time, DeBakey's work on the artificial heart was drawing to a close. Time after time, his animals had died from the same panoply of causes: infection, hemolysis, right-heart failure. Finally, DeBakey said there was no point in pushing the experiments any further and completely changed direction to work on ventricular-assist devices.

The Turn Around in Calf-Survival Times

Progress with artificial hearts had been going slowly when Kolff hired Olsen in June 1972. Olsen quickly established protocols and standard operating procedures, covering everything from the time the animal came into the laboratory through anesthesia, surgery, all postoperative monitoring, and even autopsies, insisting that everyone follow his directions.

One morning he and the team opened a calf's chest, preparing to put the animal on the heart-lung machine, then waited for the Dutch surgeon, Dr. Jay Volder, who was missing.

"He's not coming," said a veteran technician who had participated in more than a hundred implants. He said to Olsen, "Let's put the heart in ourselves." Otherwise all of the instruments and the heart would have to be washed and resterilized, and the calf would have to be sutured closed or terminated.

"I don't think I can do it all," Olsen replied.

"Sure you can. I'll help," some offered. All the people in the OR chimed in, "Go for it, Don."

"Okay," said Olsen. "We'll do it." And they did—without a flaw.

On the second day following the planned surgery, when Volder came in, he was jokingly told, "We don't need you around anymore. We did it, and look, the calf is standing up, feeling fine." Volder did not come late to an operation again. Olsen returned to being the assistant for him and other surgeons.

The Turn-Around Heart Design

That fall of 1972 as a medical-school freshman, Jarvik was spending several hours a week on heart design. He was in the lab one day when Kolff announced, "We

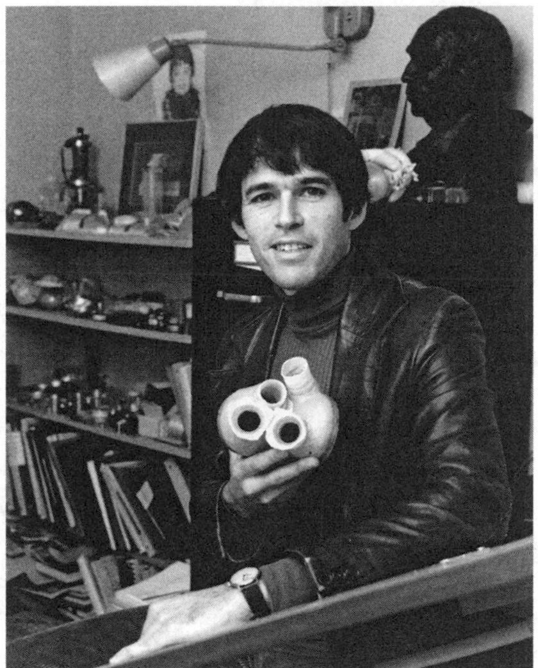

Robert Jarvik worked on artificial hearts while attending medical school.

have lost the lead. In Cleveland Nosé has the new survivor record. One of his calves lived for seventeen days." Still working by himself, Jarvik thought he might overtake Nosé if he concentrated on the geometry that he was sure held the clue to success. Olsen suggested that Jarvik examine the dimensions of a calf's chest. The bovine cavity is elliptical, longer from front to back, narrower from top to bottom and side to side. Kwan-Gett's heart, however, was more or less round with the metal bases of the hemispheres abutting like two halves of an orange joined together.

Who said it was best to have those metal bases at the center of the heart? Was that the most efficient use of chest space? Did the very shape of the heart interfere with blood flow into it? Why not use a design that was more elliptical like the chest cavity? It was time, Jarvik decided, to turn things around. Kwan-Gett had designed his heart like a divided sphere with two separate ventricles united by strips of Velcro. Jarvik designed a model with two independent chambers but wedded them into the shape of a knotted bow tie with the bases at opposite ends and the ventricles touching in the middle and fastened by Velcro. To achieve his ellipses, Jarvik slimmed and lengthened the ventricles.

He did not regard this as an invention. Rather, he was adapting the basic diaphragm model Kwan-Gett had developed. Also helping Jarvik was the advent of new polymers and adhesives that gave him an opportunity to make new design changes. Jarvik observed surgery several times to understand the implant procedures while designing his new heart, but he never participated.

Olsen modified the surgical procedure developed by medical doctors. They did the midsternal split the way it was done in humans, which resulted in a deep incision with several complications in calves. The artificial heart's left ventricle was implanted, deaired, and started in order to pump the blood returning from the lungs. Then the right ventricle was implanted. Then both ventricles were pumped with slowly increasing pressure and heart rate to take over circulation while the animal was weaned off the heart-lung machine.

The first implant of the new heart with the smooth blood-contacting polyurethane surfaces took place in a calf. Initially the calf refused to eat, and Olsen's alfalfa slurry had to be pumped into him twice. Pneumonia flared on the third postoperative day, so the staff administered antibiotics plus nasal oxygen. On the afternoon of the fifth day, Kolff examined the calf and concluded that the animal was about to die. He called Olsen at home and, even though it was Sunday evening, asked him to come in and terminate the calf. "I want it out of the lab by tomorrow morning," he said, "because I'm bringing in a very important benefactor."

When he reached the lab, Olsen met the experiment's principal investigator, Dr. Hartmut Oster, a German physician doing a residency. With Oster was his wife, Traudel, who had become as involved as he was in the calf's fate. When Olsen told them Kolff had asked him to terminate the calf, the Osters pleaded, "Can't we do something?"

Realizing how much the calf meant to them, Olsen said, "Well, maybe I can try something. If it doesn't work, I'll have to do the autopsy before Dr. Kolff gets in tomorrow morning." Then he hurried out to buy some Vick's VapoRub. Putting a teaspoon of it in hot water to create a vaporizer, he treated the calf with the medicated steam. When he left for home at midnight, he instructed the Osters to keep replenishing the vaporizer. Returning at 5:00 AM, Olsen found the calf eating hay, drinking water, and showing no signs of pneumonia.

At 8:00 AM, Kolff came in with his guest. In the hall outside the animal room, Olsen could hear him telling the benefactor, "We had a calf with an implant, but because of pneumonia, we had to terminate it." Walking through the doorway, Kolff saw the calf. "Well, there has apparently been a change," he said in surprise. As he let the visitor examine the animal he asked Olsen, "What happened?"

Olsen answered, "An old veterinarian's trick."

After more than two weeks, the calf weakened and died due to thrombus on the right-side inflow valve.

Jarvik asked, "How about the fit? Did the heart sit well in the chest?"

"Very well," Olsen answered. "It didn't crowd any vessels."

The lab's books recorded that the calf lived eighteen days and twenty hours. That was just a shade longer than Nosé's calf; the team had accomplished its goal of regaining the calf-survival record. Exuberantly Kolff told the government that Jarvik's device was "our most successful heart."

The New Surgeon

For some time, Olsen had been the chief assistant during the heart implants. The OR technicians, generally infallible judges of a surgeon's skills, liked what they saw. His autopsy stitches were done in near-metronomic style with the same tension and identical spacing.

Olsen invited Kolff to lunch one day and told him, "Our team is not successful in keeping calves alive. Doctors Nosé at Cleveland and Pierce at Penn State are both good, well-trained surgeons, and their implant success rate is better than ours." He asked Kolff to hire a better-trained surgeon so Utah could be competitive. Kolff informed Olsen that he was sticking with Volder.

Some months later, when Kolff recognized his veterinarian's surgical skills, he took Olsen to lunch. "I want you to be first surgeon," Kolff said.

"That would be a mistake," Olsen responded. "I don't have the right union cards. I'm not a heart surgeon and have very little experience. All I've done is watch the good and the bad and learned from that."

"There's no doubt in my mind you can do it," Kolff replied emphatically. And that settled the issue. It was September 1973.

When Olsen was reviewing the autopsy records, he noticed the presence of unusual bacteria. How had these bacteria invaded the system? He reviewed the standard operating procedures, including using a midsternal incision to crack the chest open. With the anesthetized animal on its back, an electrically powered saw split the sternum, the chest's central bone. The two sides were then spread apart to access the heart. In human beings, this procedure is easy because the bone is relatively thin.

In calves, however, the sternum must support more weight and is two to three inches thick. Not only is it much harder to saw through, but it requires a much longer healing time. The chest wound was a perfect portal for bacteria after surgery. Moreover, the calves lay directly on their incisions, further hampering healing and making it difficult to maintain sterile conditions.

Olsen knew that Kwan-Gett and others had sometimes tried another technique called a right-lateral thoracotomy. It took more time and was difficult, but he was convinced it would promote recovery and minimize bacterial complications. "Let's do some experimenting," he said to Lowana Reese Finch, the OR supervisor.

Laying a calf on its side, he prepped the skin on the right chest, then cut a lateral incision over the fourth rib and removed it. He then spread the space between the third and fifth ribs to create an adequate surgical opening. He scissored out the heart, attached a Jarvik-3 (J-3) model, closed the wound, and propped the animal chest down. The incision was visible on the animal's side, free from any contaminating contact with the surface under it. Satisfied the thoracotomy worked, he said to the surgical nurse, "Lowana, okay. This is how we'll do it from now on." Within one and a half years, the lateral approach had been adopted by all medical doctors implanting artificial hearts in animals in the United States and many foreign labs.

Another step forward was the resolution of the DIC problem, the blood-clotting condition that had once threatened the implants. After DeVries speculated that DIC was killing the experimental animals, Kolff asked for a full-scale investigation by the director of the medical center's coagulation service, Dr. Edward J. Hershgold, a blood specialist with impressive credentials. Like DeVries, Hershgold was unable to confirm DIC's presence, though there was indirect evidence. In any event, because the animals had greater survival with the new heart designs and materials, their bodies exhibited an inexplicable ability to combat enemies. They began compensating for the coagulation, neutralizing it by making adjustments. For all practical purposes, the Artificial Heart Research Laboratory could forget about DIC.

The facilities in the old army barracks were extremely cramped and out of date. If an implanted calf survived, it had to be housed in the surgery room, which limited the number of implants. Even with the run-down facilities, spirits and energy were high. Ideas were hatched, and some flew. Comradery was quickly established, and often the international group of researchers and technicians met for lunch on a volleyball court between the buildings.

They also sometimes took more rigorous treks together in southern Utah. On the weekend of May 3, 1973, Kolff and fourteen of his staff members were on a jeep trip to Canyonlands National Park. While they vacationed, Building 512 back in Salt Lake was in flames. Fire broke out in the hall of Kessler's heart-molding shop in the middle of the frame structure. The blaze quickly spread through the OR, the instrument room containing the expensive computer

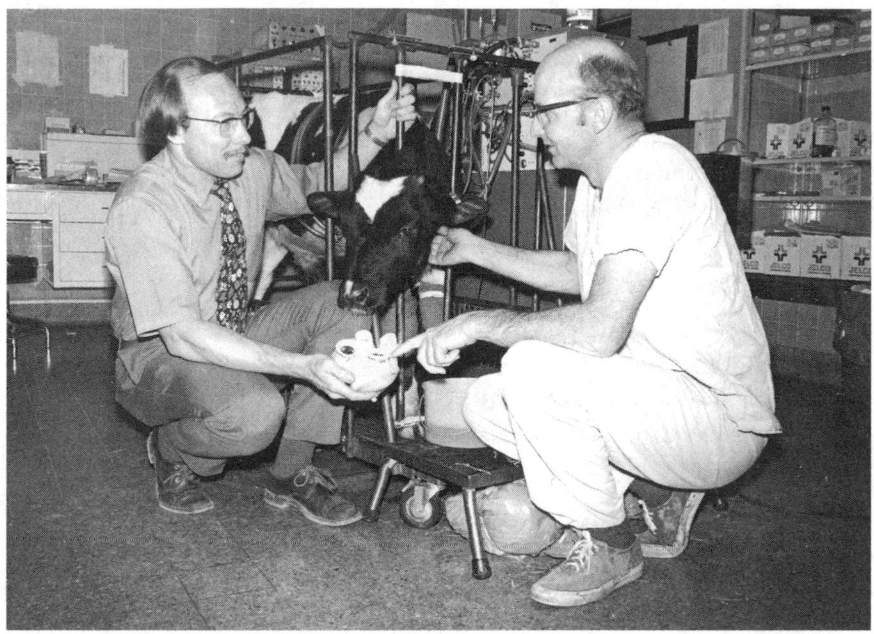

Tom Kessler (*left*) and Dr. Don Olsen discuss a recovering calf after an artificial-heart implant.

setup, and the machine shop in the center of the building. Tanks for oxygen and other gases blew up, shattering windows. Firemen managed to save the two end sections, but smoke and water damage were extensive.

The fire was barely out when Mary Johnson was notified at home. Just the day before the fire, she had finished typing an important report to the Atomic Energy Commission. Planning to give it to Kolff on Monday, she had left the only copy on her desk in the building's north end. Hurrying to the lab, she told firemen, "I've got to get in there. I must see if a very special report on my desk is safe." They waved her in. The report was smoky and water soaked but intact.

Jarvik had also skipped the trip. When he rushed to 512, he decided that much of the equipment gutted or damaged in the fire could be replaced. The molds for making the J-3 heart were unharmed, though even if they had been ruined, he knew he could always make new ones. And the important records documenting the results of each implant, stored in one of 512's end rooms, were also safe, but they smelled of smoke for many years. Fortunately no animals were then housed in the lab. Unable to pinpoint the fire's cause, both state and city fire marshals opened arson investigations but concluded that there was not enough evidence to finger a firebug. The damage was hundreds of thousands of dollars.

As cleaning began, the lab staff remaining in Salt Lake City arranged for emergency headquarters. They moved to another barracks, Building 518, which was directly east of Building 512, relocated desks, and rented typewriters and a copy machine to continue their research. When Kolff and the others returned on Monday morning, they were able to get right to work. Kolff was calm, asking only if anyone had been hurt. Told there had been no injuries, he said, "Well, then we must get on with what we have to do." He salvaged what he could. His major loss was his personal collection of older artificial hearts and other memorabilia.

The heart-lung pump and the crane for lifting animals were stained with soot but usable. So were a machine for recording scientific animal data and a number of compressed-air heart drivers. The insurance check, about $311,000, was intended to replace lost equipment, but Kolff used it to pay for additional personnel and animal experiments.

He then made an item-by-item list with photographs of what the lab needed and pleaded with individual manufacturers to donate their products. What was not donated, Kolff told his staff to build or borrow, hoping these loans would become gifts. Only as a last resort did he buy equipment, using funds from an emergency appeal he had sent to private industry. Olsen was successful in obtaining two Bird ventilators from company owner Forrest Bird. Kolff told federal bureaucrats that no mere fire was going to interrupt him. Reporting to the NHLBI on the "temporary setback," he ended with typical bravado: "We are considerably closer to a clinically implantable heart."

One big task was to keep staff morale high. Kolff's Division of Artificial Organs and the IBE had projects involving artificial hearts, kidneys, eyes, arms, ears, and blood vessels. The full- and part-time staff had swelled to 125. About half worked in the university's engineering building, but the rest had been burned out of 512.

Another challenge was to find a new home for the animal experiments at a price Kolff could afford. The team attempted to implant a heart in a calf in space the Animal Resource Center made available, but it was far too small. Use of the nearby Utah Biomedical Test Laboratory was explored, but the rent was far too expensive.

New Facilities

Olsen was aware that St. Mark's Hospital, one of the city's oldest medical institutions, was moving into a new building and vacating its timeworn, red-brick quarters on the northwest side of Salt Lake City about twelve minutes from the

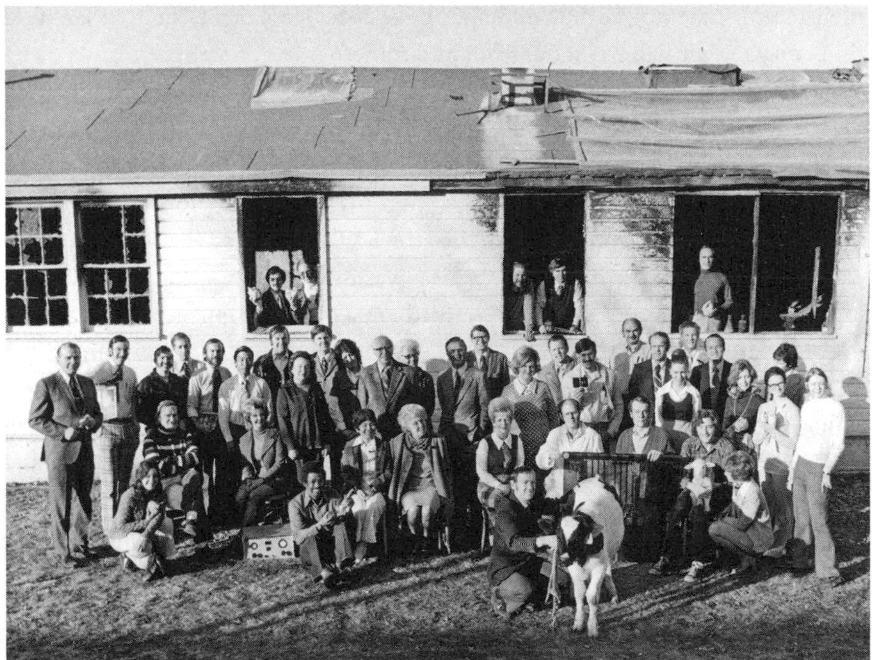

The Division of Artificial Organs team members gathered in front of burned-out Building 512.

university. He talked to the chief engineer, Harley Bloomquist, who had worked in the building for forty-two years and regarded it with great affection. Olsen suggested that if the Division of Artificial Organs moved into the surgical wing, it would prevent vandalism. Bloomquist agreed and told him to call the hospital's administrator, T. J. Hartford.

When Olsen visited Hartford, the administrator was preoccupied with supervising the hospital's eleven-mile move. Undeterred, Kolff became most persuasive. Hartford finally promised, "I'll talk to the board," and Kolff knew some of the board members. Within two weeks, a lease was signed for the entire surgical wing: twenty-five thousand square feet, ten times the size of Building 512. There were six operating suites and room for offices, and the rent was only two hundred dollars a month. The best part was that Olsen convinced Bloomquist to work as a consultant and manage all of the support equipment within the building.

There was a catch. Because the building might be sold to investors who wanted the entire structure, the lease had a thirty-day eviction clause. Kolff had no choice but to accept it, though it made him nervous whenever outsiders showed up. "Every time I see these characters with their hats on, big cigars in their mouths, looking at the building, I have a sleepless night," he told Janke. "I think maybe they will buy it out from under me."

Janke merely commented, "He thrives on crisis."

The hospital patients were moved out in March and April, and the Artificial Heart Research Laboratory moved in during June and July 1973. Some of the engineers did not wish to unpack their things because of the short eviction time, thinking they would soon be out on the street. Olsen assured them that the only way he would leave the building was if he was dragged out kicking and screaming. They could consider themselves already dug in for the long term. Reassured, everyone unpacked and began to make a new home in the roomy building.

Later in the summer, after St. Mark's Hospital had moved everything it wanted, the Artificial Heart Research Laboratory got whatever was left, but it was mostly junk: some old surgery lights, bookcases, and laboratory benches. Allocating space and deciding where the various laboratory activities were to be located in the spacious five-story building was challenging. Kolff insisted that some rooms be set aside as living quarters for national and international visitors and students working in the lab.

Locating artificial-heart manufacturing, under Kessler's direction, in the second-floor delivery rooms was an easy decision. The secluded area with ceramic-tile-covered walls was ideal for future clean rooms because of the need for filtered air. The other rooms on the second floor became hematology labs. The fourth floor included six surgery rooms, far more than needed, but only surgical-supply storage could share the space.

Olsen did not like having the four implanted animals that occasionally acquired driveline infections so close to the surgery rooms. Furthermore, the hay and feces were also contaminants. He considered moving the animals into the old laundry room on the ground floor. Kolff was adamantly opposed because the team, and particularly Olsen, would not see the animals often enough during the day. Olsen promised to begin and end the workday by coming through the animal-holding area.

All of the huge washers and dryers were moved out and sold as junk metal, as were the large sheet-folding machines. There was a trough in the floor that drained. It was not located in the best place for calf waste, but there was no money to make major changes. This space worked for many years, and the barn had several additions with separate quarantine and animal-holding areas. Several times it housed as many as eighteen calves and sheep with either pneumatically or electrically powered artificial hearts. Olsen continued to enter and leave the building, as promised, through this area until his retirement in 2010.

The End of Dacron Fibrils

For a year, Olsen had been suspicious of the fibrils used in the hearts. How could glue keep all of them attached, particularly on the flexing diaphragm? He put a fibril heart in a mock circulation system and added filters so fine they would catch almost anything floating in the water. They revealed that thousands of the fibrils had slipped their moorings, but when he examined tissue from implanted animals under a microscope, no fibrils showed. "That's not possible," Olsen said to his technicians. A polarizing light documented their presence; the fibrils glowed like bright stars in a clear western sky in the animals' brains, livers, and kidneys. They provided potential for vessel-blocking clots that left their calling card—infarctions. Moreover, as the calf Taro had verified, they were spawning grounds for infections.

Nevertheless, the J-3 fibril hearts were the lab's accepted models, favored by Kolff as the answer to clotting. In late 1973, Olsen implanted one in a calf named Tony. While the calf set another world record of thirty days, the triumph was bittersweet. To achieve compatibility, blood encountering foreign surfaces deposits a layer of serum protein. Tony's record month of life allowed enough time to form not only one layer but also a second, third, and fourth. Eventually protein practically filled the entire heart, crippling its pumping ability. Cause of death: low cardiac output. "What went wrong?" an anguished Olsen asked. "We must not have given him enough anticoagulants. Next time we'll give a lot more heparin."

On February 28, 1974, Olsen implanted a silicone heart in a calf named Kamui. The animal outlived Tony by six days. Cause of death: low cardiac output. Did that mean his heart, too, was larded with protein? Had the blood thinner failed? Olsen rushed Kamui to autopsy. The heart did have protein, but it looked unlike anything he had ever seen. For some reason—possibly the heavy dosage of heparin—it had mineralized into a hard rough crust that looked like barnacles. This was such a dramatic instance of the jeopardy inherent in fibril hearts that Olsen told Kolff, "We've got to find another material." Kolff disagreed. He said researchers in Cleveland and Boston seemed to be faring well with textured hearts.

Olsen had no alternative to propose—yet. But he knew that Kessler was also experimenting with a material to eliminate fibrils. The material was segmented polyurethane, a different version from the one discarded in Kolff's Cleveland experiments. Kessler was convinced that it was sufficiently inert biologically to avoid clots. The difficulty was that nobody knew how to mold it into a heart. He and his assistant, Gail Burkett, tried method after method with results that were disappointing but tantalizing enough to keep them experimenting. Kessler felt they were on the verge of pioneering a feasible manufacturing technique. At last, he discovered that manipulating the molding process was the answer. "Okay," he announced to Olsen. "We've got ourselves a polyurethane heart."

Jarvik noted that a polyurethane heart was a definite achievement but wondered if this plastic would be strong enough to endure the punishment of pumping 90 times a minute, 129,000 times a month—perhaps even more? In particular he worried about the diaphragm that would bear the brunt of constant flexion under air pressure. To be effective, it had to be thin and supple. Was it too thin to be durable? To learn the answer, Olsen and Jarvik tested the hearts in a mock circulation loop.

The diaphragm failed. Holes developed in the wrinkles from the repeated flexing and unflexing. If that happened while the heart was in animals, killer air bubbles could enter the blood and find their way to the brain. The two men conjectured that a diaphragm with more than one layer might be stronger. That no one had ever built a heart with a multilayer diaphragm only encouraged Jarvik. Polymer chemists told Jarvik that multilayer polyurethane diaphragms were used in other applications.

His new version of the diaphragm had two sheets of polyurethane. Concerned that the supple plastic might distend enough to bump into the ventricle's housing—reviving the old problem of crushed red blood cells—Jarvik added a layer of heat-set Dacron mesh between the polyurethane sheets to limit stretching. A heart with this system was implanted for the first time on May 7, 1974. The calf lived only nine days, but that was not cause for despair. Infection, not heart failure, killed the animal.

Barely five days later, on May 21, 1974, a male Holstein calf was brought to the fourth floor OR of the old St. Mark's facilities. His name was Burk in honor of Kessler's heart-making associate, Gail Burkett, who was leaving to have a baby. At 195 pounds, Burk was a big, bawling calf.

Technicians anesthetized him, relaxed his muscles, and inserted the respirator's endotracheal tube. Olsen sliced open the chest, took out the fourth rib on the right side, and opened the pericardial sac to attach the heart-lung pump. Removing the natural heart, he quickly sutured and wired in the J-3 heart. Then a minor crisis arose.

The tubes in Burk's heart had short bits of Dacron velour to act as sleeves where they entered the chest wall and encourage fibrous-tissue growth that would slow or block the invasion of bacteria along the drivelines and lock the airlines into position. Olsen fiddled with the sleeves. Something was wrong.

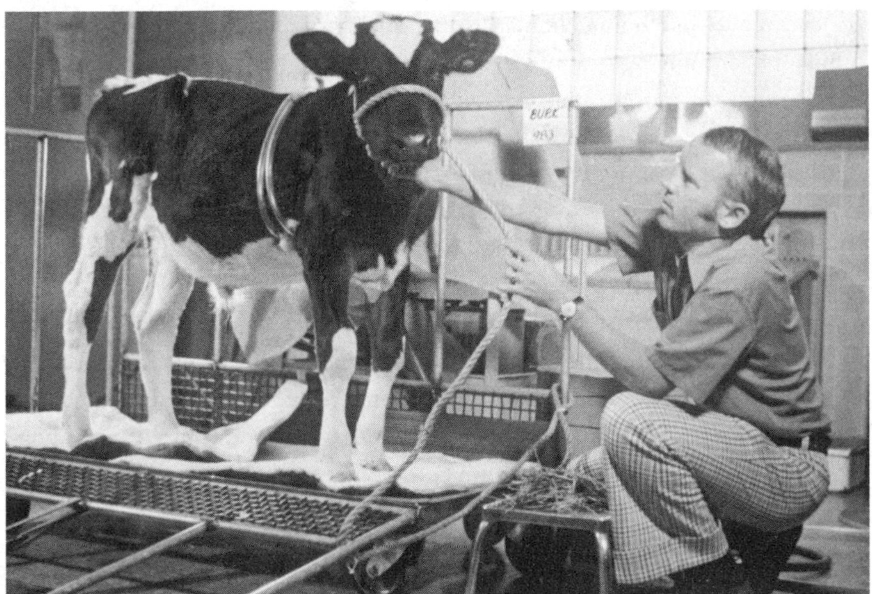

John Lawson cares for Burk on an artificial heart.

They would not seat properly on the lines. "Looks like they're useless," he said. With the limited period that animals could be safely kept on bypass, he did not have time to bring in a new heart with sleeves that worked. "We have no choice," he said. "We'll go without them." It was a gamble he had to take. With connectors he attached the tubes to the six-foot hoses linked to the air driver.

At first Burk was tentative about life with an artificial heart. Though he hadn't eaten for twenty-four hours before the surgery, he ate sparingly. He stood for no more than fifteen minutes at a time. Abruptly, Burk turned the corner. He began eating ravenously, gaining about two pounds a day. His blood chemistry, somewhat chancy in the beginning, settled down to normal. There were no signs that the heart was chewing up red blood cells.

By the start of Burk's second month, the experimenters realized he needed more exercise than merely standing in his cage. They took down the sides of his cage. While two technicians guided him, Burk walked slowly around the room, tethered by hoses to the three-hundred-pound heart driver pushed by another technician.

As prosaic as that seemed, it was a landmark in the sixteen-year history of artificial-heart research. No animal had ever lived long enough on the artificial heart to require physical exercise. The event was more than mere exercise. The men in that room knew it focused on an issue that hung like a cloud over the eventuality of a human implant: what quality of life would be possible for a human patient relying on the apparatus? Burk's walks three times a week were ponderous, slow-motion affairs and ultimately inadequate. His muscles began to atrophy. However, he was still alive on the sixtieth day after surgery.

Burk fought other battles. Without the velour sleeves, the air tubes leading from his heart did not bond with the skin. Skittering around, they irritated the tissue, leading to an infection. "Should we terminate?" Kolff asked. "He has the record at two months. I am concerned about the infection."

Olsen was less worried. "It seems to be localized. We can drain the wound. So far there is no fever. I believe we can keep him longer." Kolff didn't press the point. Burk's J-3 was designed for a calf weighing, at the most, about 220 pounds. With his big appetite, Burk was up to 277 pounds and counting. At what point would he simply outgrow the J-3's ability to pump sufficient blood?

Fears intensified when Burk's venous pressure increased ominously. His liver became perceptibly swollen, and his neck puffed up with edema, signs of right-heart failure. The technicians were worried that the diaphragm, as in the case of Kamui, was failing under the weight of successive layers of protein deposits.

Technicians fussed over a different trouble spot. Seven times they replaced Burk's air drivers for various failures. The latest also had a problem with the valve controlling airflow, denying the heart adequate power. After another substitution, the pumping resumed, the swelling receded, and the high venous blood pressure subsided.

Late in his third month, Burk took a downhill slide. When he stood, his head was held down. His temperature spiked, and there were obvious signs of terminal infection. "There is no doubt that we must terminate," Kolff said.

Olsen disagreed: "I am sure he can go longer."

"You are going to an international cardiologist meeting in Argentina next month," Kolff noted. "It would be good if you could report on Burk to them. You need a clinical report of the autopsy. Terminate—now!" So Olsen, on August 25, injected Burk with an anesthetic that killed him. The calf had survived on his heart for almost ninety-five days and twenty-one hours. Several of the calf sitters who had tended him for three months wept.

The autopsy disclosed that the heart had no barnacle buildup, although there were patches of thrombi at the diaphragm junctions with the ventricles' housing, the D-H area. A few emboli, perhaps fragments from the heart clots, were in the kidneys, but function remained normal. The infection had not been localized at the surface. With the airlines to steer them, bacteria had crept up the tubes. The pericardium around the heart was infected, and the heart had blotches of white pus. The cause for termination was listed as infection.

The J-3 model came through with high marks. Its multilayered diaphragm appeared to have functioned without flaw. “Now,” exulted Jarvik to his wife, Elaine, “I have done something that really makes a difference with the heart.” And it had. The survival time tripled. Kolff told his staff, “Burk should put to rest the concerns of some who believe the artificial heart is an impossible dream.”

World Congress of Cardiology

In mid-1974, Kolff chose to send Olsen to the World Congress of Cardiology in Buenos Aires. Dr. Denton Cooley was the emcee, and after Olsen made his presentation, Cooley—as the session chair—said, “If Drs. Kolff, Olsen, and the Utah team can keep a calf alive for three months, we can keep a human alive for a year.”

While in Buenos Aires, Olsen was invited to Liotta's office. He was now the minister of health for Argentina. Cooley was also in the office when Olsen arrived. Liotta invited Olsen to bring three or four hearts with pneumatic drivers to Argentina. He proposed that Cooley fly from Houston and the three would implant the hearts in human patients.

Olsen said, “Thank you for the confidence and invitation, but Utah cannot win either way.” The heart had been developed with federal grant money. If the patients survived, the Utah group would be criticized for taking the results of NIH-sponsored research and using them first in Argentina. If the patients died, the Utah group would be criticized for experimenting on poor Argentineans. Even though he had to decline, the invitation by these two famous individuals to implant the Utah heart bolstered his confidence.

Maintenance and Repair

Responding to an application for a federal grant, agency overseers asked Kolff to name his second in command should anything happen to him. Rather than be specific, Kolff said that the university's vice president for research would designate somebody. Not good enough, said the bureaucrats, and turned down the application.

“For heaven's sake,” Olsen said. “We worked for almost a year on that proposal. If that's all it would have taken to save the grant, why didn't you put my name down? You know I've been making all the day-to-day decisions in the animal lab.”

Kolff said he would think about it. On the next grant application, he filled in the blank space for identifying who would take over if he was incapacitated with “Don B. Olsen, Director, Artificial Heart Research Laboratory.” That was Kolff's way of telling Olsen he was now the director.

With or without the title, Olsen had work to do. Burk's results on the artificial heart had spotlighted shortcomings. There was the problem with the sleeves that had not seated properly on the airlines. Researchers in the materials section suggested covering the lines with Dacron velour, which would promote bonding with tissue with or without the sleeves. Olsen usually brought the lines straight through the bony chest from the heart. "Next time I'll tunnel them under the skin for short distances outside the chest wall," he said. "There's more tissue there to hold the lines, which provides a better chance to limit, if not eliminate, movement and infection."

Steven Nielsen, the lab's electronics and computer whiz, attacked the problem of the pneumatic drivers that had failed eight times. To the casual observer, Nielsen seemed shy. At morning conference, he generally held his tongue when he disagreed with a speaker, waiting until they could talk in private. Five feet, ten inches tall and broad shouldered, he looked like what he was: a solid man. Olsen frequently bounced ideas off him, respecting both his judgment and brains.

Nielsen had arrived in 1970 as a university sophomore working part time in Kolff's lab. Now twenty-three, with an electrical-engineering degree and the experience of a two-year Mormon mission in Argentina, he had a definite goal: to apply advanced electronics to biomedical projects. First assigned to the lab's control system for artificial kidneys, he transferred to the heart-driver project.

When Hank Wong, designer of a prototype driver that was to succeed Kwan-Gett's machine, was killed in a motorcycle accident, Nielsen built the working models. He could quote chapter and verse on the machine's drawbacks: it was noisy, unreliable, and inaccurate. Nielsen felt he could create a better driver. Following earlier designs, he wanted the linchpin of the driver to be a three-way valve that guided compressed air through hoses into the heart, allowed the air to empty, and—when necessary—applied light-to-moderate suction.

But the specific valve he envisioned—compact, easy to install, and capable of operating almost indefinitely without lubrication—was not in any catalogue. Manufacturers laughed when Nielsen outlined his specifications. It took months of searching the country by phone to locate a supplier in Kalamazoo, Michigan, who unexpectedly responded, "An artificial heart? Hey that sounds exciting. Sure! We've got a little item that can be modified to do just what you want. We call it the Humphrey valve."

Engineering technicians came in to help Nielsen build the driver. It was about the size of a shopping cart. It had thumb-wheel switches to adjust the pumping pressure, dials to monitor pressure, and outlets for compressed air. The three-way valves from Kalamazoo lived up to the supplier's praise. They worked smoothly, did not require lubrication, and were so quiet it was hard to hear the air whooshing in and out. The pumping power came from the lab's main air compressor. Sophisticated electronics brought versatility to the pumping rates and pressures, determining what fractional part of the heart cycle was allotted to taking in blood (diastole) and driving it out (systole).

In addition, the driver had backup. If the main compressor failed, the driver switched automatically to its own emergency tanks of compressed air to keep the heart going without interruption. If the electricity went off, there was a battery for emergency power. If the control unit faltered, it required only a few seconds to disconnect the air hoses and plug them into the backup driver that was always available.

As a project overseer, Nielsen could have named the machine the Nielsen heart driver, but he thought that wasn't fair, considering all the people who had contributed to it, including the designers of earlier models. "Let's call it the Utah heart driver," he said, gaining Olsen's full support.

Kessler focused on the Burk autopsy report, particularly the thrombosis at the V-shaped D-H junction of the diaphragm and the ventricle. Was that just a one-time occurrence, or was it an inherent defect in the J-3 design? A new series of implants was run. The results were chilling. In six of eight calves, or 75 percent, clotting formed in the D-H zone. It was not hard to see why. In this area, blood could stagnate, leading to formation of a clot that could break free into a thromboembolism. Unless this challenge was overcome, all hopes of using the smooth polyurethane heart in a human implant were futile.

Throughout his surgery residency, Clifford Kwan-Gett had been dropping in at the lab and renewing acquaintance. On one visit, he said to Kessler, "I've been thinking about the D-H riddle. I'm sure the trouble starts with the seam between the diaphragm and the housing. I've got an idea for a one-piece blood chamber. It could be the answer." Kessler made notes on Kwan-Gett's suggestion, which coincided with his thinking. He began teaching himself how to pour polyurethane to mold the diaphragm and the housing in one smooth, continuous layer. However, he was not sure it could be done.

"Give Me Wild Ideas"

Gerald Foote came to the lab one day with a throbbing headache. He was the California physicist whose small-pump design had earlier helped the lab overcome surface scum in the latex tanks. He went to a medicine chest to get some aspirin. Putting his thumb under the lid of the bottle cap, he snapped it off, took two aspirin, and snapped it back on. Then it hit him—the bottle cap was the

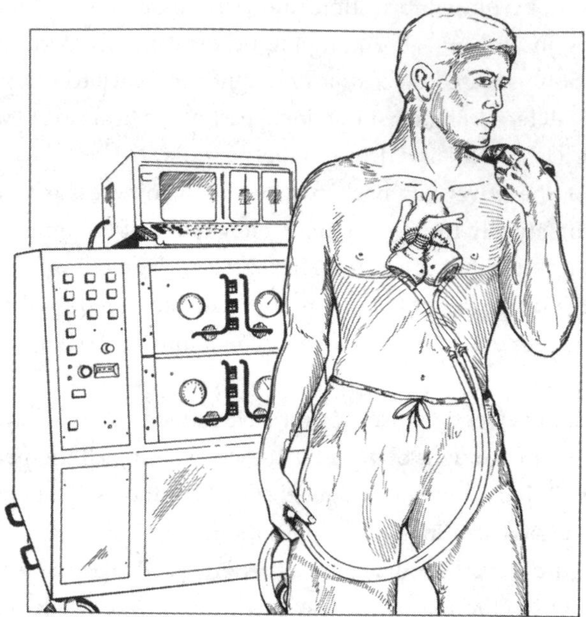

A drawing of the way the artificial heart would fit into a human chest.

answer to one of Kolff's concerns: "Surgery is best with the least time on the heart-lung pump. We are spending too long on the operating table. There must be ways to do the implant quicker." Olsen and others had timed every step of the operation. It took disproportionately long to wrap and tighten the wires where the accordion-pleated grafts fit over the heart's outflow valves, but finding more efficient connections had stumped them.

Foote's headache solved the lab's. "Think of the aspirin bottle cap," he said to Kessler. "Let's do the same for the heart—connections that snap on and off." To one end of a pair of the accordion-pleated grafts, they added semihard plastic rings that were fabricated to snap into circular grooves molded around the two outflow rings. This technique eliminated time-consuming wire twisting. The other ends of the grafts were left bare for suturing directly to the aorta and pulmonary artery.

Kessler had designed and built wide disc-shaped cuffs that were sutured to the cut edges of the atria after the ventricles were removed. He placed circular grooves around the inflow rings that fit into the atrial cuffs. They could snap the semirigid Silastic rings onto these grooves; the rings had inch-long Dacron aprons to sew them to the remnants of the two atria.

Serendipitously these quick connects provided a bonus: "Look, if we ever have to go back to replace a ventricle, it'll be just a matter of popping the hearts out and in," Foote said. But not all the surgeons appreciated the innovation; they complained that snapping the connections together with their bloody gloves on was difficult. Sometimes Kessler had to demonstrate the technique during implant surgery. However, the quick connects shaved a half hour from the surgery time.

Ideas were the lifeblood of Kolff's lab, and he expected people to keep them coming. "Even if you think they are wild, let me have them," he said. Kolff asked yet again for research ideas for a new grant proposal he was writing.

Olsen had something to propose he thought was stunning. The man-made valves in the artificial heart were often weak. They were grossly inferior to natural valves, sometimes breaking and collecting thrombi and creating four potential peril points. Olsen proposed saving the natural aortic and pulmonary artery valves, but Kolff found the idea unreasonable. "If this could be done," he said, "good surgeons would already have perfected it." In fact, a Texas surgical team had already attempted it—unsuccessfully.

Olsen and a freshman medical student who did not share Kolff's skepticism decided the idea was worth a try. They began by studying every anatomical detail in calf and sheep hearts. Then, instead of cutting the aorta and pulmonary artery above the two valves guiding blood out of the heart, they cut below them, retaining little skirts of tissue for suturing. The stumps of the right and left coronary arteries were ligated. These then snapped onto the circular grooves added to a special version of the J-3 heart from which the outflow valves had been removed.

They perfected the technique on cadaver calf hearts, but because Kolff had been so negative, Olsen was reluctant to try it in an implant. One day in 1975 while Kolff was out of town, however, Olsen took a chance with a calf he dubbed AoPA (for aorta and pulmonary artery). The hours of rehearsal paid off with a successful implant. Kolff remained on an extended trip and vacation, and AoPA was sure to be a surprise for him. In anticipation of Kolff's return, Olsen took a radiograph clearly showing that AoPA did indeed have only two artificial valves. When Kolff saw the radiograph, he was complimentary about the success.

The calf's natural valves were far more efficient and had less resistance to flow than the mechanical ones. The J-3 heart with the two natural valves had more cardiac output with similar heart-driving parameters.

An electrically powered, pusher-plate artificial heart was being developed in the laboratory to interface with a Stirling engine powered by a plutonium

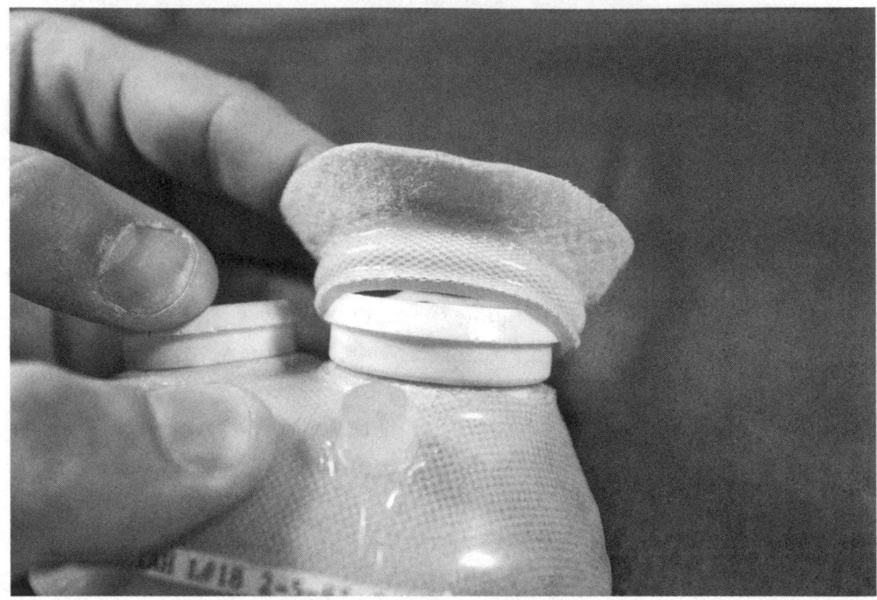

Snap connectors are used to connect the parts of the artificial heart.

isotope. That heart also had two mechanical valves for each ventricle. Olsen implanted an electric-motor-powered version of the heart in some calves, saving both natural valves. When these calves were exercised on the treadmill, the heart consumed three-to-five fewer watts of electricity to drive the heart. This was a significant power reduction. However, no other surgeons ever adopted his technique, and Olsen only used it infrequently because it extended surgery time.

To avoid the muscle atrophy Burk had suffered, a treadmill was built to exercise AoPA and other calves. The tilt and speed could be adjusted, enabling technicians to vary and monitor performance. AoPa's heart, with its mix of natural and artificial valves, maintained circulation for 122 days after surgery until quite suddenly the calf died. The cause of death was, literally, a broken heart—one of the J-3's two artificial valve discs had shattered. AoPA added another month to the survival record, but it had taken a year to get to this point.

COMDU: the Cardiac Output Monitor and Diagnostic Unit

None of the artificial-heart teams had solved a very important problem. The health and well-being of calves on artificial hearts was difficult to monitor and ascertain through performance. Cardiologists, other physicians, and attendants monitoring a human patient would need to know more about what the artificial heart was doing and how to adjust the device for maximum benefit.

Years of experience working with calves had taught Olsen that many subtle appearances and mannerisms revealed that the heart and calf were doing well. Clearly, appetite, the calf's general appearance, and performance on the treadmill suggested its well-being, but these were totally inadequate parameters for humans. To obtain arterial blood to measure blood gasses required catheters that were far too dangerous for humans. Clearly there had to be accurate physiologic measurements before the artificial heart could be accepted for human use.

What nearly everyone wanted to know was the cardiac output. Then it was important to know how to adjust the artificial heart. Many had tried, but all had failed to measure the blood flow from the artificial heart. The flow probes placed around the major vessels were inconsistent and lasted only a short time. They were square-wave flow sensors, older technology that soon became unstable.

The Utah team had long known that the volume of air exiting from the ventricle had to correlate with the blood filling it. They decided that if they could calculate the volume of exiting air, they could prove the filling volume of blood times the heart rate equaled the cardiac output. This could become the best single measurement to monitor the well-being of patients on the artificial heart.

Olsen had studied pulmonary function several years earlier in calves, including measuring the volume of exhaled air using a Fleish pneumotachograph. He learned of a newer model that measured air volume more accurately. Olsen ordered new models to measure pulmonary function on calves with artificial hearts and gave one to Nielsen to try to measure the air volume leaving the ventricle during diastole. Several experiments proved that the air-volume measurements were nearly identical to the stroke volume of the ventricle. The idea was patented and allowed technicians to identify several important features in assessing patients' blood circulation. It was impossible to obtain hard numbers for atrial pressure, but it could be calculated by the filling time of the ventricle. One could also determine hypovolemia (inadequate blood volume). The equipment, with its broad capabilities in monitoring the artificial heart's performance, was named a cardiac output monitor and diagnostic unit (COMDU).

The stroke volume of the ventricle multiplied by the heart rate gave the cardiac output. Initially the team could not record every stroke volume because the first Apple computer was only fast enough to measure every third to fourth heartbeat. Newer, faster computers could display each stroke volume. Starling's Law of cardiac output, identified much earlier by Kwan-Gett, was proven. Twelve other models of artificial hearts have been implanted into humans around the world, but only one heart has survived the clinical tests and is used today—the one monitored by the COMDU.

The Readiness Factor

Nearly two decades had passed since Tetsuzo Akutsu had opened the era of the artificial heart by telling the ASAIO the way he and Kolff had nurtured life in a dog for ninety minutes. Now in 1976, Olsen reported to the ASAIO that for the first time, the artificial heart had sustained life in an animal for more than four months. The meeting's chair, Dr. John C. (Jack) Norman, a surgeon with Cooley's Texas Heart Institute and experimenter with ventricular-assist devices, saw beyond the words to the report's implicit challenge to researchers.

When Olsen finished, Norman said he would like to have a discussion on future human use of total artificial hearts. He asked, "Who will decide about using them and under what circumstances?" The clear implication was that human experimentation with the artificial heart would thrust researchers into a world of dark and troubling ethical and moral issues. Indeed, the government had recently decreed that all human experimentation had to be approved by IRBs. The boards were required to have a variety of members specified by the government. This was to ensure both an independent appraisal and rigid standards for obtaining a patient's informed consent.

San Francisco's Dr. Benson Roe acknowledged Norman's concerns, arguing that it would be "dangerous and irresponsible for our enthusiasm over laboratory successes to be projected into the public domain until we have a complete and thorough answer to some of the questions that you have posed. Can you imagine walking around with a bunch of machinery and a compressed air tank?"

In the audience was Theodore Stanley, who had left Kolff's lab to become an anesthesiologist. He had returned to the Artificial Heart Research Laboratory as a consultant. "Rather than being emotionally upset about the thought of the heart," said Stanley, "it is more prudent to recognize that there will be human implantations. Scientists should decide under what circumstances the heart will be implanted. If they disregard that responsibility," Stanley warned, "politicians will make all the decisions."

Half-a-dozen others contributed to the debate until Norman brought it to a close by suggesting that perhaps scientific inquiry was itself a measure of advancement. Kolff did not participate, but his views were well known. In a declaration to the government, he said he had a very simple philosophy:

> I will collaborate in placing an artificial heart in a human recipient only if there is no other hope for the patient and there is a reasonable chance that he or she can be restored to an enjoyable existence. A patient must wish for the operation, and we must be confident that the

> artificial heart we offer will serve his circulatory and metabolic needs. A patient should be expected to be up and out of bed two or three days after the operation, similar to the successes in calves. He should be mobile, self-sufficient, without pain in his chest, and with far fewer restrictions than a man confined to a wheelchair.

Kolff pointed to the work of Dr. Norman Shumway in Palo Alto, California: "He did most of the investigative work leading to the early heart transplants, but now that nearly everyone else has given up, he continually improves his results. We [in Utah] may not be the first to implant an artificial heart in a human, but we will consistently work to make this possible and safe."

The Nuclear-Powered Heart

In the 1960s and early '70s, all things seemed possible with nuclear fission. It was going to provide unlimited energy, heating, and lighting for America's homes and power for her factories. If it could do that, why not let it drive an artificial heart? A feeling of euphoria swept through both the government's NHLI (later to become the National Heart, Lung and Blood Institute [NHLBI]) and the AEC. The NHLI bet millions that the atom could be harnessed to drive ventricular-assist pumps. The AEC put its money behind the total artificial heart.

The AEC scenario called for private industry to make a nuclear engine fired by its pile of plutonium that was small enough to plant inside the abdomen. Kolff's job was to build an artificial heart that could be powered by a flexible drive shaft from a miniature reactor. What appealed to Kolff was the notion of a completely implantable heart—no tethering to a bulky air driver, no wires through the chest. Jesting, he said that a man with such an artificial heart might win the 1990 Boston Marathon, provided he was not disqualified for having an unfair advantage.

By 1976 Kolff's lab had received $752,000 from the AEC to design, build, and implant what was called the ERDA heart (as the AEC's successor, the Energy Research and Development Agency [ERDA] later took over the project). His advice, however, was to go slowly with the nuclear-engine implants. He warned that if small heart-powering A-plant units were stockpiled in hospitals, the logistics of guarding them would be insurmountable. He suggested concentrating on a heart that functioned with either electricity or atomic energy. "Use it on the heart, but first run it with electrical power," he suggested. When both the patient and the heart were considered good risks, then "the nuclear engineer could come in for a second minor operation in which the electromotor is exchanged for the nuclear engine."

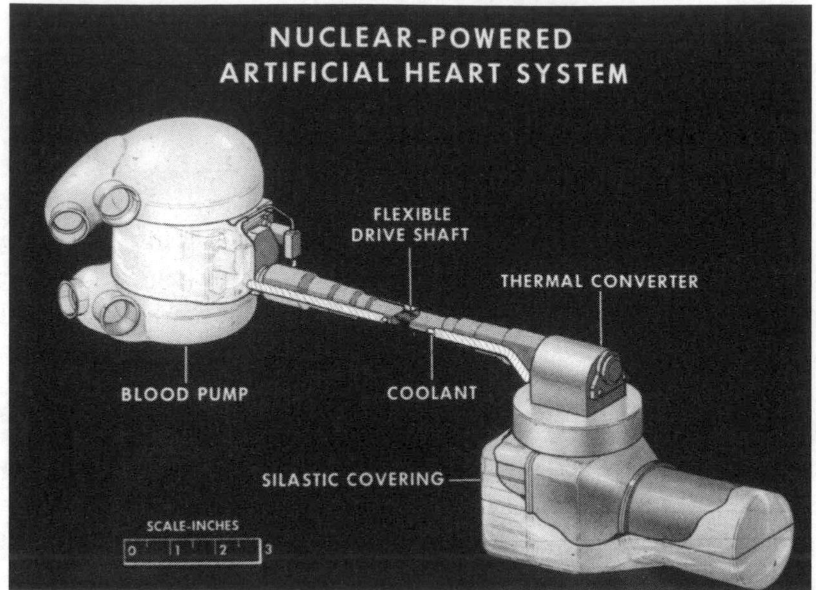

A prototype of a nuclear-powered heart.

What Kolff had learned in Cleveland was that the electrically powered heart was tricky. He relearned this in Utah. Time and again the drive shaft manufactured by a private company broke. It was also difficult to dissipate heat adequately. A major unresolved problem was balancing the two ventricles so the right one did not outpump the left one, causing pulmonary edema and death. Olsen solved this lethal problem by having Kessler build a small hole through the adhered part of the atrial cuffs. This permitted the slightly higher pressure in the left atria to move into the right one. With this adaptation, a calf was kept alive for nearly six months on an electromechanical heart.

Still, Kolff was willing to pursue a workable atomic heart, and he found it inconceivable that after nearly three years, ERDA scrapped the project. Subsequently the NHLI followed suit, but it was not technological failures that killed the atomic heart. Washington thought about people walking around with plutonium in their bellies and nervously envisioned terrorists kidnapping them, stripping out their reactors, and having the makings of a decidedly nontherapeutic venture.

Rob Jarvik Officially Joins the Team

Kolff decided to bring Rob Jarvik full time onto his research team. Jarvik had begun medical school in September 1972 and was now scheduled to graduate in

June 1976. His medical-school teachers thought he was someone who charted his own course. They assumed he would follow the rest of his classmates into an internship to qualify for a license to treat patients. Jarvik refused. He felt that being able to write the letters MD after his name, indicating he had graduated from medical school, was enough.

"I'm better off without the license," he explained. "If I don't have it, I'll have to work all the harder because I'll know there's nothing else. It never hurts to have some extra stimulus."

Jarvik approached Olsen in January 1976 and asked for a full-time job in the Artificial Heart Research Laboratory. Olsen told him that he would not hire him because Jarvik's wife and two small children needed more financial security. "You must take a residency and pass your boards to be licensed to practice medicine," Olsen advised. Jarvik responded that he had never intended to practice medicine, and furthermore, his father had recently died and left him independently wealthy. He told Olsen that he thought everyone knew that he had lost eighty thousand dollars in gold futures the previous October.

Then Olsen took a different approach. He told Jarvik that it was unbelievable that he had taken a place in medical school and deprived of an education some other student who would have made a commitment to treating ill patients. Jarvik told Olsen that if he could not get a job in Utah, he would go elsewhere. Olsen suggested that Jarvik return later in the week, and he would give him an answer.

Failing to get what he wanted from Olsen, Jarvik approached Kolff for a position. Kolff bypassed Olsen's decision, hired Jarvik, and put him in Olsen's Artificial Heart Research Laboratory. It created a nearly unmanageable predicament for Olsen.

Jarvik's personality caused other conflicts. One day Mary Johnson was as angry as only an executive secretary can be when she thinks somebody is disrespectful to the boss. In this case, the target was Jarvik. She felt the charm of his dark-haired, blue-eyed, boyish good looks had worn thin. "Can't Dr. Kolff say it is a nice day in morning conference without your asking, 'Says who?'" she accosted Jarvik. He gave her a blank stare. That annoyed her even more. "It's embarrassing!" she snapped. "Everyone is uncomfortable, including me. You're always challenging him, always asking why something has to be done this way or that. Would you please not argue with him in front of everyone?" Jarvik shrugged.

So did Kolff when Johnson complained about Jarvik's attitude. "Let him be," he said.

Abebe's Race

Cleveland provided a prod for renewed efforts in Utah. In Yukihiko Nosé's lab, a calf with an artificial heart eclipsed AoPA's record by living for 145 days. Jarvik heard about it as he was pushing plans for a new design, one he called the Jarvik-5.

Kessler had a little joke. Surveying his second-floor prosthetics center in the old St. Mark's Hospital with its high ceilings, dental-technician tools and drills, and pink tile walls, he liked to tell visitors, "And this is the delivery room." He wasn't kidding. In the old days, St. Mark's Hospital had used his quarters for obstetrics. Kessler continued the deliveries, but they were artificial hearts, not babies.

Meanwhile, after months of experimentation, Kessler was about to introduce his latest offspring—a seamless chamber to hold blood in a ventricle. "This little baby is really something," he said to the staff. "It won't get any thrombosis in the D-H junction—absolutely guaranteed. We can say that because it doesn't have one. It's a single piece—no seams, no creases where clots can form."

The seamless design was based on designs that both Jarvik and Kwan-Gett had discussed with Kessler. The seamless blood chamber was adapted to fit in the Jarvik-5 or J-5. This heart had a hundred-milliliter stroke volume. There was now genuine optimism that the lab was on the verge of consistent, long-term success, a quantum jump toward human implantation.

One of the fears generated by Burk was that a calf that lived a long time after its implant would outgrow its artificial heart. To accommodate the growth of calves in extended experiments, Jarvik made the J-5 heart bigger than previous models, enabling it to pump more blood with each stroke. He retained the J-3's two-layer diaphragm. When it came time to implant the J-5 in 1976, somebody asked, "What are we going to call the calf?" John Lawson, the experiment's principal investigator, christened the calf Abebe because he wanted the animal to go the distance. Abebe Bikila had twice won Olympic gold medals for Ethiopia in the marathon while running barefoot, the only man ever to do so.

Abebe the calf recovered quickly from his surgery. There were no blood abnormalities; his vital signs were good, and his appetite voracious. Five days after surgery, he was exercising vigorously on his treadmill. He was still doing it after three months. Despite having ballooned to 396 pounds, he walked the equivalent of two hundred yards uphill in ten minutes.

Though Abebe gradually lost muscle strength, he surpassed the Cleveland calf's record. Not until his sixth month on the artificial heart at day 184 did the signs of right-heart failure make it necessary to return him to the OR. Olsen

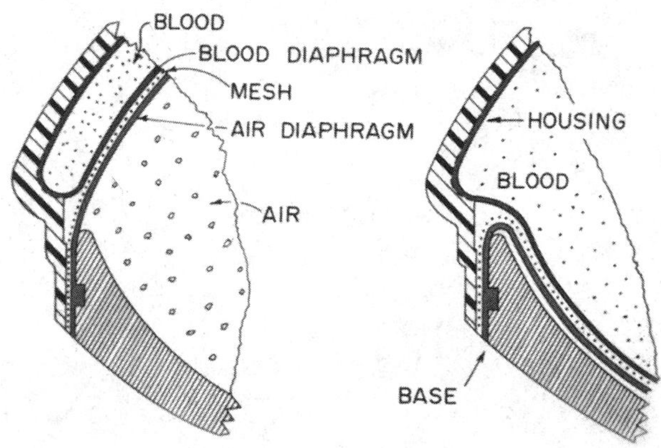

Design of the continuous blood diaphragm of the J-5 heart.

expected to find the J-5 had malfunctioned. "We'll put in another heart, maybe do a transplant," he said. Once it had been epochal even to think of getting an artificial heart to work. Now Olsen was planning to snap one out and install another.

The problem, however, was not in the heart but in the quick-connect's plastic cuff shepherding blood from the right atrium into the ventricle. Its inside wall was coated with hard, shiny tissue that almost completely obstructed the blood flow. Olsen had never encountered anything like it. He thought it looked like the pannus that people get with trachoma, an overgrowth of fibrous connective tissue. He and his OR crew succeeded in stripping away the growth. Unfortunately, because of all the surgery to cut the heart free from its adhesions to the pericardial sac, and since Abebe was on anticoagulants, he developed uncontrollable bleeding and was terminated while under anesthesia.

In the postmortem, the staff came upon another surprise. The blood-facing layers in both diaphragms were speckled with holes. The Dacron mesh, built in to limit stretching, had rubbed against the plastic for more than twenty-three million heartbeats, creating the holes. There were small knots joining strands of Dacron that had worn through the thin polyurethane. While that had not contributed to Abebe's death, it was only a matter of time before the diaphragms would have collapsed. Jarvik added a third sheet of polyurethane to the diaphragm, separating it from the blood-facing layer with graphite lubricant to stop any possibility of the layers sticking to each other and eroding.

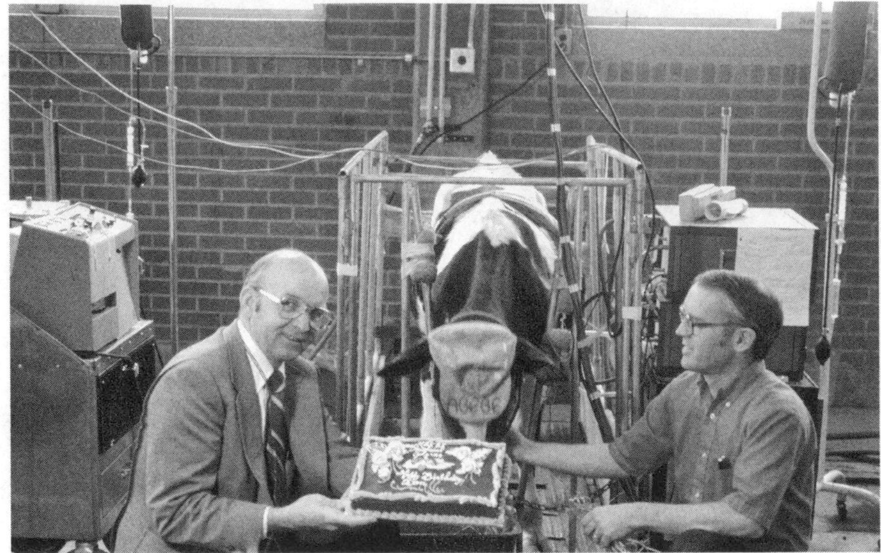

John Lawson (*right*) and Don Olsen treat Abebe to a celebration cake for his long survival.

But the question remained of what to do about the newly encountered problem of pannus. Once again, success had spawned a new challenge.

Empire Secured

Stewart S. Grow was a real-estate investor, and from their first meeting in 1977, Kolff saw him as a threat, the man who was going to evict the lab from the old St. Mark's Hospital. When Grow announced he was buying the whole building, Kolff asked, "Would you keep us as a tenant?" Grow said he would if Kolff was willing to pay fifty thousand dollars a year in rent. That was twenty-five times what the lab had been paying, but it only came to about two dollars a square foot, less than half the commercial rate in that area. Grow offered Kolff a fifteen-year lease, which the university agreed was a good deal.

Olsen had many discussions with Stewart and his two partners, Darrel Deem and Ed Rogers, who made up Marcus Associates, the purchasing group. Olsen agreed to the rent amount and offered to assist the men in filling the building with rent-paying offices or companies. They agreed in return to donate seventy-five thousand dollars a year to Olsen's development fund at the university. Marcus Associates continued donating to Olsen's development account until they sold the building for a good profit.

In late summer of 1978, University of Utah's President David P. Gardner summoned a group of people to a small hill just east of the medical center. It was an occasion that Kolff had eagerly anticipated. After the fire in Building 512 and the move of the Artificial Heart Research Laboratory to St. Mark's Hospital, Kolff's administrative offices had remained in Building 518, a wooden barracks.

The hillside meeting was proof that Kolff's long wait was ending. The meeting was called to unveil a plaque saying the building being constructed on the site would be Kolff's new headquarters, named after its principal benefactors, the Dumke family. Kolff received words of tribute: "Your artificial-organs programs," said Gardner, "stand at the forefront of their science and among the first rank of research programs conducted by universities the world over."

It was a happy occasion in sharp contrast to the earlier controversies that had marred the long-awaited construction of a new building. Following the Building 512 blaze in 1973, the Utah Legislature had set aside $600,000 to build a new structure for Kolff. With the money came a state-designated architect. Kolff hired his own architect, saying: "I have definite ideas of what the building should look like and what it should include." Angered that two architects were being paid, state officials had put the project on hold. The ensuing debate went on for two years before it was finally settled, mostly in Kolff's favor.

By then skyrocketing construction costs and design changes had added another million dollars to the cost. Kolff the fund-raiser went into action. He negotiated a $300,000 contribution from Michigan's Kresge Foundation. Then in 1975, Kolff heard that Edna Wattis Dumke, daughter of a construction-company tycoon, was thinking of making a contribution to the university to honor her late husband, Dr. Ezekiel R. Dumke, who had been affiliated with the school for many years. Kolff asked if she and her family would think of earmarking the bequest for his work.

Before answering, the Dumke family called Dr. John Dixon, the health-sciences vice president, for his thoughts about donating money for artificial-organ research. Dixon, who had tangled with Kolff on the dialysis center's location, told them he thought it was "a fine idea." After their $650,000 gift was received, construction crews moved in.

Kolff had his architect design a surgical theater on the lower floor with a large window in the ceiling above the operating table so people could observe implantation of the artificial heart in humans. Olsen was opposed for several reasons: first, the building was much too small to accommodate both the artificial heart and dialysis. He told Kolff he intended to stay in his facilities in the old St. Mark's Hospital. Second, the surgical room was too small to house all of the ancillary equipment needed to implant the heart. Finally, at this point, Olsen was an assistant professor of surgery, and Kolff's plan was discussed at some

Department of Surgery faculty meetings. The conclusion was that his stand-alone building would not permit rapid access in the event of an emergency. Nevertheless, Kolff got his observation theater, and it remained for almost seven years; then he remodeled it.

Kolff observed his sixty-eighth birthday in 1979. He had been showered with honors from around the world, written or coauthored more than six hundred articles, and had entire issues of scientific magazines dedicated to him. Both to keep him working and symbolize his international status, the university named him distinguished professor of surgery, waiving age limitations on his retirement. Responding to the congratulations of his staff, he jokingly said, "This brings both good news and bad news. The good news is that I don't have to retire. The bad news is, God help you if I ever get senile."

"Don't worry," Mary Johnson told him. "I'll be the first to let you know."

Kolff's work was far from done. He would not consider it finished until the artificial heart had been implanted in a human. "My husband," said Janke Kolff, "is in a race against time."

At the same time, a man was entering the crowded field of cardiac-failure patients. He and Kolff had wildly different origins, but he was unknowingly tracking a parallel path to Kolff's progress in artificial-heart research, not because of interest but because of the pressure of events. His failing heart continued to worsen.

PART THREE

8

Barney's Story

In a Looking Glass

Through the years it's been fun reminiscing.
I'd see your face and you'd call my name.
Now my friends are older and much wiser,
but most of us remain at heart the same...

—Lyrics for the fortieth reunion, Provo High School Class of 1939

During the summer solstice of 1979, two evenings past the longest day of the year, Barney Clark put on his favorite jacket. It was deep pearl gray, thinly striped with maroon. His shirt was white, his tie a mellow blending of compatible colors. The slacks were a coordinated gray, and his tasseled black Italian loafers were carefully buffed.

Two and a half years later, Barney would be the first human in the world to receive a permanent artificial heart to replace the natural one that was failing him. But tonight he was preparing to attend a gathering of old friends. Barney was big: six feet, three inches tall, 188 pounds, and broad shouldered. Fifty-eight years old, and two years retired as a dentist, he was meticulous about his appearance, proud of keeping his gut flat as a board.

Looking into the bathroom mirror, he gave himself a final checkout. The reflection showed the face of an all-American boy who had weathered well. No wrinkles creased his forehead, and his features were well defined. His dark brown hair, graying at the temples, silver in the sideburns, was dressed with a touch of Brilliantine. "Not a hell of a lot left on top," he mused.

Barney's eyes were an engrossing blue green with a hint of mischievousness. The lashes were long and black, the brows thick and scraggly. Barney clenched his teeth in an exaggerated grin, broadening his slightly crooked smile. He

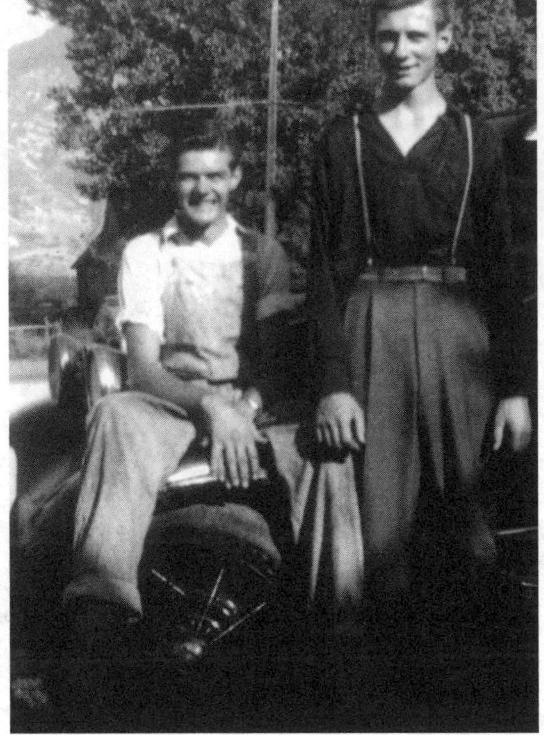

Barney Clark (*left*) and Weston Brown formed a bond as close as brothers.

was not checking his teeth. He knew they were in perfect condition. The grin was practice for an on-demand smile. "Guess I'm expected to do a lot of this tonight," he said. He was to be master of ceremonies at a quintessential American custom: the fortieth reunion of his class from Provo High School in Provo, Utah.

Satisfied with his appearance, he walked back into the bedroom. "Hark, hark!" he shouted in good humor. He struck a pose: back straight, long arms outstretched, lifting an imaginary bugle.

His wife, Una Loy, knew he was making fun of himself. "C'mon, honey," she said. "You'll be great!"

"Easy for you to say," he answered. "You don't have to get up there and make a damn fool of yourself."

On December 1, 1978, a document with legal-sounding language had arrived at the Clark home in Des Moines, a tiny suburb twenty-five miles south of Seattle. The house was an imposing Tudor with a curved entrance drive through iron gates and an acre of lawn, including terraces that swept down to a bluff overlooking Puget Sound. The paper said that because of a "forty-year succession of life's bombardments," the Provo High School class of '39 was charged with being "casualties of hour-glass-itis, also known as it's-later-than-you-think mania."

The certain signs of this, the paper went on, could include, but were not limited to, "loss of teeth, hair, eyes, waistlines, bust lines;" acquisition of "wrinkles, bulges, droops;" double-vision because of "money pressures, moving, not moving, retirement;" and "dazed nerves resulting from too much or too little grandbaby sitting." Because of "the damages suffered by such abuse," the citation demanded "relief in the form of your attendance" at the fortieth reunion in June 1979. Purpose: "to drop away the years and laugh your way to perfect health through reminiscing."

Barney and Una Loy joyfully honored the summons. Volunteering their help, Una Loy responded, "Barney and I realize that something like this is a major endeavor, and we should all do our bit." Originally the affair was to be just a dinner dance. But as the time neared in May, the planning committee, consisting in part of a lawyer, professor, veterinarian, social worker, and housewives, grew ambitious.

"Why not also have a program?" asked the class vice president, Birdie Boyer Boorman, when the group met in Provo to plan.

"Great," the others agreed. An English teacher with drama experience, Birdie offered to write a script. "We'll need a master of ceremonies," she said. "And I've got the candidate—Barney!" Why him? He had never been a class officer, nor had he been heavily into extracurricular clubs and sports. He had something else, Birdie explained. "People like him. He always seems to radiate the feeling that it's wonderful to be alive."

The others shared her enthusiasm. "Good choice," said lawyer Ray Ivey, who had been Barney's friend since grade school. "He's friendly, outgoing."

Ray's wife, Joy, recalled, "Barney could always get me to smile if I needed to laugh instead of cry."

"Let's phone him," said Birdie. "We're all here together. What more severe pressure can we put on him than that?"

Ray called, but Barney hesitated, "Well, uh." This was not quite what he had had in mind when he had agreed to Una Loy's offer to help. Then he said, "Oh, okay. How can I say no when you're down there working your hearts out? Sure, I'll do my part."

Being asked pleased him, although he told his wife, "Really, all I want to do is just go down to Provo, relax, and enjoy everybody." She understood. He did not like drawing attention to himself. There was something else. Though he was the picture of good health, his ruddy complexion and good cheer masked the fact that lately he had not been feeling particularly well.

On the golf course, he got winded dragging his cart uphill. "Something's wrong," he said. "I just can't keep up with the fellows." When bad spells of wheezing, coughing, and congestion hit him, he needed most of a morning to clear his lungs. A week before the master-of-ceremonies call, Barney had gone to a pulmonary specialist. "Do you smoke?" the doctor asked.

"I did. Quit two years ago," Barney replied. The doctor did a workup. The cardiac exam was negative, but chest X-rays and tests for pulmonary function showed severe obstructive-airway disease. He had emphysema and some asthmatic bronchitis. The doctor sent him home with a prescription for a bronchodilating drug plus an atomizer to calm his asthma. He didn't talk about it. When his wife asked him how he felt he said, "I'm fine."

The house where Barney studied himself in the looking glass on Saturday night, June 23, 1979, was the Provo home of his wife's sister and brother-in-law, Shirley and Glenn Farrer. It was nestled on a bench near the foot of the Wasatch Mountains flanking the fertile Utah Valley.

From the bedroom window, Barney could view almost all of Provo with its current population of seventy-four thousand people—four times larger than it had been in his youth. The town was much smaller than Utah's capital, Salt Lake City, forty-five miles north, but it was a matter of local pride that Provo had a higher density of Mormons. Directly below the Farrers lay the pristine campus of Barney's alma mater, Brigham Young University (BYU), the world's biggest church-affiliated university. To the west, the afternoon sun lit up 150-square-mile Utah Lake, where the old gang had gone to picnic.

The Clarks had arrived the previous Thursday, giving Barney time to attend the reunion rehearsal and both he and Una Loy to join sixteen of their dearest old friends at an intimate supper at the Riverside Country Club. Ivan and Gladys Nelson, up from Phoenix, Arizona, for the reunion, said to him at supper, "You look wonderful. Playing a lot of golf?"

"Some."

"I'm thinking about retiring," said Ivan. "How's it going for you?" he asked Barney.

"Great. Best two years of my life. Stub my toe here and there. Try to keep out of Una Loy's way. Look after some business things."

"Don't you miss going to the office every day?"

"I miss my patients, but I sure as hell don't miss dentistry." Barney's eyes twinkled. "I do kind of miss the prestige, having people say, 'Dr. Clark!' or 'Hi, doc,' and asking me for advice because I'm a doctor."

"How's your mother getting along in the rest home?"

"Hell, you know mom. Cheerful, never complains."

"Sounds just like her."

Ivan remembered Barney's mother from the time he and Barney had been in fifth grade. She was a widow with very little money, moving from relative to relative. She supported Barney by dipping chocolates in a local candy factory. Probably Barney was the only kid in their group with a mom who worked. Knowing she was not home after class, Ivan's mother welcomed Barney into her kitchen with hot bread—fresh out of the oven—butter and homemade plum jam with the pits still in, and cold milk.

"We used to tear that bread apart," Barney remembered.

"You could eat a loaf at a time." Ivan replied.

"It was delicious."

"You made my mother feel like a queen," Ivan added.

Looking at Gladys, who was Una Loy's lifelong confidante, Barney winked: "You still have the most beautiful eyes I've ever seen. And the sweetest smile."

"Oh, you big flatterer. You always were a flirt," Gladys replied. Barney laughed.

Everyone at the supper regretted the absence of one of the old gang, who the year before had also come home to Utah—to be buried. His name was Weston Brown. He was Barney's best friend. After the war, he had become a dentist, practicing in Yakima, Washington. One Sunday in February 1978, he had staggered from his apple and pear orchard near the house. "I can't breathe," he mumbled to his wife, Linda. "I think I'm having a heart attack." Doctors found no evidence but did a tracheotomy to help his breathing. When Linda visited him, he gave a thumbs-up sign. Three days later, he was dead; one of his lungs had inexplicably ruptured.

Barney was a pallbearer at Weston's funeral. The two of them had shared the pleasures and trials of being kids, adolescents, and men. They were both tall and thin with long arms and spindly legs. They were inextricably linked, two limber kids whom the girls thought "wiggled like noodles." Barney had walked barefoot for the entire length of Provo's Fourth of July parade one year, toting a bass drum while Weston banged it. He was there the night Weston met his wife-to-be. "Hell," he said. "Wes was the reason I went to Seattle. I followed him into dental school." To the two Clark sons and daughter, he was Uncle Wes.

Some weeks after Weston's funeral, Barney came home and said, "I just feel awful today."

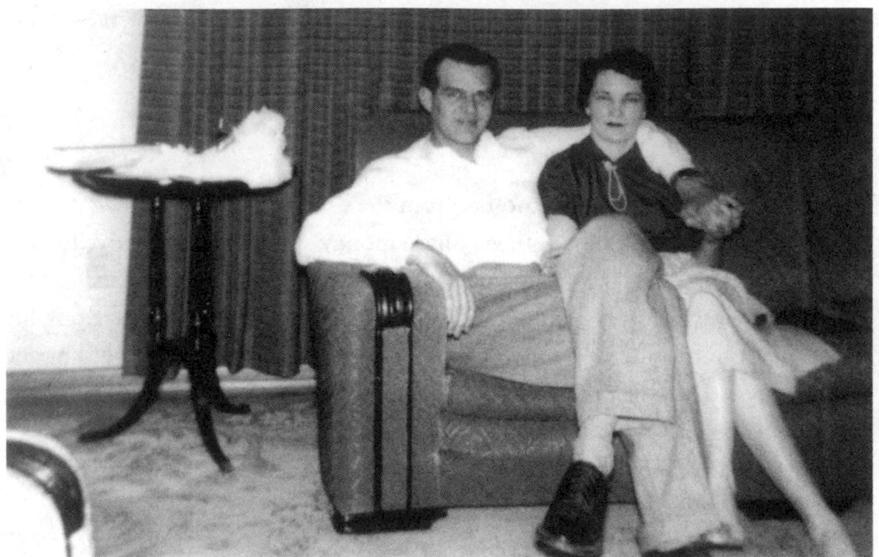

Barney and Una Loy Clark at home in 1955.

"Why?" Una Loy asked.

He started to sob as if his heart were breaking. It was the first time she had ever seen Barney cry. "I just miss Wes so much. Been thinking about him a lot. I was sitting in a café for lunch, and I just had to come home. You know, he was the closest thing I ever had to a brother. Losing Wes makes you know how short life is." When the tears quieted, Barney added, "I'm just very grateful to have the gift of life."

Everyday Love

Una Loy Clark was then fifty-eight and five feet, two inches tall. Unlike her husband, she had not grown a smidgeon since she had first seen him in seventh grade. Then he had come up to the bridge of her nose. The word for her was "pert": shining, almond-shaped hazel eyes with black brows and lashes and even features that required no makeup. She did use a rinse to keep ahead of the gray invading her curly hair. Lest anyone think this was an affectation, she was quick to say, "The brown washes right out."

For the reunion night, she wore a powder blue cocktail dress primly styled with a mandarin collar, long ruffled sleeves, and a flared skirt. It was one of the colors Barney liked on her. Often he told her, "I like women to be feminine. They're to be cherished, not to be aggressive."

Their children said, "Dad's so old-fashioned."

"I love that about him," Una Loy said. "He's my protector."

He was as particular about her appearance as his own. When his weight escalated five pounds, he told her, "That's it! Rabbit food for lunch, cottage cheese for dinner."

"Swell," she said. "Cooking's a bore."

Likewise, when she crept above the 112 pounds he liked, he cautioned her, "Honey, don't you think it's time to do something?"

"Listen, brother!" she said. "It's not the pounds. The weight's just shifted." Having asserted herself a little, she did as he advised. Not that his word always prevailed. Thinking she spent too much time at home—cleaning, sewing, tending to a hundred chores—he commanded her to "get out of the house, buy some clothes, and spend some money on yourself."

Thriftily she retorted, "I can make clothes just as good as Mrs. Joe Blow gets for $250." Sometimes, to please him, she did bring dresses home from the stores. "Which one do you like?" she asked.

"All of them," he replied, but he bet that she would take most of them back. He teased her but respected her flinty common sense. Early in his dental practice, he bought some penny oil and gas stock in Utah. Una Loy objected, stating that "money belongs in the bank."

"Okay," said Barney. "To stop you from worrying about whether there'll be money to run the house, I'm putting you on a salary. Every two weeks—just like the girls in the office—you'll get a check. We'll start with a thousand dollars a month. Out of that you'll pay all the household bills." She was proud of the way she managed her accounts. "You know what?" Barney reported in later years. "My wife has more saved than I do."

At home they laughed a lot, frequently when her tongue outraced her mind. To her a faux pas became a "phoo faw." "More poetry than truth in that," she would say.

He lovingly told her, "Your concoctions endear you to me." She kept on using them. Not that he was immune to tongue twisting. He pronounced aluminum as "a-loon-a-mum."

"Honey," Una Loy would say, "It's a-loom-i-num."

"No, it's a-loon-a-mum."

He had large hands with long, powerful fingers. When they sat watching TV, he made a game of pinching what she called her "pointy finger." "Ouch," she said. "That hurts my nose."

"You're just wired up wrong," he kidded.

They were not sentimentalists. Neither one could remember their wedding date and never thought about it until an anniversary card arrived from Una Loy's sister-in law, Barbara Mason, in Salt Lake City.

"It's on the seventh," he said.

"No, it's on the sixth," she countered. Then she had to get out her Book of Remembrance, where the marriage certificate said, "March 6, 1944, Provo, Utah." "Doesn't matter," they told each other. "We believe in love every day."

"How do I look?" Una Loy asked when she came into the room where Barney was talking with the Farrers. She had arrestingly beautiful legs, trim ankles, supple calves.

He appraised her appearance. Putting an arm around her, he squeezed and said, "I love this old girl." That was the limit for any public display of affection. "It embarrasses me to see couples that hang onto each other and smooch," he always told her.

Such down-to-earth attitudes were reflected by his fascination with writers such as Zane Grey and Louis L'Amour. Self-deprecatingly he said, "I know some people think it's a little simple, but they relax me, and I don't have to do any thinking." She teased him for the "high quality" of his reading, but he continued to enjoy tales of the West's outlaw trails, where the heroes stood tall, shot straight, and rode with the wind always at their backs. Barney said with a grin, "And those books know how to treat sex. They stop with a kiss and leave something to the imagination."

"But you like James Bond movies and books," Una Loy said.

"That's foreign intrigue."

"Violence scares me," she said. She also was unsettled by Sean Connery's frolicking in agent 007's bedroom scenes. Turning away from the screen, she gasped and said in a stage whisper, "Oh, Barney, do you believe that?" He, and everybody who could hear her, chuckled.

Barney admired John Wayne, Jimmy Stewart, and Gary Cooper. He and Una Loy named their firstborn Gary, and she thought Barney was like Stewart in his slow, deliberate speech. She also thought he looked like Wayne in his early thirties. Both of them were magnetized by the aura of patriotism and masculinity projected by the Duke, impressed by his five courageous years of walking around with half a lung, fighting "the big C." They were packing for the reunion trip when they saw the headlines: "John Wayne Dead of Cancer." America had lost a folk hero.

Tom and Dick

In their Provo homes that night, two men had to smile at the reunion tomfoolery they had allowed themselves to be talked into. One was G. Tom Purvance. At Rotary luncheons, he identified himself as "the only Catholic, Democratic veterinarian in all Utah." For the program, he was to wear a high-school band uniform while playing, hopefully straight-faced, a one-note French horn solo to "Night and Day." He had undergone emergency surgery to bypass four blocked coronary arteries but still worried about angina attacks.

The other was Joseph Richard Murdock, a botany professor with two nicknames: Dick or Butch. He was more than six feet tall, weighed 250 pounds, and had captained the Provo High football team. Yet he was to don a tutu and jump out of a make-believe cake.

Tom and Dick had met at the rehearsal two days earlier. "Going to be good to see Barney again," Tom said. "Lost track of him after the war. Bet we take right up where we left off."

"He is that kind," Dick agreed. "You're just friends immediately. It doesn't dim with time." Tom had been in the Provo High Bouncers Club when Barney was its president. In New York, Chicago or Los Angeles, such a club would have been hooted down as a gathering of finks. In Provo the faculty chose twenty boys and girls each year because they were popular and respected and could keep order at dances and assemblies.

"Barney was a gentleman, but you didn't push him around," Tom said. He was there the day famed American athlete Jim Thorpe talked to an assembly. In the front row, three boys were unruly, disrespecting the presence of perhaps the world's greatest athlete. "If you don't stop giggling," Thorpe said, "I'm going to quit my presentation." Instantly Barney was there. Tapping their shoulders, he beckoned them to the door. The miscreants did not argue; they simply got up and followed him out to the applause of the other students.

"He never did anything halfway," Tom said. "Gave his heart to everything he did." He paused, looking at Dick's burly frame. "I remember him on the football field, trying to tackle you. You must have outweighed him by a hundred pounds. It was as if he had run into a truck."

"He wasn't a great athlete," said Dick, recalling it had taken Barney three years to make the football team as a second-string end. "He was always out there, taking the bruising of the scrimmages, running his patterns. Wouldn't quit, just hung in there," Dick said admiringly

"I never saw him back away from a fight," Tom added.

"Used to be a lot of that after dances and the games. Barney was a good man to have alongside you. If you were in trouble, he'd put his head in a buzz saw for you."

Meanwhile, Barney was in the Farrer living room, tapping his foot. Una Loy had slipped back down to the bedroom. "Una Loy?" he finally called, his voice booming. "You ready? Or shall I start the count?" Not waiting for an answer, he began, "One … two … three …"

She knew that using her name instead of "honey" was a warning. "Oops, I had better get my act together," she said. Running up the stairs, she fussed, "What have I forgotten?"

Taking her by the hand, he said, "Let's go. What's the matter? Worried about your lipstick? You know it'll be gone in five minutes." She looked at him. The smile was back on his face. Lipstick was a private joke. She was one of those women whose lipstick—no matter which brand she tried—seemed to vanish almost as fast as she put it on. When they were out in company, he often whispered, "Go put your lipstick on."

Escorting her to their Buick Riviera, he opened the door for her. It was a courtesy he always showed her. Even as a teenager, his manners had been impeccable. He was the one boy who stood for his elders, helped women with their coats, and walked them to the door. His friends' mothers told each other, "That Barney Clark is a very polite, well-behaved boy." As usual, he saw that Una Loy was settled into the car, closed the door, and got in the driver's side.

Starting the Buick, Barney said, "I kind of miss the old Lincoln." He was referring to a 1974 Continental with the power and legroom he liked. Generally he drove it, but he could not chance it on the nine-hundred-mile Utah trip because of newly developed glitches. He was impatient with car troubles. Because he lived in a home that was spotless and ran smoothly, he expected the same from his automobiles.

"Remember how the Lincoln reeked when you got it?" Una Loy asked.

"Yeah, the guy who owned it smoked cigars. It took me three months to get rid of the smell. Funny thing about that guy—a Japanese working for a Japanese company—he had the car about six months. Then his bosses found he was financing it on the expense account. Hell of a fuss over that. They told him to turn it in and get himself a compact car, preferably Japanese." Barney acquired the Lincoln when one of his golfing chums, a Ford dealer, told him it was a good buy. Bringing it home, he assured his wife it was a "real investment," though he confessed he didn't like the color.

"Looks tan to me," she said. "What do you call it?"

"Shit brindle brown," he replied mischievously.

As Barney and Una Loy drove down the Provo bench on that balmy evening, the sun drenched the rocky tips of the Wasatch Mountains, the Mormon pioneers' "eternal hills." To the south was Provo Peak, still snow topped in June. To the north was Mt. Timpanogos, towering at 11,750 feet, the mountain local

Indians had called the "sleeping princess." Caught in its shadows, Provo Canyon was starting to surrender to the night.

Up that canyon was Sundance, the seven-thousand-acre ski resort and home of the Sundance Institute and actor Robert Redford. He had bought it after falling in love with Utah's grandeur when filming *Butch Cassidy and the Sundance Kid.*

"I heard something interesting today," Barney said to Una Loy. "Business people fighting Robert Redford seem to be losing. Looks like they won't get the canyon highway straightened."

"I think he's keen," she said.

"Yeah, like his movies. He's natural. There is nothing phony about him."

Talk of the canyon reminded Una Loy of a summer Saturday evening long ago and a windy, bumpy ride the two of them had taken in the rumble seat of Weston Brown's Model T Ford. She tugged Barney's sleeve. "What's going on?" he asked.

"I was just thinking about the first time you kissed me."

"Oh, ho?"

"We weren't neckers, you know. We were very proper."

"I know."

"I believed that you didn't kiss anybody unless you were really, truly going to marry him. In fact, if you just let a boy kiss you, that was really, really bad."

Barney smiled. "Okay, you tell me what you think happened that night."

"We came up the canyon, we stopped, and all of us got out to take a walk. You said to me, 'C'mon, we're going back to the car.' We got into the front seat, and you put your arm around me..."

"Yes..."

"That much was fine with me. You said something, and I turned to you, and you kissed me right on the mouth!"

"What do you think of that kiss now?"

She mimicked a schoolgirl's giggle. "You tricked me!"

"Yeah, but once you found out it was inevitable, you settled right back and enjoyed it. And that's all there was—one kiss."

"I struggled for just a second," she sighed. "I thought you were so handsome, so clean. And I don't know what I would have done if you had really pursued me. I liked you; I really did."

"I loved you," he said. "I always did, but I thought you were Lee's girlfriend." He was referring to Lee Preece, one of Barney's friends that Una Loy was seeing more than any other boy. "In high school," Barney explained, "I didn't have an awful lot of self-confidence. I didn't think I was as good as the others until I went into the army. After I became an officer, I started to feel better about myself."

It always surprised her that he had ever felt inferior. She guessed it had something to do with his father's violent death and what he regarded as the taint of being poor. While other kids in their group had had happy-go-lucky childhoods, Barney had had to work in menial jobs to bring money home. "I was ashamed," he said.

"I don't know why," she answered. "I thought it was neat, your helping out your mom and all." But when Barney hadn't pressed his case with her, she had married Lee. Three months after their wedding, Lee had gone overseas as a reconnaissance pilot in Burma. Ten months later, she had gotten a telegram. His P-38 had gone down, and he was dead. Nine months later, Barney, by then a second lieutenant and a bombardier, had married Lee's widow, the girl he had always loved.

Frank and Norma

On that reunion night, a Provo accountant named Frank Gardner and his wife, Norma, were rushing to the Elks Lodge. They were hosts for one of the Class of '39 tables, and they wanted to get there before their guests arrived. "That Barney," Norma said. "He can crack you up every time. Feed you those hunky-bull stories and then just sit there howling."

At the country club supper the night before, Barney had loved being back with his old friends, telling stories about Una Loy, their kids, and his favorite foil—himself. Eyes rolling, his laughter ranging from a deep baritone to a child-like cackle, he put himself down with the skilled timing of a Jack Benny.

"Here's one for you," he said to Frank and Norma. "It's our wedding night, and we're driving to the Hotel Utah. I put my arm around her. I ask, 'Are you nervous? Are you scared?' And she looks up at me and says, 'Why should I be scared? You're just like my big brother.'"

Barney paused. "Now that," he said, "that really made my day!" Una Loy, who overheard the story, burst out laughing. She knew the story's last line, one that he hadn't included. After her big-brother remark, Barney had said, "You won't think I'm your brother very long."

Someday

As they headed for Sundance, the Utah Valley stretched out behind Barney and Una Loy. At that time, the valley still had wide vistas and tidy farmlands framed by the far-off mountains; there were few homes and buildings. To both of them, Provo would always be the home of their hearts, yet they also longed to travel.

"Someday," Barney said, "I'd like to see New England in the fall. Or maybe we could take an ocean cruise."

He was fascinated by the sea. Once, when they had vacationed at an Oregon resort, he had stood for the longest time watching waves crash onto the rocks below him, letting the spray mist his face. "Looking out there makes you think of the entire world and its problems, of everything in it," he commented.

"When you get right down to it, we're really kind of small and insignificant," she replied.

Off to their right tonight, Barney and Una Loy could see the seven-year-old Provo Temple with its single graceful gold spire and panoply of white panels. He knew she had yearned for a temple wedding. They had been married in a civil ceremony, but Mormons have a celestial rite. Couples go to the temple to be sealed, bound together not just until death but for all eternity.

Barney did not meet the requirements for that. Though he tithed and obeyed most of the church rules, he was neither a regular churchgoer nor faithful to the Word of Wisdom. According to this teaching, Mormons shunned tobacco and strong drinks—alcohol, coffee, and tea. Barney was a backslider, a Jack Mormon. He relished a good cup of coffee and thought a piece of heaven was an ice-cold martini. When he and Una Loy went out, he enjoyed a cocktail before and after dinner. That led to his absence from Sunday services: "I am not going to do that on Saturday night and then go to church the next day," he explained.

They talked about it. "I know you're worthy," Una Loy said. "You're loving, and you care about people. You're honest."

"I'm sorry, honey," Barney told her. "I know what you want, but. . . ."

She nodded. "I know that someday we'll go through the temple. And you'll decide when you're ready." Neither of them, in the summer of 1979, knew how fast the time was running out.

9

A Boy with a Dad Going Nowhere

The childhood shows the man,
As morning shows the day.
—John Milton, *Paradise Regained*

On the Road

Like many native Utahns, Barney Clark could trace his ancestry to the migration of Mormon pioneers to America's Great Basin. From 1847 to May 10, 1869, when the meeting of eastern and western rail lines at Promontory Point, Utah Territory, ended the official pioneer era, some seventy thousand Saints plied the 1,100-mile Mormon Trail to gather with like-minded church members. One in ten died on the way. It was an historic era unparalleled in American history, and those who undertook the rigors of this hegira were doggedly determined, a prickly bunch motivated by a sense of destiny. They were, in the parlance of early Mormons, "coming home to Zion."

They gathered first in the Midwest states of Missouri and Illinois. But conflicts with non-Mormons led to lynchings, fires, and constant political harassment. No government stepped forward to assure their rights to freedom of religion. Coupled with the dangers of cholera and other fatal diseases of the era, the effects of having to relocate frequently, poverty, and the challenges of frontier life, church leaders were inspired to travel to the unsettled West as a safe haven.

At Fort Bridger in what later became Wyoming, the first company of pioneers encountered mountain man Jim Bridger. He had trapped for furs in what later was northern Utah and knew the territory. When Brigham Young told him he and his group were headed for the valley of the Great Salt Lake, Bridger responded, "Mr. Young, I would give a thousand dollars if I knew an ear of corn could be ripened in those mountains." Undeterred, the pioneers continued on.

Young, who was ill with "mountain fever" when they reached their destination, had yet to emerge from the canyon into the valley, but his associate, Apostle Wilford Woodruff, had made a short foray to the destined spot. Later, Woodruff wrote, "I turned the side of my carriage around, open to the west, and President Young arose from his bed and took a survey of the country. He had seen the valley before in a vision, and upon the occasion he saw the future glory of Zion and of Israel, as they would be in the valley of the mountains. When the vision had passed, he said, 'It is enough. This is the right place. Drive on.'"[1]

When—in late July 1847—the vanguard company reached the Salt Lake Valley, Bridger's assessment might have seemed accurate. The only trees grew along the banks of the numerous creeks streaming from the mountains to the east. The creeks ran to the bottom of the valley and into the Great Salt Lake, a body of water similar to the Dead Sea in Israel. However, the valley's hardpan clay soil proved productive when watered by the pure water from the mountain creeks. Within hours potatoes had been planted. In a short time, the pioneers had developed an irrigation system that became a model for many arid areas.

Answering Young's call, the Mormons came by the thousands during the next decades, some in wagons, others pulling handcarts, and many on foot. The graves that formed a grim border along their way were a testament to their courage. Only the strong survived.

Among those who sacrificed familiar surroundings and family connections to make the trek was Barney's maternal grandfather, Sidney Smith Bailey. After converting to Mormonism in England, he uprooted his wife and son and, after crossing an ocean and half of the American continent, the family rolled west in one of the wagons attached to an early wave of pioneers. They arrived in the Great Salt Lake Valley in 1850 but almost immediately headed south to a greener valley bordered by a freshwater lake. A year earlier, Young had sent thirty families to what evolved into Utah County, directing them in "farming, fishing and instructing the Indians in cultivating the earth and teaching them civilization."

The colonists almost walked into a massacre. The place they earmarked for their fort by a wide stream feeding into Utah Lake was the annual gathering place for twenty-thousand Ute, Paiute, and Shoshone Indians. To avoid bloodshed, the pioneers moved their wagons south of the river. What the natives called Timpanogos, the Mormons renamed Provo, honoring mountain man Etienne Provost, who years earlier had survived an Indian massacre to become the region's foremost fur trader.

Because he was industrious, thrifty, and a good farmer, Bailey fit right in with his fellow settlers. His farm prospered, and within ten years, he had acquired more land and was preparing to build a home to replace the shack where the family had survived the initial years.

As their situation improved, Sister Bailey suggested they find a young girl to help with the housework. Bailey knew just where to find her—in church. Her name was Ruth Baker. She, too, was a native of England and had been baptized into the Mormon Church there. Wanting to join the migration to Zion, the Bakers had scraped up enough money to buy one passage on a ship bound for America. The son, James, was supposed to make the journey, then raise the funds to bring the remainder of the family, a common emigration pattern. However, James had fallen in love and didn't want to leave.

"Send me," said Ruth. She was ten years old. Her parents enjoined her to "be faithful, be prayerful" and sent her with other British converts headed to Utah. At Lawrence, Nebraska, they joined the fifth church ox train, traveling to the Kingdom of God with seventy-five wagons and five hundred people.

For two months, Ruth walked most of the Mormon Trail because the wagon to which she was assigned was overcrowded. During much of the day, she nursed an ailing woman, and at nightfall she joined others in gathering sun-dried buffalo chips to fuel the cooking fires. Though tired, discouraged, and homesick, she endured the blustery mountain storms and other hardships of the trail.

When they arrived on October 1, 1863, one of the men in the group told Ruth that he would give her room and board until she was old enough to marry him. Such arrangements were common in the Mormons' polygamous society, but it was not what Ruth wanted. The father of the family with whom she had traveled saw her crying and invited her instead to "go with us to Provo and be our little girl." She was living in Provo and earning money as a housekeeper when Brother Bailey asked her to be his wife's helper. She considered Bailey "a fine gentleman," so elegant she dubbed him Sir Sidney, so she accepted his job offer. Eighteen months later, Bailey's wife drowned when their wagon upset in the flood-ravaged Provo River. Within two months, Bailey married Ruth, not yet fifteen and thirty years his junior.

The marriage expedited Ruth's long-held determination to bring her family to Utah because Bailey provided money for their passage. Her father, stepmother, and her brother, James, and his wife joined them in Provo. Ruth and Sidney had nine children. Her daughter Ruth married John Wright McAdam, who later became a mentor and beloved Grandpa Mac to Barney, although he was, in fact, the boy's uncle. When Sidney was seventy-six, Ruth had a last child, Ethel Irene Bailey, Barney's mother. Sidney died when she was just six months old.

Doughty pioneer Ruth was left with a house but no money. She turned to nursing to provide for her children. Relatives cared for little Ethel. When Ruth grew progressively deaf and could no longer work, Ethel, then fourteen, took a part-time job in a confectionery stuffing prizes into candy boxes. She graduated from high school and wanted to earn a degree from BYU but could not afford it. She dropped out to support her aging mother by dipping chocolates at the Hansen Candy Company.

Ethel was fun loving, perhaps too high spirited for her McAdam brother-in-law. When she went on dates, he had one of his sons keep an eye on her. "They watch me like a hawk," Ethel complained to her mother. While grateful for the family concern, she wanted more freedom. When she was twenty-two, she met Moroni Jensen Clark, the only son of Daniel and Christina Eliza Jensen Clark, Mormon converts who had immigrated to America in the 1880s from England and Denmark.

The Clarks, however, were not churchgoers and were not accepted by some Mormons. And if the Clarks had assumed that naming their son Moroni after the Book of Mormon angel would make him religious, they were disappointed. He refused to use the name and became known to friends and acquaintances simply as Clark.

He was born in a Montana railroad town of the type that Brigham Young warned against for its rowdy ways of smoking, drinking, and gambling. The Clarks moved to Provo, a community where religion was the principal tie, when young Clark was eighteen. He attended BYU, then went into the army. As a result, his notion of a good time was not a Saturday night social.

Clark charmed Ethel, but her chaperon, cousin Vearl, reported, "It's hard to tell about him." In her frame of mind at the time, that made Clark even more appealing to Ethel. After what she described as "an up-and-down" courtship, he proposed. "Only one way to do it," she said. "We'll run away." They went to Salt Lake City and were wed by a judge on November 4, 1919. They moved in with her mother so Ethel could continue to care for her.

On January 21, 1922, Ethel gave birth to a son. They chose not to call him Moroni after his father but instead named him Barney Bailey Clark. Sometimes Ethel joked that the name had popped up because the Barnum and Bailey Circus was in town, but in fact, she simply liked the sound of Barney.

Barney grew up knowing little of his paternal grandparents except that his grandfather had died in Idaho and his grandmother had "sort of disappeared." He became part of his mother's family. He lived in Grandmother Bailey's home and remembered her as a sweet-smelling, white-haired lady who was very hard of hearing. He had to tell her when callers knocked at the door and then repeat their comments by shouting.

Clark became a traveling salesman and was home no more than two or three weeks a year. When he did come home, he usually had fifty cents for his mother-in-law. "Buy something nice for your afternoon tea," he would say. Then it became Barney's task to run to the store to buy her "bit of cheese." At his age, this was a big responsibility, and he later said it made him feel "warm all over." Ethel was glad Clark was kind to her mother but annoyed that the fifty cents he gave his mother-in-law was often the only cash he brought home. She continued working at the candy plant to support Barney and her mother.

Late one Sunday afternoon, when the McAdams had driven Grandmother Bailey to a son's home, she was in the middle of a lively game of dominoes when she began to act strangely. "Grandma, it's your turn," another player said, but her turn was over. A stroke had hit, and three days later, on April 8, 1926, the courageous pioneer who had set her childish footsteps on a new course in America's West was dead at seventy-three.

In 1929 when Clark was home for a few days, the little family went for a drive. On the east side of town, a mile or so from the McAdam home, Ethel pointed to a house. "That's our house," she said.

"What do you mean our house?" Clark asked.

"Well, I bought it."

Clark was astounded. It looked like a dollhouse with a kitchen, living room, bedroom, and unfinished basement. It also had a screened porch. "Where did you get the money?" was the logical question from a husband who knew he had not provided it.

"Saved some and got a little bit from what Mom left. I had enough for the down payment. It's rented to cover the mortgage."

"You figure on moving in here?"

"Some day."

To Have the Strength: The Depression

"Chaotic" is the word that best describes Barney's childhood. There was little continuity as Ethel tried to provide a home while dealing with the vagaries of Clark's gadabout lifestyle. Sometimes Barney was left with relatives so Ethel could travel with her husband. She feared that if she did not go to keep the books in order, he certainly would be fired.

In 1928 Barney was six, and the family was in Billings, Montana. It seemed a rough town to the little boy from Provo. Small, skinny, and somewhat quiet, he was in the first grade. He already had attended school in Idaho that year. Each time he went to a new school, other students seemed duty bound to challenge the new kid. He did not mind the scratches, bruises, ripped shirts, and dirt that came with fights. What bothered him was getting beaten up so much. His father was seldom around to see the effects, but one late winter afternoon, he was.

"Well, seems like you got slaughtered," he said. "If you don't stick up for yourself better than that, I'll give you a lickin' myself." Then his tone softened. "You don't have to win every time, but you've got to give it everything you've got."

His father's words contained no practical advice, however. It was up to a red-haired Irish kid named Mike to do that. Mike, a couple of grades ahead of Barney in school, looked tough, and Barney figured he would be a good instructor. "You can fight good," Barney told Mike. "Will you teach me?"

Mike looked him over. "Maybe," he said, "but if I do, you have to go to Catholic Mass with me. Barney had never attended another church, but if weekly Mass was the price for learning to defend himself, that was fine. Mike taught him the fine points of fighting: "Keep your hands up, get your feet moving. And hit him before he hits you."

Two months later, Barney was in yet-another town—Casper, Wyoming—and being razzed by another kid. Barney was ready and gave as good as he got. After that no other kid wanted to take him on. "Did the best I could," Barney reported to his father. "Atta boy," Clark said. "Nobody can ask for more."

Life with his parents roaming the western states while Clark peddled Calumet baking soda was pretty boring for Barney. The towns had different names, but they all looked the same: a country store, weather beaten, its paint flaking, the front yard decorated with an old hand-operated gasoline pump.

One particular old store they pulled up to Barney had seen before. Clark ran a comb through his light brown hair, patted Ethel's shoulder, grinned at Barney, and jauntily climbed out of the car. "You and the boy can wait while I go in," he told her. Clark was known as a "jim-dandy salesman," but it was better not to have a wife and child in tow.

"Come on," Barney's mother beckoned. "There's a real fine ditch running down there by the fence. Let's see what we can find."

"I'll get me a boat," the boy said, running to find the right stick to float downstream. Watching it rocking out of sight, he said to Ethel, "Know what? I wish I had a brother." Ethel knew Barney was lonely. His father was not much of a companion. She could remember only one occasion when he had expressed love to his son. That was the night Barney had awakened from a scary nightmare and started to crawl into their bed on Clark's side.

"What are you doing?" his father asked.

"It was a real bad dream."

"What was it?"

"A tiger was coming to get you."

"Aw, come on in here, son." Clark pulled him under the covers, wrapping his arms around him as Barney snuggled close. The next day, the child told his mother, "That was the most wonderful thing. I felt so safe." It was such a unique moment with his father that he never forgot it.

Sometimes he got to go to a movie, and Barney liked them, even if he'd seen them before. Tom Mix, Hoot Gibson, and other celluloid cowboys were his favorites. His parents bought him a hot dog or hamburger and parked him in the theater while they had dinner. They ate out every meal. At first that was a treat for Barney, but the glamour wore off with repetition. He had no one to talk to. Noticing that his father left a tip, Barney decided it would be fun to take part of it. He got away with this misbehavior several times until his dad caught him. Then the boy got his worst spanking ever.

Eventually Ethel realized that life on the road wasn't ideal for a little boy. She decided to take Barney back to Provo, where he moved in with Grandpa Mac and his wife, Ruth. Ruth was twenty-six years older than Ethel, and Barney called her Grandma Ruth. Their house was just two doors from his late grandmother's home.

The McAdams were a solid, stable family with a large, single-story red brick home with a screened front porch. The house was just blocks from the main intersection of town—Center Street and University Avenue—where the Provo Tabernacle was the pride of the community. For many years, the McAdam peony plot was called "the best-kept garden in town."

For Barney it was a homecoming. He knew the kids and was in awe of no one, including George Crum, who was two years older and three inches taller. George tried to test Barney, and they both shed some blood before Mrs. Crum separated them and made them friends over cookies.

Father Figure

Barney learned respectability from the grandfatherly McAdam, who was Provo's assistant postmaster. Grandpa Mac was also bishop of the Provo Sixth Ward of the Mormon Church.

Grandpa Mac and Grandma Ruth had plenty of room in their home and hearts for Barney. Their three children were grown and gone. Grandpa Mac's ideals were embodied in an annual award he established at Provo High School in 1921. It honored a student who excelled in athletics, sportsmanship, and scholarship. It was the school's most prestigious award.

Grandpa insisted on good manners. Before Barney came to the table, he had to wash his hands and comb his hair. If he misbehaved, Grandpa Mac's bushy black eyebrows shot up. If Barney ignored this look, Grandpa Mac held out a fist with the thumb extended, like an umpire wordlessly throwing a player out of the game.

Young Barney received his religious training from Grandpa Mac, who had blessed him as a newborn baby in a standard Latter-day Saint rite. He sat on the front row in church with his back straight and his head up. "Mom, I don't dare move my eyes one way or the other," he complained to Ethel.

But there were plenty of good times. "Sonny," Grandpa Mac would say, "looks like you need a new pair of shoes." Within a day, the shoes appeared. He took Barney to baseball games and bought him ice cream cones, too.

"He keeps his promises," Barney said. "He never lies to me." McAdam loved the boy. He told his wife and Ethel, "He's got the making of good stuff."

While Barney settled into a better life in Provo, Ethel continued to travel with Clark. Barney spent time with them periodically. On the weekend of May 1, 1931, he joined Ethel in a small apartment in Pocatello, Idaho. Clark was due home from a trip to Wyoming. Ethel told Barney, then nine, that he could stay up to greet his father, who did not arrive in town until midnight.

However, instead of joining his family, Clark went to the home of one of his best friends from Provo, Lawrence J. Innes, who was having a small party. Clark had a pint of whiskey in his pocket, and Innes and his friends thought he already was mildly tipsy, though not obnoxious. When Clark went to the kitchen to mix himself a drink, he overheard Innes say to another guest, "Ever seen Clark while he's drinking? He can be hard to handle."

When guests began leaving, Clark stayed until Innes told him, "You'd better go, too, because we're going to bed."

Clark went to his apartment, where Barney and Ethel were waiting. He slammed the door shut. When Ethel tried to greet him, he brushed by her. His eyes were blazing with anger. Barney watched his father rummage in a linen closet until he found what he was after—a loaded Smith and Wesson .38-caliber special.

"Call Larry," he shouted at Ethel.

"Not with a gun in your hand. I won't call until you put it away," she told him. He promised that he would, and she called Innes. "Ethel wants me," he told his wife. "I'll be right back."

As soon as Innes came in, Clark growled, "Larry, what did you mean by what you said about me?" Innes ignored his remark, walked by Clark to where the frightened Barney was standing, and patted the boy reassuringly on the head.

Barney's father took out the gun and pulled the trigger three times. One bullet ripped into a wall. A second hit Innes in the arm, and the third in his abdomen. Terror stricken, Barney watched Innes crumple to the floor.

Ethel rushed to the telephone. "There's been a shooting!" she told the operator. "Call a doctor; call the police!" Grabbing Barney, she ran out of the apartment. Clark loaded fresh cartridges into his gun. Then he crawled out the bathroom window. A block and a half away, he put the gun in his mouth and pulled the trigger. The bullet tore through his palate and into his brain, killing him instantly. Innes was also dead.

The coroner's conclusion, as reported in the local newspaper, said Clark had been "temporarily deranged through intoxication."

McAdam family members drove to Pocatello to bring Ethel and Barney back to Provo. A day later, Clark's body arrived. Grandpa Mac presided over the funeral services.

Ethel and Barney stayed that summer with the McAdams while she fought to reorganize her life. She found an apartment, and the Hansen Candy Company rehired her to dip chocolates. During her lunch break, she earned a hot meal for herself and Barney as a waitress in a friend's restaurant, Cupboard Lunch. Some nights young Barney woke to find her crying in bed, clutching Clark's hat. The boy put his arms around her and snuggled close. He didn't know how to comfort her, which made him feel insecure and incompetent. "I feel so bad," he thought. "I love Mom. She's working so hard to keep us together, and I don't know what I can do to help."

These were big issues for a little boy to handle. He resolved to make something of himself. "I'll have to do it on my own," he realized, "but I don't know if I've got the strength."

In Franklin Grade School, kids sometimes asked Barney, "Where's your dad?"

"He's dead," he replied succinctly.

Often he walked to school with Ardyth Jensen, the girl next door. She liked Barney because he never teased her for being chubby the way the other boys did. They had a music class together. Knowing how Grandpa Mac loved to lead the singing in the Kiwanis Club, Barney appreciated music, but he could not carry a tune. The students all said their music instructor was the meanest teacher in the school. Once, scolding a boy in front of the class, she knocked him down with a chair. Only one student had the courage to help him up and protect him from further blows: Barney. Walking home that afternoon, Ardyth said, "That's neat, what you did. I'll bet you'd make a good doctor."

With Vearl

Barney was keen on pranks. On one occasion, he and his friend George sneaked into their absent landlady's apartment. Barney sprinkled a layer of crushed soda crackers over the sheet of her bed. Then he got a glass of water and poured it over the crumbs, creating a thick, gooey mess.

George didn't see Barney in the neighborhood for a while and assumed his partner in crime had been found out. Actually they got away with their "crumby" crime. Barney was really in New Jersey, visiting Grandpa Mac's son, Vearl McAdam. Vearl had started as a telephone lineman and risen through the ranks to become an executive with General Electric in New York.

He invited Ethel and Barney to spend some time with his family in River Edge, a New Jersey bedroom suburb. Barney had finished his school year, and a trip to the East would be a welcome change, Ethel decided. Vearl sent the money for their train fare. He was aware that Ethel had lost her meager savings when a bank had failed. He had a special liking for her because she had helped save his marriage.

As a young man, Vearl had served a Mormon mission in New York's Lower East Side, Wall Street, and the Bowery. His wife, Thelma, had stayed in Provo with Ethel. Thelma was a new convert to the Mormon faith and still a bit of a high flyer. Vearl heard that she was straying, Ethel sent a letter and advised him, "Don't jump to conclusions. Wait until you get back."

When he returned to Provo, he and Thelma still had some rocky times, and Ethel eased the path, talking to them and working to keep them together. Later, Vearl told her, "I don't know what I would have done without you being there."

In the River Edge home, there was always a big bowl of apples, oranges, and bananas on the dining-room table. Barney looked but didn't touch. Thelma, who loved to cook and prided herself on her gracious hospitality, couldn't understand it. "What's the matter?" she asked. "Don't you like fruit?"

"I didn't know we were supposed to eat it," he replied. "I thought it was just to look at."

"Barney, just help yourself," she assured him. Afterward she had to keep bunches of bananas on hand because they disappeared so fast.

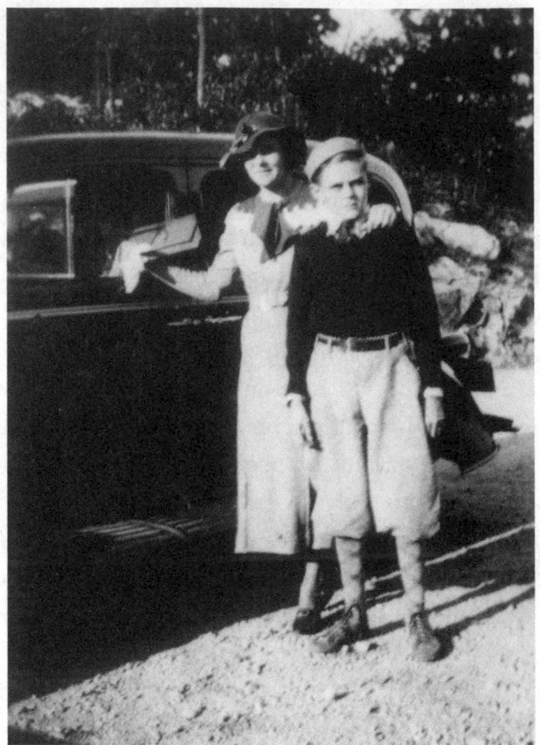

Barney in his famous knickers with his mother, Ethel.

Thelma also told Barney he was welcome to invite his friends to their home whenever he liked. She kept a supply of chocolate-cream cookies, which Barney had never tasted. Once he got into that habit, the cookies became another high-priority item on Vearl's shopping list.

At Vearl's home, people dressed for dinner. Decorum was important. Barney learned to stand when his elders entered the room, to say, "Yes, sir," and "No, thank you, ma'am." He even went with Vearl and Thelma's daughter, Beverly, to take ballroom dancing lessons. Occasionally Vearl took Barney to New York, leading him through the Lower East Side where he had served his mission. They went to Wall Street, and Vearl showed the boy his office.

Barney was the son Vearl had never had. He wanted to help shape him. "You will never amount to anything unless you are a gentleman," he advised. Vearl was always gracious toward women. "You must always remember women are to be loved and cherished. Not fussed over but made to feel important," he told the boy. Barney thought of his mother. That was not the way she had been treated.

As the summer dwindled down, Ethel prepared to return to Provo. Grandpa Mac had already enrolled Barney in seventh grade in Dixon Junior High School. Vearl urged her to stay longer: "There's a school within walking distance of our house. Barney can go there. I really would like it if you stayed with us."

Ethel agreed. Barney was twelve and a little small for his age, but he was old enough to care about comparisons between himself and his new classmates. Most of the New Jersey seventh-graders wore knickers while he was wearing long pants. He pleaded for knickers. Ethel said no, but he continued to wheedle. Finally, the day came when he went to school in his new knickers.

Despite the haphazard comings and goings of his childhood, Barney never had to repeat a year in school. Not brilliant in his studies, he still managed slightly better-than-average grades.

With Christmas coming, Ethel told Barney to be practical. "If anybody asks what you want," she said, "tell them you want house slippers." On Christmas day, with everybody around the tree, Vearl picked a present for Barney to open. Stripping the wrapping, he found a box labeled "slippers." Inside were house slippers. A bit later, Vearl handed him another present. It also was labeled slippers. Barney did not open it so fast. When he did, it held roller skates. From then on, all his presents were marked house slippers, but each one was a special gift: a wristwatch, a wool scarf, and a jacket. It was Vearl's idea to tease him. "This is the best Christmas I ever had," Barney declared.

Ethel was less happy. She felt that life with Vearl and Thelma was like being in the homes of other relatives. "We have no independence," she told Barney. "Nothing belongs to us. We can't do what we want when we want." She also found it difficult to get along with Thelma. She thought Thelma put on airs, showing off the way she and Vearl were now society, entertaining the best people, wearing the right clothes. Ethel felt like the poor relative from the country. "We're going back to Provo," she told Vearl.

"There's something I want to talk to you about," he responded. "Would you think of letting us adopt Barney?" Ethel was stunned. Give up her son? After all they had been through? It was unthinkable. "Think of this," Vearl argued. "We could give him so much. I can send him to college, make sure he has a good start."

"No," she answered. "I want Barney with me." Then she began soul searching: Was it selfish to keep Barney? Could she be robbing her son of a secure future? After asking the questions, she pondered, prayed, then packed and prepared to return to Utah. "He needs his mother" was her final answer.

Note

1. "Faith was also the moving power behind Brigham Young. I often reflect on the tremendous faith he exercised in bringing a very large number of people to settle this Salt Lake Valley. He knew very little of the area. He had never seen it, except in vision. . . . he knew almost nothing of the soil or the water or the climate. And yet when he looked upon it, he said without hesitation, 'This is the right place, drive on.'" B. H. Roberts, *Comprehensive History of the Church of Jesus Christ of Latter-Day Saints* (Salt Lake City: Deseret News Press, 1930), 3:224, quoted in Gordon B. Hinckley, "The Faith to Move Mountains," *Ensign*, November 2006, 82–85.

10

To Grow Up in Provo

So many worlds, so much to do,
So little done, such things to be.

—Alfred, Lord Tennyson

In early March 1934, Mr. Swensen called the seventh-grade music class to order in Provo's Dixon Junior High School. Swensen had red hair and a sandy moustache. Although he was formal, his students liked him. Ten minutes later, there was an interruption. A message came from the principal's office, followed by a boy in gray, tweedy knickers. Reading the note, Swensen said, "Students, this is Barney Clark. He is from New York."

Because Dixon drew students from several grade schools in Provo, most of the youngsters did not know Barney. In Utah boys wore long pants, so the knickers intensified the impression that Barney was an easterner. He did not mind. Perhaps girls would be impressed. At noon, though, he met kids who had gone with him to Franklin Elementary School: Ray Ivey, whose home was near Grandpa Mac's, and Ivan "Ike" Nelson. They introduced him to Lee Preece and Weston Brown. During the school year, these four had become a tight group, proclaiming they were "one for all, and all for one." Girls had tagged them "the four musketeers." Now Barney became the fifth.

"Barney's a pal," Ray said. That endorsement did not keep Wes from asking, "How come you've got those funny britches?"

Barney shrugged. "Mom got them in New York." That night at Aunt Nell's, where he and Ethel had moved, he said, "They gave me guff about the knickers. Can't I get something else?"

"Sorry, you'll have to wear them. I can't afford anything else right now," his mother answered.

Una Loy

Barney's outfit was also the subject of conversation that night in another Provo home. Effervescent Una Loy Mason was describing what she had seen in Mr. Swensen's music class: "Mom, the cutest boy came in today. He's from New York." In minute detail, she described exactly what he wore.

Ireta, her mother, laughed at her daughter's detailed description. "I can see that boy just as plain as day," she said.

"If you can, then you know he's four or five inches shorter than I am," Una Loy sighed. Height was a difficulty in her life. She had sprouted above her mother and older brother and was scared she would grow as tall as her Grandfather Bell, the family's six-foot-plus giant. "Please, Heavenly Father, don't let me be that tall," she prayed at night.

In the Mason home, it was hard to forget Grandfather Bell. In the main hall was an old-fashioned photograph depicting him as a resolute, righteous patriarch, sheltering his diminutive wife under his arm. They had bravely withstood the rigors of the frontier.

All Una Loy's ancestors, who had embraced Mormonism in England, had crossed the plains to Utah in the early 1860s in oxen trains and on foot. They settled in the mountain valleys north and south of Provo in towns named Heber, Richfield, Aurora, and Glenwood. Amid Glenwood's rolling hills and high plateaus, one of their descendants, lanky Herbert Bell, built a great house from gray and black stones. It was near a running stream with water so pure it was a delight to drink. He sired fourteen children, among them a daughter named Ireta. She marched to a different drummer. While her sisters were learning to bake, she hid behind the sofa reading. In those days, a seventh- or eighth-grade education was considered plenty for girls, but the spunky Ireta rode eight miles in fair or foul weather to earn a high-school diploma with honors.

She loved to write poetry and short stories and dreamed of being a writer. Also she sang and danced in the church road shows that traveled from ward to ward. In Aurora one night in 1916, she spotted the handsomest boy in the whole world in the audience. Nudging the girl next to her, she vowed, "I am going to marry him." After the show, she boldly introduced herself to George Dewey Mason. Equally smitten, he came courting with a mare and buggy, calculating that was more romantic than his father's car, which the old man drove like a horse. He kicked it and swore at it, bellowing, "Whoa! You damned old fool."

Ireta and Dewey Mason were married in 1917. A year later, their son, Ferral, was born, but when their daughter made her appearance on Mother's Day in 1921, Dewey was on a church mission. Seeking a unique name, Ireta asked Grandfather Mason. "Call her Una!" he boomed. "I love that name."

"I don't understand it! I won't do it unless you think of something to go with it."

"Why not Loy?" a friend said for no apparent reason.

At the church blessing ceremony, Grandfather Mason said, "We give her the name Una. What's her other name?" he asked Ireta in a whisper everyone could hear. When she told him, he shouted, "Oh, for hell's sake!" then added "Loy."

Una Loy was two years old when her father returned from his mission. She couldn't stand this stranger and called him "that man." It took months before she called him Poppa and came to adore him. She was an engaging little chatterbox. When she was four, after helping Lavone Howard churn ice cream, she proclaimed, "Lavone's wonderful, and I'm going to marry him."

"You can't, honey," her parents said. "He's your cousin."

"Then I'll never marry anybody because I just love Lavone," Una Loy declared.

In her home, there was abundance of love. Ireta and Dewey were always hugging and kissing each other and the children. Ireta told Una Loy, "You're the best Mother's Day present I could ever have."

In 1926, when Una Loy's younger sister, Shirley, was eighteen months old, Ireta nudged Dewey off the farm and into the city to learn a trade. Starting as a janitor, he advanced rapidly to manage Singer Sewing Machine's Provo store. There was enough money to pay Ireta as a seamstress, whipping up sales by demonstrating how easy the machines were to use.

With the extra money, she could indulge her old passion for the stage. She sent all three children to top-notch dance instructors, and Una Loy and Ferral became the Ferraloys. They tap-danced professionally in vaudeville and theaters and appeared for free before Provo High School assemblies, BYU gatherings, and the people Una Loy called the "little poor souls in the red house on the hill." That was Provo's euphemism for the Utah State Hospital for the insane. One of those souls was Eliza Clark, Barney's paternal grandmother, who had disappeared into the institution seven years earlier.

On stage and off, Una Loy always looked just right. She pressed her clothes constantly, prompting her bemused mother to protest, "Una Loy, you'll wear them out."

"No, I won't; you know how careful I am." Ireta had to agree that her daughter was conscientious. She was invariably elected a class officer. She had an ingenuous perkiness. Long before the school's Friday night dances began, her program was completely filled.

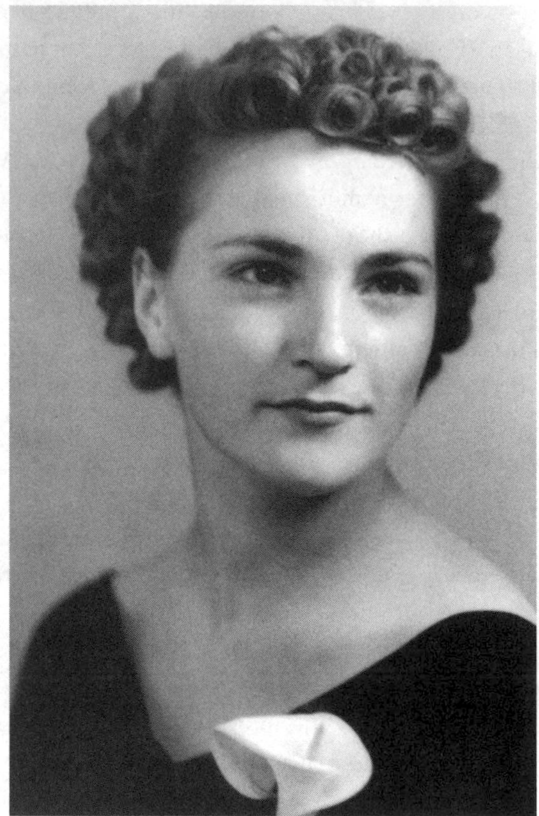

A high-school photo of Una Loy Clark.

Friends

Barney imagined that his dancing had a touch of elegance; after all he had been taught in the East. Dixon's weekly dances were a social event. Almost everybody came. Usually the music was recorded, but occasionally the school shelled out twenty dollars to hire a four-piece band. Often while dancing with another girl, Barney winked at Una Loy. When he switched to her, she asked, "Who are you winking at now?" What surprised her was that she was a little jealous.

Another night he gave her a peck on the cheek. Coquettishly she reported that to the boy she had come with, Lee Preece. "That makes me mad," Lee said.

Una Loy soothed him by saying, "He doesn't mean anything by it." She told her best friend, Gladys Dixon, "That Barney Clark is a flirt."

"I kind of think so, too. Barney and Ivan came over to see me and my cousin Louise. We were outside talking when, guess what? Barney tried to kiss her. I said, 'Sock him, Louise, sock him!'"

"Did she?"

"No, and he didn't kiss her, either!"

"Well, I like him." Una Loy sighed. "I just wish he'd stop winking at other girls when he's dancing with me."

Barney's playboy image was only a façade. Having to live with relatives and denied the security of a working father, he suffered from low self-esteem. His self-assured air intensified when he had to go to work at a young age. At the candy factory, he packed prizes in boxes just as his mother had done years before. Then George "Pop" Hansen, the owner, promoted him. Barney began making "all-day" suckers, even though he was so short he had to stand on a stool to dip into the tall vat of confection syrup.

Hansen and his wife offered their young employee clothes their son had outgrown. "Only if you let me pay something," Ethel said. Recognizing her pride, they accepted small amounts. Barney made a game of searching every pocket of the pants and coats, hunting for overlooked nickels and dimes. Sometimes he hit the jackpot and found a quarter. Jubilantly he exclaimed, "Finders keepers, losers weepers."

Barney earned movie money by traipsing around Provo with a sandwich board advertising current attractions. He got passes and a small salary, but he paid the price of feeling silly. If he saw any of his friends, he ducked into doorways.

He looked forward to days when Grandpa Mac announced, "Sonny, I'm playing golf today. Want to be my caddy?" The pay was a quarter. Caddying was an act of love because it let him spend hours with his idol. Barney studied him, mimicking his mannerisms. Grandpa Mac let him hit a few balls. "Not bad," he said to Barney. "You might like this game." He gave him his old golf clubs.

Grandma Ruth scolded her husband, "You spend too much time at golf. Why can't you spend Saturday with me?"

Grandpa Mac's eyebrows flashed the usual storm signal. "I need the relaxing," he said without smiling, and that was that.

Usually these scenes took place in the kitchen, Barney's favorite room. In the winter when he came home from school, Grandma Ruth opened the oven door and said, "Come on, Sonny, get your feet warm."

Then she brought out a jar of peaches and hot bread, watching, delighted, as he tore into the feast until he groaned, "I'm about to burst."

One day when Grandpa Mac was not playing golf, Barney went on a mountain outing with some of his pals. Also along was the school bully, an intimidating, thick-chested kid. Ike had handed over candy and money to avoid a run-in with him. The kid was bossy on the hike, telling the others where to go, what to do. He got on Barney's nerves. Finally, Barney said, "I am not going to take this anymore. We are going to have it out right now." With that, Barney whaled into him. They traded punches and rolled in the dirt before the others pried them apart. That was the last time the bully bothered anyone.

"You tamed him down," Ike said to Barney. "None of us had the courage. What you did took guts."

Barney and classmate Wes Brown had become best friends. They were forever joshing each other. About to enter the ninth grade, Wes still kidded Barney about his funny britches and the way Wes had conned him into lugging his drum for the Fourth of July Parade.

Laughing, Barney lied, "Aw, go on! I just felt sorry for you. You were too weak to do it yourself!"

The joke was on both of them—the boys had the same skinny build. As they began to grow, they matched each other inch for inch. They were only shades apart in coloring. Wes's hair was light brown, and his eyes were light blue. By the ninth grade, the pair were inseparable. Whenever the girls spied Wes's Model T, they knew either he or Barney was behind the wheel.

The boys drove the car across town to case out a dance held by their archrival junior high. They were drawn to a girl with ivory skin, jet-black hair, and dark brown eyes. She was one of the smallest girls in the whole room. Her name was Linda Spackman. "Hello, Stubby," Barney said. Linda decided she liked Wes.

Wes's father bought and sold hay and wore overalls. He found it hard to say no to his son. Wes often pleaded, "Hey, Dad, you got a dollar I can borrow?"

Knowing it would never be repaid, his father sorrowfully answered, "Wessie, aren't you ever going to learn how to be a lender instead of a borrower?" Then he pulled out his old black purse, jiggled it, stared into it, and commented, "I don't have much in here, but maybe, Wessie, I can find a dollar." More often than not, there was also a little extra change for Barney.

Barney often stayed overnight in the Browns' new brick home, a neighborhood showplace. Coincidentally it was next door to the Masons. "Wes," Barney frequently said, "let's go see Una Loy."

It was winter of Barney's final year at Dixon and getting close to the Girls' Day Dance, and Ardyth Jensen still had not asked anybody. What about Barney? He did not seem to have any special girl. The next time she saw him, she asked, "Barney, are you going to the Girls' Day Dance?"

"Ardyth," he said, "you're my friend, my really good friend. Will you do me a favor?"

"Sure."

"Please don't ask me to the dance. Don't make me say no. I am really hoping Una Loy will ask me." He waited for the invitation, but it never came.

Changes and Challenges

Ethel was still chasing the elusive thing called happiness. She began dating, causing mixed emotions in her son. While it seemed strange to have a mother going out with men, Barney also told Wes, "It would be nice if something worked out for her. Mom's had a real raw deal." She went through training to become a beautician, but the shop closed, so she went back to dipping chocolates and waitressing. She got enough money to rent them an apartment. Barney now had a dog, Mickey, a fluffy white terrier Grandpa Mac had given him. When Barney was at school, Mickey tagged along with Ethel to the candy plant, curling up in a window well where she could see him through the glass. He had a built-in lunch alarm. When he got up to stretch, Ethel said, "Noontime." Her watch confirmed it.

Ethel and Barney had little arguments. When she lectured him one day, he countered. "Now, Mom; c'mon, Mom, you don't really mean it."

"I'm serious," she said, and resumed trying to get through to him.

Barney, in a playful mood, kept saying, "Aw, Mom; c'mon, Mom...." Ethel was getting mad. Then he picked her up, put her on the couch, and—with the knuckles of two fingers—lightly tweaked her nose. Her anger dissolved in laughter.

Ethel finally met a man on whom she pinned her hopes. He worked for a railroad in Salt Lake City. She married him and lived with him while Barney stayed at Grandpa Mac's. She could see Barney nearly every day because she commuted to Provo, holding onto her candy job. In the summer, Barney went to Salt Lake City to be with Ethel and Frank. It was a Barney Ethel had never seen before. He moped around, leaning against walls, door frames, even bureaus.

"Can't you stand straight?" Ethel asked.

"I'm so tired," Barney complained. Most days he sprawled on the bed, popping orange licorice jelly beans and reading Tarzan books. At summer's end, she understood the lassitude. He had grown at least three inches. Back in Provo, he started high school and boarded with an aunt.

"You're going to need a coat," Grandpa Mac said. "Go down to the store where your cousin Harold works and get yourself one for winter."

Barney picked a sharp-looking forest green blazer with camel lapels. "That's not warm enough," Harold said.

"Let me take it. If Grandpa Mac doesn't want me to have it, I'll bring it back," Barney promised.

"Take it back," Grandpa Mac said. "You'll freeze in that."

"Please let me keep it. I'll wear it with a sweater. I really like it." Something in the boy's tone caught the older man's attention.

"Well, all right this time. I'll get a heavier coat. Keep the jacket, but you will have to work off the price." To pay for it, Barney tended the peony beds and dug out the new potatoes planted between the flowers with gusto. A railroad let him try tapping ties to maintain the tracks, but he wasn't strong enough. He did janitor work at the candy plant and took any odd jobs he could find.

Because he had to husband his time, he did not have much chance to indulge in school activities, although the teachers observed that he was well liked and responsible and chose him for the Bouncers Club. In the early fall, he scheduled his work to leave afternoons open, trying to make the football team. Barney did not have the look of a football player. With his skinny legs, he was storklike, long and lean. Part of the drill was for him to block Butch Murdock, a two-hundred-pound lineman. Barney spent a lot of time lying flat on his back, staring at Butch after he knocked him over. "That Barney," Butch said, "He gives 110 percent every time." However, the coaches thought he was too gangly and cut him from the varsity, holding out hopes of "maybe next season."

Ethel's husband lost his job, and there was no way they could afford to stay in Salt Lake City. She asked her tenants to vacate the little house she had bought in Provo. The bankers holding the mortgage assured her they would not foreclose if she at least paid the interest. It was $9.75 a month. Barney paid it with the money he was making as a stock boy at Woolworth's. He never missed a payment.

His stepfather gave up looking for work. Every day Frank sat at the kitchen table, brooding and drinking. Often he grabbed the dog, Mickey. Holding him over the steps leading to the cellar, he threatened, "This dog is as good as dead."

"He didn't do anything to you," Barney said. Frank never dropped Mickey.

Barney told his mother, "Frank can be a nice guy, but when he drinks, he's mean."

"He is depressed," Ethel said. One noon Barney returned home before his mother. As he opened the door, he smelled gas. Hurrying through the sitting room, he looked through the kitchen door. His stepfather was there with his head in the oven. Frank was dead.

The Game of Life

In the little house, the living-room couch made up into a bed for Barney. Wes, Ivan, Ray, and Lee were always dropping in, and when Ethel got up in the morning, she never knew how many pairs of feet she would find hanging out the ends of the bed. The boys frequently were up long past midnight, talking in hushed voices to avoid bothering her as they spun their dreams. Barney was plain and direct: "I want to make a lot of money and make it quickly. I'm not going to work a day past fifty-five."

"How are you going to do that?" Ike asked.

"Work, work, work. Whatever I do, I want to be the best," Barney said.

Every Christmas Pop Hansen had a special assortment of candy nicely packaged so men could buy a box for their families. Barney asked, "How about my taking some candy out and trying to sell it?" He thought it might be an easy way to make extra money.

"Well, sure. I'll let you do that."

Barney hurried to the post office. Grandpa Mac, the assistant postmaster, bought some, then introduced him to the other workers. They hustled sales all over Provo. "Mom," he said, "I got an order to give Pop he won't believe."

Unfortunately, Hansen could believe it. His salesmen complained that before they could start selling, some young kid had been there first, grabbing all the business.

"Barney," Pop Hansen said, "I didn't know you'd be so gung ho. We will let it go this year, but you can't do this again."

That spring Ethel did not have enough money for the water bill. To pay it off, Barney got a job reading meters. The day came, however, when he realized he and the other crewman were working the northeast neighborhood where Una Loy and her family had recently moved. When they got to her house, Barney asked his companion, "Uh, would you do the meter here?"

The man shook his head. "Naw, you're younger. You jump out." Barney was mortified that Una Loy might see him. This wasn't the image he wanted to create. He was trapped, however. Approaching the meter, he saw the front door open. Una Loy had seen him through the window and was rushing to greet him. He got down on his knees, eyeballing the meter, trying to disappear into it.

"Hi, Barney."

"Hello." Blushing, Barney got back in the truck as fast as he could. Una Loy was bewildered. Why had he been embarrassed?

Later, at a picnic with the kids at Pleasant Grove, she told Gladys about the meter: "Barney was so strange. I don't know what got into him. He wouldn't even talk to me."

"Ivan says Barney really likes you."

"He never asks me out."

"Of course not. Would you, considering Lee?" It was true that Lee Preece did seem to be on her doorstep a lot. "You ought to send him home," his mother told Ireta. "Don't let him hang around and bother you."

"Mrs. Preece, I am so happy to have a boy like Lee here," Mrs. Mason assured her. Lee was short, muscular, and good at sports. Barney respected him and often visited his home; his mother felt complimented by the way he attacked her potatoes and gravy. Girls thought Lee was serious; "he acts five years older than other boys," they said. In his high-school yearbook, Una Loy wrote, "I admire you for your high ideals, and that you will always be as good and thoughtful as you are now is my constant prayer. If you ever need me, I'll be happy to help you."

At the picnic, she confided in Gladys that "he's dear, and I care for him a lot." Then she added, "He's possessive, though."

"Barney says Lee is his friend, and he doesn't want to 'cut his grass.'"

"Oh, that's silly. You know I go out with other boys, including friends of his," Una Loy said. They gave up trying to solve the mystery of blushing Barney.

At the Timpanogos golf course, the subject was girls. Barney had a job doing the night watering, and friends buzzed over to see him. One—LeGrande "Grandy" Young—was a junior-year transfer to Provo High. He had first seen Barney on a street near school, joking with a bunch of girls and fellows. "Gee," he said, "I'd like to get to know that tall guy."

They got together at the boxing club, training several nights a week. Though outmatched, Grandy sparred with Barney, who was eight inches taller and forty pounds heavier. Basically shy and somewhat self-deprecating, Grandy liked to be around his new friend; he enjoyed Barney's sense of humor.

Grandy had a crush on Una Loy and had taken her to several dances. He said to Barney, "She's so pretty. I'm crazy about her." His talk made Barney uncomfortable.

At the golf course, Barney worked all night dragging heavy rubber hoses, much like fire lines. Each area got a two-hour soaking. During that time, Barney could do what he wanted. Some evenings he drove out with friends to Provo Canyon's "hot pots," where warm water welled up to fill craters. The pool where they swam was fairly big, more or less rectangular, and covered by a roof. In their run-and-swim tag game, they raced along the edges. When they reached the corners, they had to dive in, swim across, and try to tag someone.

One night class president Frank Taylor was chasing Barney and thought for sure he would catch him at the corner of the pool. To get a swimming start, he dived in, popped up, and waited for Barney. But there was no splash and no

Barney anywhere on the side of the pool. Mystified, Frank got out. Only then did he discover that Barney wanted to win so badly that he had jumped up, grabbed a rafter, and swung out of sight. The ploy was not a total success. "I'm bleeding," Barney said. A giant sliver had jammed through the webbing between his left thumb and index finger.

"We'd better get you to a doctor," the other kids said. They sped ten miles through the canyon to the hospital in Heber, where an emergency-room doctor removed the sliver and bandaged the hand. It was Barney's first trip to a hospital, his first surgery.

He played it up. "It really hurts. Doctor said not to get it wet." Taking the hint, the gang stayed for hours, setting the hoses for him.

The next afternoon Frank met Barney downtown. The bandage was gone. "You did a real Tom Sawyer on us, didn't you?" Frank asked

Barney grinned. "It healed quickly."

In the fall of their senior year, Butch Murdock was the football team's captain and Reed Nilsen was its all-state fullback. "Hey, Barney," said Butch when he saw him at practice. "Glad to see you're out again." This season Barney vowed to make the varsity team. Other players usually just walked the ten blocks to the field. He ran. The coach applauded when he came early and practiced catching passes. He stayed late, blocking and tackling. This year the coaches did not cut him, assigning him to second string. The first team was the best Provo had had in years; the players had a chance to win their division and advance to the state championship if they beat American Fork.

It was the fourth quarter, and Barney was playing. Provo trailed, 12 to 6. The quarterback called for a pass to Barney, thinking American Fork would be concentrating on ground plays. Running to the right, then cutting left, Barney broke into the open fifteen yards from the defender. Nilsen assured himself, "He will catch it. We'll be tied. Then if we make the extra point, we can win the game." Transfixed, he watched the ball spiraling to Barney.

It hit his hand, then his chest, and fell to the ground. Barney kicked himself all the way back to the huddle. Nobody blamed him. "Forget it," said Captain Murdock. "It's all right." Barney didn't think so. Provo lost its spark and the game.

The next day Barney went over to Grandpa Mac's. After twenty years as a Mormon bishop, the older man was used to dealing with people who hurt. "I really goofed," Barney said.

"I know. I was there."

"I feel bad, especially for the team."

"Sure. But everyone has problems, Sonny. It's how you handle them that matters."

"What do you mean?"

"It's attitude. You can let setbacks throw you, or you can accept that life has ups and downs. Every day it tests you, asking if you can be a graceful winner. We're here to learn, to grow, and to move on. Buck up, Sonny." Barney felt much better when he left.

Young Love

Lee Preece's family had moved to Salt Lake City, so he wasn't around Una Loy as much. Barney started visiting her. They strolled to the park, where they could sit and talk. Once he borrowed Grandpa Mac's car and drove her to American Fork for a root beer. The gas cost ten cents, and another dime paid for the drinks. They went to some Friday night dances, double and triple dating. After one outing, the gang dropped them off at her house. "Would you like to go for a walk?" Barney asked. "It's so beautiful." The moon was full. Provo was mantled in snow. For two hours, they walked, holding hands, immune to the chill, and he was content to be silent.

Never able to let the conversation lag, Una Loy said, "Hello? Hello?"

He squeezed her hand. "I like that," he said.

Barney called Una Loy early one Saturday morning. "Mom and Wes and I are going to Salt Lake to look at a used car for me. Would you like to go?" She said yes, though the call surprised her. What earthly use could she be in buying a car? She did not even know how to drive. The four of them packed into the front seat of the Model T roadster. Barney drove with his mother in the middle, and Una Loy sat on Wes's lap.

This was the first time Una Loy had met Barney's mother. "She's so attractive," Una Loy thought, admiring Ethel's dark brown hair, creamy complexion, and smart way of dressing. She was gracious, although Una Loy could see she was upset. "I can't help you with this," Ethel told Barney, referring to financing his car.

"Sure, Mom. If you sign the note, I will make the payments," he assured her. When they arrived at a used-car lot, he said, "Mom, you and Una Loy do what you want. Wes and I will look for a car."

"Are you hungry?" Ethel asked the girl.

"Not really," Una Loy replied.

"Let's have a sandwich." Una Loy ordered the most inexpensive sandwich for lunch. She wished she had brought her purse so she could pay herself. After they dawdled for an hour, Ethel called a friend and asked if they could visit. "She doesn't know what to do with me," Una Loy guessed.

When they returned and saw the clunker Barney had chosen, Ethel shook her head. Grudgingly she signed the note. The car was awful and barely made it down the highway. The voltage-regulator warning light kept flashing, frightening them that something was about to burn up.

"I don't know about this car," Ethel said. "Do you think we'll get home?" Barney's confidence was shaken, but eventually they reached Provo. That night Ethel blasted Barney: "I don't want you to buy a car because you can't afford it. Nothing would do but that Una Loy had to come up with us. You knew I wouldn't make a fuss with her there."

"No, Mom, honest, that's not it," Barney protested.

The next day the car stalled right in the heart of downtown with Barney and Una Loy in it. "You steer," he said; "I'll push." As he did, the motor suddenly came to life. Not knowing how to drive, Una Loy could not synchronize clutch and gas, and the car jerk-jerk-jerked down the street. Barney had to laugh. All he could see through the rear window were Una Loy's tiny pin curls bouncing as if she were on a trampoline.

Barney spent a couple of days tinkering with the car before asking a mechanic to look it over. "This," said the man, "is an absolute piece of junk." Fortunately Barney was able to talk the used-car lot into taking it back.

It was winter of 1939, and Barney and Una Loy had gone to a movie. Lee chose that night to visit from Salt Lake City. Informed by her mother where they were, he found them and sat next to Una Loy. She could tell he was pouting, acting like a jilted suitor. "I'm going to South America," he announced and stomped out.

That baffled Una Loy. "I am not going steady with him," she reminded herself. "I'm not doing anything wrong. He's sweet, but he is just so serious." In a couple of days, Lee returned, his heart patched; he wanted her to be his girl. Una Loy felt that way, too. "Lee and Barney are the only boys I care for," she said to Gladys. "I don't know which one I like best."

Wes and Linda took Barney and Una Loy to Provo Canyon, where Barney kissed her for the first time. When he did not ask her out again, she asked him to the Girls' Day Dance. They had a glorious night. Her mother had made a new, off-the-shoulder, yellow formal with a bouffant skirt. Barney wore a dark blue suit and looked really handsome. They danced every set.

Because of a late spring snowstorm, Barney would not let Una Loy walk up the stairs to her front door. He gallantly picked her up and carried her. At the very top, he slipped, and they tumbled into the snow. He helped her to her feet. In the porch light, she saw he was blushing.

It was graduation. The seniors' last social event was an all-day picnic at a mountain resort. Barney was in a quandary. He wanted to take Una Loy, but he was worried that would hurt his friend Lee. What he needed was advice. On the street, he met Una Loy's brother, Ferral. "I'd like Una Loy to go with me to the picnic," Barney confessed.

Two years older, married, and about to go on a church mission, her brother said, "Well, why don't you ask her?"

"I can't on account of Lee."

"Why don't you let her decide?"

"I just love her dearly, and I will!" He hurried to the office where Una Loy was a part-time secretary.

"Will you go to the picnic with me?" he asked

"Oh, Barney, I am truly sorry," Una Loy said. "Two nights ago Lee asked me to go with him."

11

Real Men Go to War

*A man travels the world over to find what he needs
and returns home to find it.*

—George Moore

Where did the intersections in Barney's path diverge to bring him in 1982 to such a critical place in U.S. history? Was it merely a logical progression on his journey through life, chance, or the hand of some higher directive that placed him on the threshold of momentous history from time to time? One of the major changes in his journey resulted from the dire need for income.

Barney's mother, Ethel, had rented a little house in Ogden, north of Salt Lake City, to take a job at Hill Field, known today as Hill Air Force Base. Barney stayed in Provo, determined to pursue his college education and acquire a profession. He was accepted into BYU. Barney was willing to work hard to earn enough money to pay for his education, but that proved difficult.

Vearl sent money for his freshman year, but Barney rejected more help. He still worked in the stockroom at Woolworth's and watered the golf course at night. He stood on scaffoldings and ladders, washing down walls and ceilings in BYU's buildings with a harsh cleaner called Dic-A-Doo. "It splatters on your arms, and they feel like they're on fire," Barney complained to his mother.

Some of his earnings went for payments on his latest car—another beat-up, temperamental jalopy. Its engine sputtered more than it purred. When the motor died, he had to rock the car, sometimes singing it a lullaby until it started. His friend, Wes Brown, complained, "Barn, you can't carry a tune in a basket."

Barney didn't mind. Patting the car, he said, "This baby loves me."

There was also a girl in his life, the woman who later headed the reunion committee, Birdie Boyer. She was a Provo High and BYU classmate. Her father, a widower, was an osteopathic physician whom Ethel sometimes dated. Birdie had light brown hair, soft brown eyes, and a winning smile. At Provo High, Birdie Boyer, Una Loy Mason, and Gladys Dixon had been named the three "personality girls." Birdie was elected senior-class vice president while the slogan, "For a better administration, vote the Mason-Dixon line," won top student-body offices for the other two girls.

BYU's freshmen elected Birdie their "typical girl." In Provo High, Barney had gone to a few of his gang's picnics and dances with her. In college she was his main date at parties in Bricker, considered the classiest social group, BYU's version of a fraternity. Birdie often visited Ethel, spending hours talking with her. Ethel grew fond of her and thought that someday Birdie might become her daughter-in-law.

In February 1941, Barney announced to his mother that he was enlisting in the National Guard. "It's like I'm going backward," he said. "Getting no place. I want to get out of your hair and support myself. The guard's going to be federalized, and I'll draw army pay, be able to make the car payments, even put something aside. And besides," he added, "I can do a year in the guard and be free from the draft." There was no doubt which unit he would sign up with because many other Brickers were already in the guard's medical detachment in Provo, "pill rollers" assigned to the 145th Field Artillery Regiment. The medics ran their outfit something like a BYU social group, voting on members they would accept to maintain their tradition of being "the best and the brightest."

On March 3, 1941, the National Guard was federalized into the regular army. After some drills and lectures, the Utah unit, consisting of twenty-five medics and 125 artillerymen, was ready to go to the army's 40th Infantry Division camp at San Luis Obispo, California. The men's mood was good. This was an adventure. The guns of war were booming almost everywhere else in the world, but on that day in Utah, few thought the conflict would touch America.

All of them marched the six blocks from the armory to the Provo railroad depot. A snapshot captured Barney's determined grin, the jaunty tilt to his cap, a jacket too big at the waist, and sleeves three inches too short. A Model T Ford festooned with banners saluted the warriors. Driving it, Butch Murdock kept the horn honking to mark this momentous occasion. At the station, the soldiers were enveloped in a ritual typical of small-town America. About five hundred relatives and friends waited, fathers soberly shaking their son's hands, mothers embracing them, and best girls kissing them good-bye. They hoped all would come home safely.

Ethel hugged her son, and Grandpa Mac and Grandma Ruth wished him Godspeed. Looking at them from the train window, Barney realized they were his Gibraltar, his touchstone of security and happiness. They had done what they could for him; the rest of his life was up to him.

Accustomed to the limited perspectives of the Intermountain West, Barney found it hard to grasp the sheer size of the 40th Infantry Division's camp at San Luis Obispo. The division had nine thousand more men than the entire population of Provo. To house them required seven thousand tents spread over acre after acre. There were a parade ground and a gunnery range, fire stations and terrain for maneuvers, frame office barracks, and a huge theater tent.

The men of the 40th were citizen soldiers drawn from the National Guards of California, Nevada, and Utah. The Beehive State's units had histories of service dating to the 1849 Gold Rush days, wars of the nineteenth century, and the chase after Pancho Villa in Mexico, as well as the San Francisco earthquake and fires. During World War I, the guards were melded into the army's 40th Division, the famous Sunshine Troops.

Barney's duties with the medics were not very rigorous. When the artillerymen went to work with their 70-millimeter guns, he and others set up what amounted to a first-aid station. Once they informed commanders of their whereabouts, there was rarely anything to do, so most read, napped, or played cards. Being sedentary was not Barney's style. He wanted to be doing, using his mind and body to accomplish something. "What can I do?" he asked battery commanders. Startled by a soldier volunteering for extra work, they told him to help dig the trail for the gun battery.

At first his tent mate, Grandy Young, who had joined the guard with him, thought Barney was working for brownie points, trying to impress the battery bosses. "You know the code," he said to Barney. "Never volunteer for anything."

"Understand, Grandy, I'm doing this so I learn something. I want to know everything I can." LeGrande was the shortest of the medics, Barney the tallest. Standing side by side, they were the unit's Mutt and Jeff. Young watched Barney, noting he did everything with intensity, whether it was penny-ante poker, digging out ground balls while playing first base, or sparring in boxing. And a thousand times or more, Barney told him, "Grandy, someday I'm going to make a million dollars."

Wishing that he could be more like Barney, Grandy said, "You're the most success-driven guy I've ever known. Thing is, you might have to pay a high price for it."

"I'm willing," Barney said.

Barney had introduced himself to beer and a little liquor at off-campus Bricker gatherings. He liked an occasional brew. He knew that even Grandpa

Mac had drunk a glass of beer now and then before the Mormon Church had cracked down on the practice, but Barney had no role model for what entered his life in San Luis Obispo: tobacco.

He and Burke Jennings, another Provo boy, sat around a table in camp experimenting with cigarettes. Choking and laughing, neither could decide who looked funnier or more unnatural. Barney pincered the Camel cigarette between his right thumb and index finger, huffing and puffing sharp, short draws and blowing the smoke out as fast as he could. Smoking, Barney thought, was just a game.

As in all military camps, practical jokes were the defense against tedium. On one occasion, when a tent mate was asleep, Barney nailed his shoes to the floor and then sounded the alarm. Bounding from his bed, the hapless victim jammed his feet in his shoes and was locked in place.

A second prank was the hotfoot, a super-duper, 100 percent, extravaganza version. If they caught Barney napping, the men smeared shoe polish around the edge of the shoe he was still wearing, then stuck a lit match in it. The first jabs of heat woke Barney. As the polish caught fire, the searing heat ran around his shoe like an arc of pain. He jumped up, legs flailing, trying to stamp out the hurt. That only fanned the flames, making it all but impossible for him to get his foot out of the shoe. Everyone stood there, paralyzed in laughter.

Barney took it pretty well. Striking a pose of mock bravado, he smiled and shook a finger at them. "You shouldn't do that," he warned them. "You're dealing with the Great BC!!" Later in the shower, Sergeant Williams Newell noted Barney's natural endowments. In half-joking astonishment, he said, "I see the Great BC."

Barney's pay was twenty-one dollars a month. Every payday he mailed seventeen dollars back to his mother to keep up the payments on the clunker he had left behind. He was definitely planning on having it available when he finished his one-year service. In November 1941, Barney got a shock. By a single-vote majority, Congress extended guardsmen's duty for at least another year. He was furious. "Those sons of bitches!" he burst out to Grandy. "They can't take another year out of my life!"

But they could. Anger gave way to coolly calculating how he could adjust to the new circumstances. The first thing was to tell his mother to sell the car. He would not need one for a while. Then he had to decide where he wanted to go in the service. Other medics had already transferred to join the United States Army Air Corps. Fliers were the glamour boys, rewarded with officer's pay and perks. That appealed to Barney, but before he could do anything, new orders sent him, and many others in the regiment, to a place called Plum.

A Place Called Plum

Barney's life journey continued along unexpected pathways, often placing him in unusual situations. Some of the surprises were downright unpleasant in a most immediate way.

On Sunday morning, December 7, 1941, U.S. Army Private Barney Clark was seasick. His mouth tasted foul. He was on the troop transport, the *USS Tasker H. Bliss,* bound in a southwesterly direction from San Francisco to somewhere in the Pacific with the code name Plum. Having lived all his life among mountains, Barney had no sea legs. Nor did any of the 150 other boys from Provo, Utah, serving with him in the 40th Infantry Division. In fact, since leaving the port fifteen hours earlier, queasy stomachs and upchuck were the rule for many of the nineteen hundred soldiers on board. "Hey," Barney said to Sgt. Newell, "the army feeds me, then I feed the birds."

At noon—when they were four hundred miles to sea—Barney noticed the *Bliss* making a sharp 180-degree turn. Lifeboat drills were held. "What's up?" he asked.

"Beats me," his sergeant replied. Soon thereafter guards were posted to be sure everyone continued wearing a life preserver. Orders were to shut off all personal radios by nightfall. The ship was to be blacked out. The captain revved up the engines, plowing the *Bliss* ahead at twenty-four knots, faster than its generally accepted limits. No announcements from the bridge explained the mysterious moves.

Unknown to the men, Pearl Harbor had been attacked, and their ship was beating a hasty path back to its mainland port. The Hawaiian Islands had been bombed by the Japanese on what President Franklin Roosevelt called "a day that will live in infamy." America was at war. The boys from Provo then learned what code Plum meant. It was the Philippines. In due time, Barney and the others would have reached Manila Bay and Corregidor, the next targets for the Japanese. Instead, they needed to return to San Francisco.

The *Bliss*'s condition was decidedly precarious. When it left port, the United States was officially at peace, and the craft carried no bombs or antiaircraft guns. It had no naval escort. It was alone in an ocean that offered no hiding place. If the Japanese could strike Pearl Harbor, could they also hit even the American mainland? If they did that, wouldn't the troop-laden *Bliss* be a sitting duck? With the engine pushed to the ultimate, grinding out every last possible knot of speed, the steam pipes chattered. The ship limped ahead. Then came the word: "The captain has reason to believe Japanese subs are trailing the *Bliss*."

If Japanese subs were tracking the *Bliss,* they fired no torpedoes. On the afternoon of December 8, 1941, with the engine crew stretching out the last wisps of power, the ship at last docked at San Francisco's Pier Three. "How long are we here?" the medics asked Sergeant Newell.

"A week—maybe ten days. Then we go out again." So the finagling began, trying to invent reasons for leaves to go back to Provo for a few days to see sweethearts and families on what could well be their last visit home. Understanding their feelings, Newell stretched things to accommodate his men. Barney, however, stayed in San Francisco.

Across the bay, Tom Purvance, one of Barney's friends from the Provo High Bouncers Club, received a phone call. Tom had been in the medics but had been discharged so he could take a defense job at the Mare Island Naval Shipyard. He had kept in touch with the unit and visited with friends when they were in San Luis Obispo. The caller was Williams Newell. He said the Provo contingent on the *Bliss* had some shore passes for San Francisco. "You've been here for months. You know the town. Show us the place," Newell said. Purvance escorted Newell, Barney, and a cluster of others to Chinatown, the city's ultimate tourist trap of legend, intrigue, and loose ladies.

"Hey, big boy," a street prostitute shouted to Barney, "lookin' for something? Whatever it is, I got it." Barney's face turned deep crimson. Some of the ladies were more aggressive. They took hold of the men's arms, enticing them, promising "a time you'll remember." The rather conservative Utahns politely declined their favors.

Purvance suggested they visit the Streets of Paris, a nightclub that had three blondes who—while undulating—stripped down to a G-string and pasties. All that skin on parade was too much for Barney. He was sitting next to Purvance. Turning to him, he said, "Tom, I'm ready to die now. I've seen everything!"

Three days later on December 16, the men were on the *USS Monterey*, a peacetime excursion ship hastily converted to a troop carrier. Also aboard was a cargo of a thousand bombs. "If a torpedo gets us," Newell said, "it'll be some blow off." They were, as he wrote in his diary, in the "first contingent of troops to leave our native shores since the declaration of war." This time they were not alone in the Pacific. Destination: Hawaii.

Newell chronicled their departure:

> 5:00 PM—The ship is slowly going into place behind two other liners, the *Matsonia* and the *Lurliner*, the naval escort of three destroyers, and one light cruiser with two airplanes mounted on it, [which have] slipped out into the bay and are waiting for us.
>
> 5:30 PM—We are getting well under way very fast by Alcatraz and the San Francisco waterfront.

> 6:00 PM—We pass under the Golden Gate Bridge. There will probably be no turning back now. So we are getting a long, last look at the good old U.S.A. with all its freedom and glory we love so much.

This time on the ocean, Barney had his sea legs from the start. Many others were not as lucky. Barney carried lots of towels and buckets. Again there were rumors Japanese subs were chasing them. Some patrol sighters even reported spotting the hulls, but fortunately there were no attacks. When land was sighted the day before Christmas, Barney and the men crowded the decks to see what was to them a strange, but welcome, sight—islands with lush foliage and desolate volcanic craters thrusting toward the sky.

He Wants to Be a Fly Boy

The exultant shouts on reaching Honolulu, with its view of steep hills strung with small houses, were short-lived. In port the medics got sad news. The outfit was to be split up, part going to headquarters, and the rest to an unknown beach where fortifications were being set up to defend against hostile forces. Barney drew beach duty. In January 1942, he turned twenty. Though he preferred being out with the guys and hunting things to do, he stayed around the barracks to write letters to the folks: Grandpa Mac and Grandma Ruth, Uncle Vearl and Aunt Thelma, and Birdie and Wes.

His place on the sand was called Ewa, a plantation eight or nine miles across the island from Pearl Harbor. During the mornings, Barney went with the battery physician on sick call: dispensing pills, making chart notes. After that his time was his own, and there was plenty to kill. Usually Barney and a medic pal, Moyle Harward, hitched rides to a nearby recreation center with a swimming pool. The beaches were for military installations, not surfing. During the nights, they saw movies at a naval unit.

To Barney smoking was still a game. In the back of an army truck with the canvas down, he and others vied to see who was best at lighting a cigarette while traveling at least thirty-five miles per hour. He tried to avoid inhaling too deeply, spewing out the smoke in short, fitful gusts. He figured a pack of cigarettes a week did him fine.

Barney and the other medics kept hoping the unit would be reunited, but one day the top doctor, who had been with them ever since Provo, said there was no hope of that. "Maybe you better look around," he suggested. "Try for the Officer Candidate School, maybe the U.S. Army Air Corps, something like that." Barney put in to be a pilot, passed his physical, and then waited. And waited. In late spring, orders directed him to Santa Ana, California, for the start of flight training.

Before Barney left Hawaii, he talked twice to Wes by phone. Though Wes had joined the Brickers with Barney, his father had insisted that he remain in college and not follow Barney and the others into the National Guard. The friends' conversations focused on two big events in Wes's life: the engagement party for him and Linda on December 7, 1941, and their wedding set for ten days later.

"About the party," Wes told Barney, "you didn't miss a thing. It was the deadest thing you ever saw. Nobody said congratulations. All conversation focused on the Japanese attack on Hawaii. It was just, 'Have you heard? Have you heard?' Everyone crowded around the radio." After his marriage, Wes sent a letter outlining his military plans. He said that he, too, was aiming for the Army Air Corps. The letter reached Barney in late winter. It also contained news about Una Loy. She and Lee Preece were engaged. Barney took that in stride. He had had nearly three years to get used to the idea that they would be a married couple by the time he returned.

After the death of her father about a year and a half before her high-school graduation, Una Loy had gone to work as a secretary for a title and trust company. Because Dewey Mason had always been thrifty, and Ireta sold clothes for Lewis Ladies Store, it was not essential that Una Loy have a job. Still, she wanted to help out. One Saturday in the summer of 1941, she planned to take the train to Salt Lake City to see Lee. Her boss asked if she could stay a few extra hours. He was under pressure to get out some papers and needed her to type them.

"Sure," she said, then called Lee to tell him about the emergency.

"Are you sure that's the reason you're not coming?" Lee asked.

She said, "Yes."

"I'll be right down," he told her.

That puzzled her. "There's no need," she said. "I'm just working."

When he showed up at the title office, she said, "I don't understand what you're doing here."

"You don't know why I'm here?"

"No, I don't."

"You mean you don't know about last night?"

"No, I don't know about last night."

He looked sheepish. "Well," he said, "this friend and I, well, there were these two girls, and well, we went out with them last night. I thought you knew and that was why you wouldn't come to Salt Lake today," Lee lamely finished.

Una Loy was crushed. She would never have expected something like that from Lee. Anybody else she could understand. She burst into tears. "Well, that's the end of that," she said. "If you think I am going to marry somebody who can't even be true when we are supposed to be going steady..." She was further distressed when she thought, "And I gave up going out with Barney!"

Lee left but called later. "I'm truly sorry," he said. "I really love you. Can you forgive me?"

"I'll have to think about it," Una Loy said and began to cry again. His pleading went on for days. So did her weeping. But in a couple of weeks, Una Loy agreed to go steady again.

Ireta Mason was happy to see her daughter smiling again. During the recent upset, Ireta, too, had thought about Barney. She missed him. He was fun to have around and so polite. Ireta remembered that, "when he'd come to call on Una Loy, he would always stand up when I came into the room, help me with my coat. All the same, Lee's a wonderful boy, and Una Loy obviously loves him," Ireta concluded.

That fall Una Loy enrolled in BYU. She was the first to admit to others, "Sometimes I have a very difficult time making up my mind about things." It did not take her long to decide how she felt about college. She hated it. She had gone only to please her mother and be with Gladys. After two quarters, Una Loy dropped out. "Momma, I wouldn't hurt you for the world," she said, "and I've always listened to you. Please understand why I'm quitting. I don't see any sense in going to school—studying chemistry, geometry, things I'll never use. All I want is just to get married, be a mother, and have my own home."

On the evening of the Pearl Harbor attack, Lee rushed to Provo to tell Una Loy he was enlisting. "It's my duty," he said, "and I'm going to try for the Army Air Corps." Then he said, "You know I love you. Will you marry me?"

"Yes," she said. That Christmas he gave her an engagement ring. One rule of the air cadets bugged Lee: no marriage until he had his wings and commission. "Why should we wait?" he asked Una Loy. Three months shy of finishing his training, he and Una Loy, her mother, her brother's wife, and the Preeces drove to Ventura near his base in southern California. On April 21, 1941, a Mormon bishop married Una Loy and Lee. Their honeymoon lasted three days, and she took a bus back to Provo.

They met again in July for his graduation on California's Mojave Desert. Once again she rode there with Lee's parents. This time Birdie Boyer also was a passenger: Birdie was there to meet Barney, who came from his California ground-training school at Santa Ana. The two young women waited at the base together, wanting to look their best. Barney came with Lee to greet them. It felt like old home week to him. He was extremely glad to see everybody. Then he and Birdie boarded a bus for Los Angeles.

War compresses time. Una Loy and Lee had only three days before he had to be back on duty. She had just arrived home when Lee called. "I've got great news," he said. "I'm being sent to Colorado Springs for advanced training. I can take you with me." He had a 1939 maroon Chevy coupe that they called Dopey because he had stuck a decal of the Disney dwarf on one window. He picked her up in Provo, and they drove to Colorado, where they rented a little basement apartment. Una Loy made curtains, fixed up the place like home, and cooked her stuffed pork chops, which Lee said were "the best I ever ate."

In only three months, new orders assigned him to reconnaissance duty on a P-38 fighter plane. Una Loy knew these flights often made pilots vulnerable to attack. Stripped of all weapons, these planes were powerless to return enemy fire. Lee's excitement revealed that flying was "just about the most important thing in his life." The day came when she went to the Colorado Springs railroad station with him. The need for secrecy prevented him from telling her where he was going. As the train left, she began to cry. Una Loy had a premonition she could not shake: "I'll never see Lee alive again."

Shack! Shack! Shack!

Barney sailed through the pilot ground school at Santa Ana, preparing for nine months of flight training at Santa Maria, a hundred miles away. He was there only a few weeks, then found himself back in Santa Ana, where he ran into Foch "Ben" Benevent, a Provo friend, who had been stationed at Ewa with Barney and left for the Army Air Corps some months ahead of him. He was surprised to see Barney.

"How's it going?" Benevent asked.

"Ben, I'm washed out," Barney replied, disappointed.

Benevent did not ask for details. He had gone through pilot training and knew that half the cadets did not make it through the program. Usually there was no clear-cut reason for their failure. More often than not, it was just the luck of the draw. "What now?" he asked.

"Well, you know the great BC," Barney smiled. "I'm doing fine, about to start bombardier training." Benevent looked at him closely. Barney did not seem overly depressed over not becoming a pilot. In fact, he seemed in remarkably good spirits. Clearly he had put the pilot business behind him. On December 5, 1942, he completed his California stint. His graduation certificate said, "This is to testify that B. B. Clark has been awarded a special commendation for cadet group commanding officer in the Air Force Preflight School as a bombardier navigator…" For the first time, Barney began to feel good about himself.

Deming, New Mexico, boasted that its water was the "purest in America." What Barney discovered when he arrived for bombardier flight training was a windswept town of four thousand on a dusty plateau seventy-five miles west of El Paso, Texas. During World War I, Deming had hosted a cavalry training center. Now it was the site of Deming Army Air Field, new home of the training center just moved from Phoenix.

The skies were soon alive with planes from sunup to sundown. Barney was assigned to the primary training ship, AT-11, a twin-engine, twin-rudder, tail-dragger plane. Instead of the usual aluminum nose, there was a see-through plastic dome, giving bombardiers a total view of their targets.

At the center of each bombing range was what the troops called a shack, a cone-shaped pylon surrounded by whitewashed markers indicating the distance. The bombs were six-inch canisters filled with sand and tipped with enough explosives to trigger a burst of smoke on impact. When the bombs either smashed into the cone or came close, someone cried, "Shack! Shack! Shack!"

Lieutenant John Elliott, a pilot who took bombardier students on numerous AT-11 runs, was experienced in spotting good ones. He liked the intensity he saw in Barney. After a few flights, he complimented Barney, "You're all business. It's a pleasure to fly with you." Crouching in the dome, Barney had control of the plane for the last thirty seconds of the run. His bombsight adjustments steered the ship. Maneuvering until the sighting device's crosshairs were perfectly lined up, he signaled, "Bombs away!" Better than 85 percent of the time, his effort was followed by the welcome shout, "Shack!"

Barney never wasted his or the pilot's time, a trait Elliott applauded. Other students hovered over the target, worried about whether they would get a hit, and told the pilot, "I'm going to pass." Then Elliott had to go around so the cadet could try once more. Sometimes he had to fly hours past his scheduled time while a shaky-fingered kid, fearing a low score, debated whether to drop his bombs. "But not Clark," Elliott reported. "He gets out there, gets the ducks lined up, and away they go."

After his graduation in April 1943, Barney was commissioned as a second lieutenant and expected an assignment overseas. Instead, the school's officers gave him the highest tribute they could pay. They made him a bombardier instructor. Elliott told him, "The only ones they keep are the top of the line."

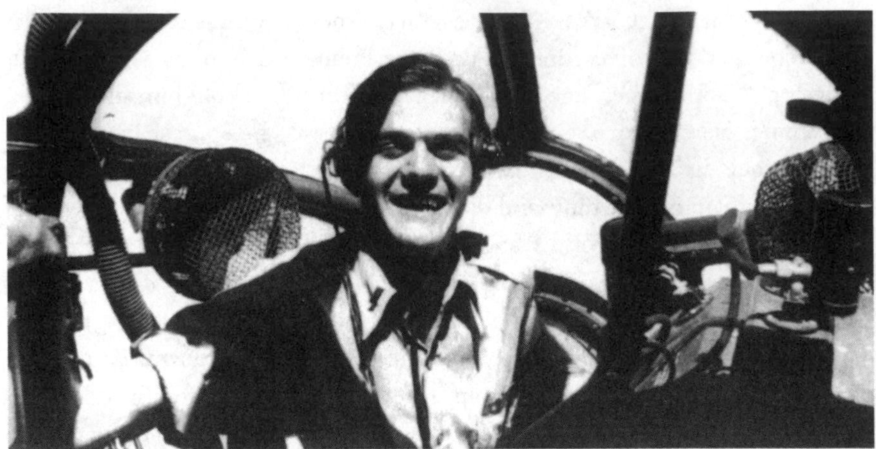

Barney Clark during his training as a bombardier.

When Barney started instructing, he requested that Elliott be on his teaching runs. "I've learned," he said "that it makes a big difference to have a pilot who flies the aircraft properly. It sure helped me." Now that Barney lived in the officers' quarters, he and Elliott became good friends. Elliott and fellow pilot Bob Derrington looked forward to the times when Barney dropped by to visit.

"Deming could get pretty dull," Derrington said, "but Barney leaves thumbs up with his laughing and joking."

Elliott agreed, adding, "You'll notice, though, that he's always a gentleman." The Deming yearbook, *Hell from Heaven,* printed a picture of Barney sporting a rakish grin.

Barney regularly had to visit the field's statistical offices to check his students' ratings, usually with a girl named Fernie Shill. She was dating Barney's best pal at Deming, a redheaded, sophisticated instructor from Chicago. The men jointly owned a dark blue convertible, and Fernie's dates were usually with both of them. Barney's smoking always tickled her. "You look like a young kid just starting to smoke," she said, laughing hilariously at his rapid-fire puffing on cigarettes clutched gingerly between thumb and index finger. Since she was a Mormon, she occasionally took him to church.

Some weekends Barney drove her to Mesa, Arizona, so they could stay with her folks. "I love your family," he said. They reciprocated, saying Barney was like a gracious, polite son. Among those who took to his "cute American look—hair sort of butchy, hat riding in a funny way" was Fernie's sister, Lois.

"Barney," said Fernie, "is like a brother. He's just the sweetest big old piece of whole wheat bread."

Next of Kin

Lee, meanwhile, was in Southeast Asia commanding a P-38 reconnaissance squadron. He flew so much he was convinced he had grown calluses. "And I don't mean on my feet," he complained. He thrived on the flying. The tough part was writing letters telling relatives that their sons or husbands were dead or missing in action. Already three of his men had been killed. Lee wrote a personal note to Ray, one of his Four Musketeers buddies, confiding: "As friend to friend, this war is definitely not fun. It may sound strange coming from me, but frankly I am fed up with the war: India, China, rain, mud, sickness, death...."

In the face of all that, Lee said, his comfort was in reliving the old days: the parties, the dances, and the picnics. He wrote, "We really have a great crowd, and I might add with a great deal of pride that we have probably stuck together as a group much longer than usual school cliques. But why not? We probably had the best one ever founded." He added a wistful postscript: "Any attempt to entertain my wife will be sincerely appreciated."

Lee wrote to Una Loy that all he ever prayed for was to be able to return to her. Knowing it would please her, he said they would have a temple wedding in Salt Lake City, including his parents and his brother and his wife. He and Una Loy would be "sealed for all eternity." Lee grew progressively franker about life in China, Burma, and India. He didn't want to worry her, but he said, "The monsoon rains are endless."

Back in Provo, Una Loy was working for the Selective Service. Her boss was her brother's father-in-law. Every day she went home for lunch, hoping never to find what she feared: the letter or telegram confirming her premonition on the Colorado Springs railroad platform. When the telegram came in July 1943, however, it was not delivered to the house. Knowing the family, the telegraph-office manager called Ireta. Ireta asked Una Loy's boss to drive her home. Ireta took Una Loy by the arm and led her to a chair. "Darling," she said, "Lee's plane went down. They presume he's dead."

Una Loy walked to her room. She was still sitting on her bed, clutching Lee's picture, when Gladys, summoned by Ireta, came in. Una Loy was sobbing. "If I just knew where he was." The letter merely said that Lee's plane had gone down in a monsoon and the military was making every effort to recover the body.

Una Loy began meeting regularly to have lunch, do needlepoint, or play cards with Gladys and other friends whose husbands were away. She endeared herself to them, always asking how they were and whether there was anything she could do for them. But when they asked her how she was, she found a way to focus on them. Thinking about others was her way to deal with grief. That fall Una Loy received a dozen red roses. Inside was a sympathy note. The sender apologized for his tardiness. He had just heard about Lee. The card was signed "Barney."

Courtship

In mid-December 1943, Barney was aboard a training flight that ran into bad weather and had to land at Hill Field near Ogden. Blizzard conditions were expected to last a couple of days, so the crew took some time off. Barney saw his mother in Ogden, then took a bus to Provo to spend time with the McAdams and also visit Birdie. On Sunday afternoon, he called Una Loy. She had been living in Salt Lake City with the Preeces. On this day, however, she was visiting her mother. When Una Loy came to the phone, he said, "It's Barney. I'm in town. Can I come over and see you?"

"I'd love to see you," she said.

"I've got to get back to Hill tonight."

"The Preeces are coming to take me back to Salt Lake. I'm sure they wouldn't mind if you rode with us that far. Then you could take a bus to Ogden."

"I'll be right over," Barney replied.

When he arrived, she thought, "How handsome he is in an officer's uniform!" They talked about Lee and old times, what Barney had done in the service, and about her work. As they talked, she sensed a change in him, a new feeling of self-assurance and decisiveness.

The Preeces came. They said they would be happy to give Barney a lift back to Salt Lake. At their apartment, Mrs. Preece said, "It's late. Why don't you both stay here tonight and go home in the morning?"

"Thank you, but first I'll have to call and see what they say at the field," Barney replied. He was told that there was no reason to rush back. The next morning Mrs. Preece cooked an old-fashioned breakfast. Una Loy called her boss to say she would not be in, so she was free to spend the day with Barney, talking about nothing and everything. It was amazing how much they had to say to each other. They had dinner that night with the Preeces. Somebody suggested they see a movie. The theater was crowded, and they had to pair off to find seating. Secretly Una Loy was glad to be sitting alone with Barney.

The picture had hardly started, however, when Barney said, "Let's bag this place, get out of here." Barney checked to see when the movie would be over. "We have two and a half hours," he told Una Loy. They began walking through the snow. He told her, "I'm going out with someone in Arizona. Her name is Lois. It's nothing serious. She's the younger sister of someone who's going with a

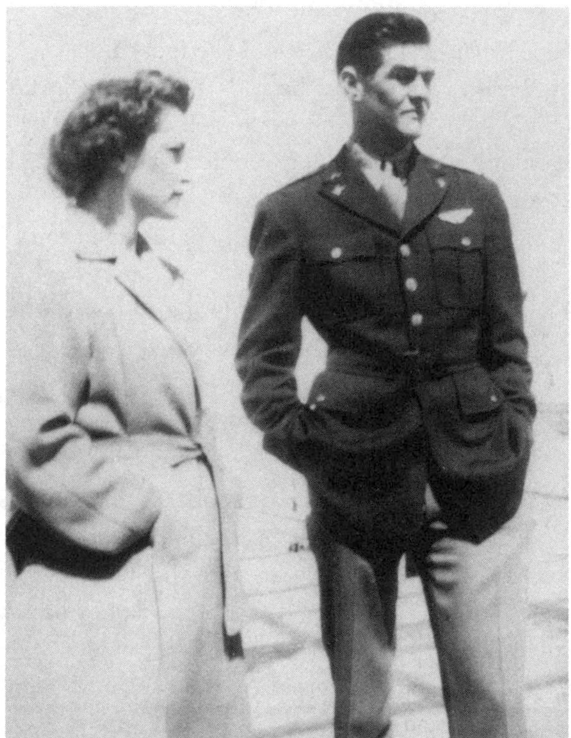

Una Loy and Barney Clark during his service in the air force.

friend of mine at Deming. She's really young, fresh, and a sweet little thing. Gets tickled by everything. I'm giving her a watch for Christmas."

"And you don't care for her?"

"Sure, I care for her. But I'm not romantically involved."

Una Loy asked, "How's Birdie? How are you two getting along?"

"Well, fine..." He hesitated, wondering how to explain it. "There was this thing last Christmas," he said. "I asked one of her friends what to get her. She said a cedar chest. I got one for her. Afterward, she said that if her mother were alive, she'd make her give it back. Some people think you give a chest only when you're going to get married. I didn't know that. She was going with other fellows. And, well, when I saw her this time, it wasn't the same for either one of us."

Barney took Una Loy's hand. They walked and talked. "Una," he said, "it's time to get back." Barney suggested they all go for ice cream.

"We're tired," Mrs. Preece said. "Drop us off, then you take the car." Barney drove into Salt Lake City's hilly Avenues neighborhood and parked. Below them the city lights on the valley floor sparkled through the snow. It was magical.

"It's like a jewel," Una Loy said.

"Una," he said, "you're as pretty as ever." She looked up, smiling. He put his arm around her. "I really care for you," he said. "Remember the first time I kissed you? When Grandy used to come out to the golf course and tell me how crazy he was about you, it bothered me. But I couldn't say anything because of the way I felt about you."

She said, "I always thought you were a flirt. I didn't think you were serious."

"Una, I was serious. I am serious."

Quietly she said, "Sometimes I think I could almost love you."

He grabbed her and kissed her. "I know I love you. I always have. I wasn't going to tell you. It's so soon after Lee. I didn't know if you cared anything for me."

"I do," she said. She snuggled against him as he drove them back to the Preeces.

The next day Hill Field was still snowed in. Barney did not have to check in until late afternoon. He said to Una Loy, "I feel like I've got to go and see Mom. I've been here all this time. Why don't you come with me?"

Mr. Preece offered a car. "We've got two. Bring Una Loy back here; then you can go to Ogden by bus."

Ethel was glad to see Una Loy. Barney let their small talk continue a bit before he said, "Una, would you excuse us?"

"Why, yes," said Una Loy, somewhat mystified. Mother and son left the apartment, and when they returned, Ethel was visibly shaken.

On the drive back to the Preeces, Una Loy commented, "Your mother seemed upset."

"Yeah. She was. I told my mother I am in love with you."

"You mean she isn't happy about it?"

"It isn't that she's not happy. She and Birdie are very close. She thought that Birdie and I would get married. It's not that she doesn't like you," he assured her.

Una Loy began to worry. Maybe Barney did not love her at all. Maybe he was on the rebound. Maybe she was only lonely because of Lee. Maybe they were rushing into something. "Well," she told herself, "we haven't done anything that can't be undone. We're not engaged. Maybe it's a friendship love, and I can accept that." She didn't say anything the rest of the way home.

Hill Field officials indicated that Barney's flight was cleared for takeoff the next morning. At the door, he said he would write. Una Loy admitted to herself that she loved Barney.

After Christmas Barney wrote to say he had given the watch to Lois and she had loved it. Una Loy thought there was something funny about that. "He says he loves me, but he didn't send me any gifts. That's okay," she said, laughing at herself. "I didn't send him anything, either."

Barney's Letter to Ireta

Barney sent a letter to Una Loy's mother six months after his friend Lee was reported missing:

January 13, 1944

Dear Mrs. Mason:

Unless you've already talked to Una Loy, you're undoubtedly wondering the occasion that brought this on. I hardly know where to start, so I'll be as truthful as possible and tell everything I know.

First, I'm in love with your daughter and I guess I have been since seventh grade and have never really known it for sure until two weeks ago.

Una knows of it and apparently she doesn't mind. Few people know of it for I don't want anyone to think that I'm disrespectful to Lee, for I know it's been too short a time since Lee's death for people to understand. I've never thought more of any boy than I did of Lee. I respected him more than any of the crowd for joining the service before his call came and putting his duty before his personal life.

It's hard to explain on paper or any other way, but love seems to strike at any time it feels like it, instead of waiting for the conventional or convenient time.

I don't think anyone will be able to take Lee's place in Una Loy's heart, but I'm surely going to run a close second if I possibly can. She and I have talked of marriage and I am lucky enough to be able to say that if circumstances and fate are willing, at some future date I will be able to claim that I have the best little wife on earth.

I surely hope you don't disapprove. I've always thought a lot of you, Mrs. Mason, and I know it's been a tough deal to raise your family after your husband died. Especially hard to see each one marry and having to worry about them continually. With one son [Lee] lost, and two [Ferral and her daughter Shirley's husband, Glenn] in the army, and your living alone, I know your hours are filled with wonder, worry, and questions of why. I surely hope and pray that this will not hit as close to you again as it already has.

There are a number of problems to be hurdled before I can ask Una Loy to set a date. Among them is the war. I'm held here [in Deming] for a year as an instructor and cannot apply for combat until the first of May. I could stay longer, perhaps even for the duration, but I shall not. I am planning on leaving as soon as my year's up. Mother has asked me to stay here as long as possible but my conscience is not satisfied with my part and share of the fighting and I am determined to ship across.

Many people cannot see my viewpoint. It is something I must do to square myself in my own mind, so it shall be done. Because of this, I shall not consider marriage until this fool world has a sense of security again and the fighting is done.

As for the place I'll take in civilian life, I don't know. But I believe in work and determination to get what you are after. And I have both at my beck and call. And if I come back and am whole, I am sure I can find a place in the postwar world.

I guess this whole deal sums up as being very unsettled except for the one important thing. I am deeply in love with Una Loy. As long as that point is clear, the others will find their own solution.

This has been a solemn letter, I know. But I feel solemn this evening. It is miserable to long to see and be near someone, but not be able to do anything about it. I have three days['] leave coming and I will ask Una Loy to come to Albuquerque in about two weeks, which is when my class [of students] graduates.

But I am leaving it to her to make the final decision because I realize that her work is a problem, and I wouldn't do anything in the world to hurt Mr. and Mrs. Preece. And I am dubious as to how they will take it.

That is about the whole story of my feelings and problems, so I will sign off for now and promise a more cheerful letter next time.

Love, Barney

After Ireta read the letter, she sent it to Una Loy in Salt Lake City. Her note said, "Take good care of this and be sure to bring it home."

Valentine's Day

Una Loy and Barney could not make arrangements for the Albuquerque trip, but they exchanged letters. For Valentine's Day, she sent him a leather shaving kit. That night he called her at the Preeces to say thanks. He also asked, "Will you come see me in Deming?"

"Well, how long do you want me to stay?"

"Well…"

When he did not say anything, she said, "Did you hear me?"

"Yes. Uh, I don't want you ever to go back."

She wanted him to say something more than that. "What do you mean?"

"Just what I said. I'm in love with you, and I want to marry you."

Una Loy paused, somewhat restricted by being in the Preeces' presence. Then she said, "Well, that would be nice."

Barney said, "I really love you. Of course, it hasn't been long since Lee died. I'm worried about the Preeces."

"Me, too," she told him.

The next day his bouquet of early spring flowers arrived. He wrote to her, "Sweetheart. I bet you didn't sleep a wink last night after me dropping that bomb on you about marriage. But I just heard your voice and decided all of a sudden that life is too short and risky, and you don't know what is going to happen—and we should take our chance at happiness while we can. Please come to Deming, and we can discuss it."

Una Loy got off the train in Roswell, New Mexico, wearing her mother's fur coat. It was an expensive, stylish coat that fit her just right. Barney ran down the platform to greet her. "You're beautiful," he said. Picking her up, he hugged and kissed her. He did not care who saw them. Then he led her to his latest car, a black 1940 Mercury sports coupe.

Barney had reserved a hotel room for Una Loy in Deming. He was at the base all day, and when he came at night, he always brought somebody from the field with him. They ate, sat around talking in the lobby, then went for a ride while he showed her this place or that. But they did not talk about marriage until she had been there four days. Then he asked her, "Do you still want to get married?"

"Well, yes, I guess. Yes." She laughed. "It's not like I've been courted," she said. "But I love you."

"I'll request a leave," he said. "I'll pick you up tomorrow, and we'll go out to the base, and you'll have your blood drawn, and I'll get mine done."

After they had fulfilled the requirements, he returned to the hotel lobby, wearing a sad expression. "Honey," he said, "I don't know how to tell you this."

Immediately she feared something had gone wrong. "What?" she asked warily.

"Just because a test is positive once doesn't mean it's true. Sometimes they make a mistake," he continued.

"That can't be!" she exclaimed. "It just can't be."

Finally, he broke out laughing. "I was just kidding." He was starting a pattern that would last through the years.

With a five-day pass in his pocket, Barney drove them to Provo. Some miles short of the town, the voltage regulator burned up. Next the generator failed. "Damn," said Barney. After buying replacements, he had exactly six dollars left. "Um, Una," he said. "I'm just about broke. If you pay for the license and the ring, I'll pay you back with my next check."

He drove his betrothed and her mother to Salt Lake City so Una Loy could buy a wedding dress. She bought the first thing she could find that fit. It was a black, street-length dress with razor-thin piping around the neck. "I hope Barney likes it," she thought.

The wedding was a time for sentiment. "You've always been here for me," Barney said to Grandpa Mac. "I want you to marry us." The ceremony, with Barney in his dress uniform, took place on the snowy night of March 6, 1944, in front of the cheery fireplace in the McAdam living room. The only guests were Ethel and Ireta, Grandma Ruth, Barney's Aunt Nell, and a woman friend of Ireta's. Each had a small slice of wedding cake; then Barney and Una Loy left for their wedding night.

In the Hotel Utah

Barney had a plan: a romantic dinner in the Hotel Utah's Starlite Gardens rooftop dining room in Salt Lake City. But with snow clogging roads, it took them three hours to get to Salt Lake. The restaurant was closed. "It's the coffee shop," Barney said. She ordered chicken salad, and he had a turkey sandwich. Since he had spent his last six dollars on her orchid corsage, Una Loy paid the check. Then they went up to their room.

Barney hung up their coats and his jacket. "Honey, do you want to use the bathroom to get ready?" he asked.

"No, I'll be all right out here. You go ahead."

When he closed the door, she took off the black dress and slipped into a feminine pink negligee with slippers to match. She smiled, recollecting she had spent more time choosing them than her wedding dress. She washed her face with cold cream and then got into bed. Five minutes went by, then ten. From the bathroom, there was no sound. "He's scared," she thought. "What are you doing?" she called.

Barney emerged fully dressed, unable to stop laughing.

She sat bolt upright. "What's the matter?" she asked.

"I've been waiting all my life for this, and *I can't get my pants off!*" His military belt was jammed. "I tried everything," he protested. He was laughing uncontrollably. "You'll have to help me." He got out his pocketknife. Together they cautiously cut the belt in half. It was past midnight.

12

A Brighter Future

Work is love made visible.

—Khalil Gibran

Firstborn

In Deming Barney rented what Una Loy regarded as a funny little room in a private house. It had a bed, chair, chest of drawers, and almost no walking-around room. Barney did not like the bed. It was so short that his feet hung out the end, and the metal frame caught him at the ankles. When he woke up after their first night back in Deming, his ankles were puffy. "I can't stand this," he said to Una Loy.

Within a day, he found another room for rent, one that had a double bed. "Now, that's comfort," he said. Unfortunately, the place was available only for a week, and then they moved to their third Deming home. It was a large front room in a home that people in Deming called a "shotgun" because all the rooms were in a straight row and a single shot would pass through every one.

Una Loy told Barney one night, "Before you go overseas, I want to be carrying your child."

He frowned, not liking the idea. "If something happened to me, you'd have the burden of the baby. No, I don't want that."

"I still want your baby," she said.

Two weeks later, when he came from the base, she met him at the door. "Barney!" she said, obviously excited. "I went to a doctor today."

"Oh?" His voice was guarded.

"He says I am pregnant!" Barney was stunned. "I'm so thrilled," she said. "It's what I want."

"He's sure? So soon?"

"I missed my period, and I went to him, and he said definitely."

"I didn't know it would be this easy." Momentarily confused, he had trouble grasping her news. "I always thought you had to practice."

"We don't have to practice," she said.

"You got your way, didn't you?" he asked, but there was no bite in his words. He was smiling, obviously feeling good.

Before his marriage, Barney had been in the habit of dropping in to visit his pilot friends, John Elliott and Bob Derrington, and ending the day with coffee and a cigarette. Before leaving to go back to Una Loy one day, he asked, "Would it be okay if I kept a toothbrush and some mouthwash here?"

"Hell, yes," they said.

Grinning, he explained, "My bride doesn't know I smoke. I'd like to get the tobacco off my breath." He brought a brush, toothpaste, mouthwash, and some tins of Sen-Sen. After that he never went home without spending five or ten minutes vigorously deodorizing.

"There's a party at the officer's club this weekend," Barney told Una Loy. "Good chance for you to meet the fellows and their brides." They sat at a table with other officers. Most of them had something to drink. Some were smoking. It was a point of pride to Una Loy that her husband did neither. She had little experience of such parties, but by and large, she enjoyed the people.

"Excuse me," she said at one point. "I'm going to the ladies' room." As she came out, she glanced at their table. Barney had taken somebody's cigarette. She saw him hold it, inhale, and blow the smoke out. As he finished, he glanced in her direction and saw her staring at him. Abruptly, she turned and went back into the ladies' room.

"Would you mind going after my bride?" he asked another girl at the table. Una Loy was crying. Barney quickly went to her, steering her to a side room where they could be alone.

Between her sobs, she said, "I didn't know you smoked."

Barney took her hand. "I'm sorry," he said. "I didn't really mean to deceive you, but I knew that telling you about smoking would make you unhappy." Seeing her cry hurt him. Trying to soothe her, he said, "I don't expect to smoke the rest of my life."

"You never used to smoke when I knew you before," she said.

He put an arm around her. "When you're in the service," he said, "you live each day for that moment. You don't know if you're going to be alive the next morning. And you do things you wouldn't ordinarily do." When she kept crying, he asked, "Would you have married me if you had known I smoked?"

"I don't know," she said. In a minute or so, she took his hand. "I love you," she said. "And yes, I would have married you." Now his smoking was a fact of life.

Sometimes, when they were snuggled in bed at night, they talked about their child-to-be and what they would do after the war. "When we were kids," said Una Loy, "you used to talk about wanting to be a doctor."

"Yeah," he said. "Medicine's always appealed to me, but back then it was just a dream. Never thought I'd have the money for tuition. Only thing I could think of was asking Uncle Vearl for a loan, and I didn't think that was right. Now they're talking about a G.I. Bill of benefits for veterans. If Roosevelt signs that, I'll have the money. I'd really like to be a doctor."

"If that's what you want," she said, "then that's what I want."

Barney wanted Una Loy to know more about the AT-11s where he spent so many hours. "Honey, you've never been up in a plane. How'd you like to go for a ride this Sunday?" he asked her.

Though she was four months pregnant and a little scared of flying, she was game. "If you'll be with me," she said, "I will be fine."

He got special permission to take her on a flight with a pilot friend. In the air, the pilot, wanting to make Barney look good, asked, "Do you want to take the controls?"

"Sure," said Barney. He motioned for Una Loy to follow him up to the jump seat behind the pilot. He was piloting when suddenly she wailed, "Barney, I'm going to throw up."

"Gee," he said. "Don't vomit here."

She sensed it would be terribly embarrassing for her to throw up in front of his friend. She got up and started toward the rear of the plane, and he immediately relinquished the controls to follow her. On the catwalk, she became dizzy. Losing her balance, she stepped down into a bomb bay. Its door flew open. Barney lunged forward to pull her back to safety.

"Damn! Damn!" he said angrily. "That was dumb. Why did you do that?" He was white as a sheet. She was too scared to answer and forgot to throw up. "Let's head back," Barney said to the pilot.

On the ground, she asked him, "Why did you get so mad at me?"

"I guess it was fright," he answered. "I didn't know what I was saying." He put his arm around her. "All I could think of was how would I ever explain to your mother that you fell out of my plane."

He did not tell her about the eerie parallel to what had been a fatal mistake. Elliott was with a pilot on a night mission when he heard another flier calling in a very emotional voice, "Deming tower! Deming tower! This is Army 213. I just lost a cadet out the bomb bay!"

Elliott said to the ground crew when he landed, "Funny how that could happen." The crew explained the cadet had been walking on the fuselage catwalk separating the two sets of bomb bays when he dropped his flashlight. "He bent down to reach for it," they said, "and he just fell out of the plane."

This was an accident that still greatly bothered Barney. He knew the cadet should have been better trained what to do while he was in the air. Having Una Loy so close to making the same mistake gave him chills for months.

Barney was home in Provo on a five-day pass in January 1945 when the baby was due. He saw that Una Loy was feeling blue. They had been waiting four days, eating up his leave while the baby took its time. "I'll take you out to dinner, honey," he said. "Then we'll go to a movie."

Una Loy indicated anything was better than just waiting. The restaurant was a greasy spoon: heavy on the fats, light in the price. Both of them ordered fried chicken and cottage potatoes.

In the movie, Una Loy said to him, "I have a tummy ache; maybe it's the chicken." A bit later, she said, "The stomach pain is getting worse." He took her to Ireta's house because she said she would rather wait at home than in some hospital, confined to a bed and not able to walk around. They had been at Ireta's only a short while when she said, "I think we had better go to the hospital."

A snowstorm hampered the trip. They finally arrived, but Barney was afraid she would give birth in the elevator. After a quick exam, the doctor chastised, "Why didn't you come sooner? I don't know if we'll even get her to the delivery room." The delivery was rapid with little pain. Una Loy wanted a girl; Barney hoped for a boy. Their child was a son, and they named him Gary Barney Clark.

The next morning—knowing Barney was going back to camp for deployment overseas—the doctor let him put on a gown and hold Gary, an unusual procedure for that time. An hour before his bus was to leave that night, Barney returned for another look, this time through the nursery window. It was so soon after the birth that Gary's head was still slightly misshapen. When Barney arrived, two women were laughing and talking about Gary. "Isn't that the funniest looking baby you ever saw?" one asked.

Barney blew up. "He may be funny looking," he said, "but he is all mine." He stormed into Una Loy's room to tell her, "I was so disgusted I just turned around and walked away. I really didn't know I had fatherly pride."

Seven months later, on August 14, 1945, Barney sat in a briefing room on Guam. He and other members of Flight Crew 33 were learning about the day's mission—their first combat. The Akita oil refineries on the Japanese island of Honshu were the targets. The covey of eighteen B-29s making the run would

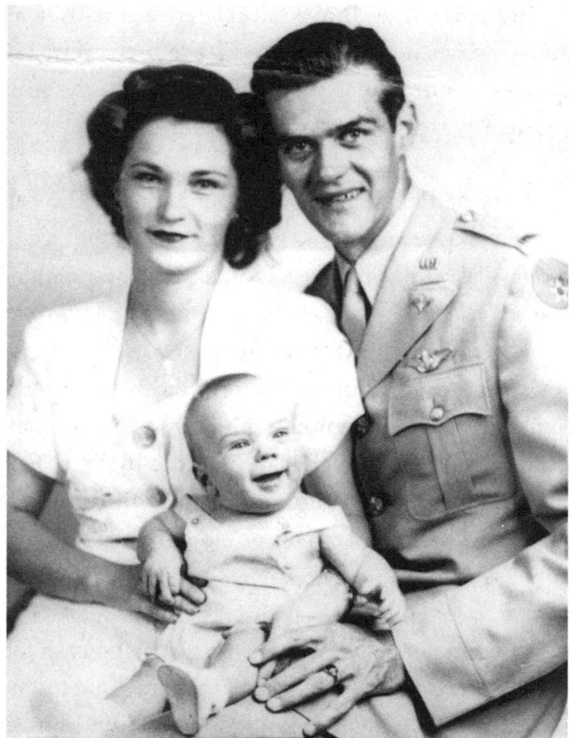

The Clarks with their first son, Gary.

be flying at twenty-seven to thirty-five thousand feet, doing high-level, radar-precision bombing. The briefing officer said the mission was not yet ready to go. With Hiroshima and Nagasaki still reeling from American atomic attacks, it appeared the enemy was about to surrender. "You're to be ready," the briefing officer said, "but the mission is on hold pending further word."

Crew 33, with Barney in the bombardier perch in the plane's nose, was ready at 4:30 PM. None of the men felt tense. "Let's play bridge," said Barney. The navigator pulled cards from one of his drawers. He, the two pilots, and Barney played for forty-five minutes. Then the command came for the planes to take off and pause over Iwo Jima to confirm that the Japanese had not surrendered. The word there was that "the war is still on."

The big bombers went into radio silence for the flight to Honshu. At their high altitude, the trip was eerily without incident. No Japanese made the slightest attempt to intercept them. Barney's B-29 was fourth over the refineries. The mission was a big success. With 80 percent of the bombs on target, the oil plants and storage tanks erupted in mountainous fires and clouds of smoke.

On the return trip, the planes broke radio silence at Iwo Jima. "It's all over," said the operator. "The Japanese surrendered." The B-29 crews asked what time the surrender had been announced. The war was already over when they had let their bombs go. Still, it was a happy moment for Barney and the crew. They were going home.

Una Loy and Gary had been living with her mother. The baby looked like Barney—the same blue-green eyes, dark brown hair, and distinctive brows. Gary was lively but very cranky; he cried a lot, especially at night. That bothered Una Loy because she feared it disturbed her mother. Ireta was working and dating; she often came in late and needed her sleep.

When Barney returned, Una Loy was surprised that he made no effort to get them their own place. Having been in the military four and a half years, he said he wanted to relax and get used to civilian life little by little. For the moment, they had no financial pressures. Una Loy had banked the bridge and poker winnings he had sent home. His military pay would continue another four months. Una Loy had some savings from working before Gary was born. Their nest egg was more than five hundred dollars.

Barney started a premed zoology class at BYU, paying cash for tuition. "The G.I. Bill would pay it," he told Una Loy, "but I'm saving that for medical school." He bought golf shoes to play the Timpanogos course with the clubs Grandpa Mac had given him. He spent time with his best buddy, Wes Brown, also home from the Army Air Corps. Una Loy thought Barney was logging a lot of hours on Ireta's sofa.

This was not what Una Loy had planned. For four days, she let the steam build; then she exploded: "We're imposing on Mother; can't you see that? I want us to be alone, just us! You're just lazy!" The last three words came out like bullets. Barney did not say a word. He turned around and walked out the front door.

His first stop was a telephone booth. "Mom," he said when he reached Ethel in Ogden, "is there any chance of our renting your house?"

"I've got tenants," she said. "But," she added, "I'll see if they'll move."

Then he walked to Woolworth's where he had worked before the war in the stockroom. "I'd like to start here again," he said.

"You got the job," the manager said. Barney stayed out for a couple of hours. When he returned to Ireta's, he told Una Loy what he had done. His point was very clear—never again could she call him lazy.

They moved into Ethel's house, and he lined up a slew of odd jobs. He still watered at the golf course at night, and he began selling hot dogs at the Provo baseball park. When Christmas came, he and Wes schemed for ways to make money. "Why not try selling trees?" Barney asked.

"Great idea," Wes enthused. "I'll get my dad's truck." They had to slog through the snowy hills to reach the evergreens, then cut them and lug them to the truck; both of them were exhausted.

Once Wes slipped into a knee-deep creek. Barney sat on the bank laughing. "I'm just too tired to help you," he said, and left Wes to climb out himself.

Their sales agent was Wes's wife, Linda. "Stubby," Barney told her, "without you we'd never make a cent." She stood in front of her home hawking the trees. But after they added the gasoline and city-permit costs, they only managed to come out even.

In the summer, Barney and Wes hauled hay. Coming out of one farm, Barney shouted to Wes, "Hey! The load is crooked. It's falling off."

"Never fear," said the ebullient Wes. "I'll go around the next turn real fast and straighten everything." The load went skittering off the truck. Barney was livid. Wes got out of the truck laughing so hard he had to flop on the ground with his long legs and arms flailing. The sight made Barney laugh, too.

"One thing about us," Barney said. "We're more laughs than dollars."

Barney went to the Hansen Candy Company. He discovered that Pop was dead and his two sons were in charge. "You got anything I can do?" Barney asked.

One of the brothers, Grant, said, "Sure, for Christmas you can make clear toys." Barney remembered those from his days of making all-day suckers. They were little transparent candies: red, green, and gold figures of Santa Claus, reindeer, sleighs, and animals.

"You got the job," Hansen said. "I'll pay you by the hour."

"I'd prefer to get paid by the pound," Barney said. "The more I produce, the more I earn."

Hansen said okay. "But," he added, "no pay for the broken ones."

Barney agreed. He was gambling. Making clear toys was tricky. The rich candy syrup needed be heated to a high temperature and then poured into little molds to cool. If the molds were cracked open too soon, the figures did not set up. If left in too long, they turned brittle. He developed the art of knowing the perfect moment for freeing the candy from the molds.

Barney worked at night, often as late as 4:00 AM, which gave him only a few hours before class. The syrup's fragrance permeated him. It took him fifteen minutes in the tub to shampoo and scrub himself. Even so, when he got into bed, Una Loy said, "You smell like sweet, sweet candy."

To help make ends meet, Una Loy also worked. With a borrowed typewriter, she prepared abstracts for her brother-in-law's title business and typed manuscripts and theses for BYU professors and students. She and Barney did not go out much. Almost every night he stayed up studying for his classes. If he brought friends home for study sessions, she and Gary vanished into the bedroom. It was a big treat for her after their son was asleep for Barney to offer some ice cream. He walked the eight blocks for a pint at Keeley's Fountain and then had to run home before it melted.

Medically Speaking

Barney was very firm that his son—now past two—should not use baby talk. "Let's not teach him to tinkle and go to the potty," he said to Una Loy. "We'll treat it medically—urinate and move your bowels." One night he asked his mother, newly back from Ogden and living with the McAdams, to babysit while he took Una Loy to a movie. After they were gone, Gary said he wanted to go to the bathroom.

"All right," said Ethel. She reached down to help him onto the toilet.

"No, no!" he shouted. "I stand up and do it like my daddy." He pulled his pants down. "We boys," he explained very seriously, "have to shake our penis when we urinate."

Telling the story to Barney and Una Loy, Ethel said, "He was so proud of himself."

When Una Loy became pregnant again, she did not tell Gary about storks. Instead, she said, "A baby's growing in mommy's tummy." It was another boy. They named him Stephen Kent Clark.

Barney told her the baby's sex while she was still groggy from the ether. She wailed, "No pretty little girl for me. Just a little ugly, bald-headed baby boy."

"Oh, honey," he said. "I would never say that." Stephen was an ideal baby with hardly any tears and fuss. Though he had Barney's long eyelashes, he was blond with light blue eyes like Una Loy's family.

The new baby was two months old when Barney frightened Una Loy. He was sitting at the kitchen table with his head resting on his hand. Looking at her, he began to shake, slowly at first, then more violently.

"Barney!" she cried. "What's wrong with you?" As the shaking continued, his head slipped off his hand, and he slumped to the floor. Drool slid down his chin. "Honey!" she screamed. When she screamed again, Barney unwound from his "stroke" and burst out laughing. "Oh, you!" she said. "You're such a character."

Some days after that, while folding a pile of diapers, she heard him drive

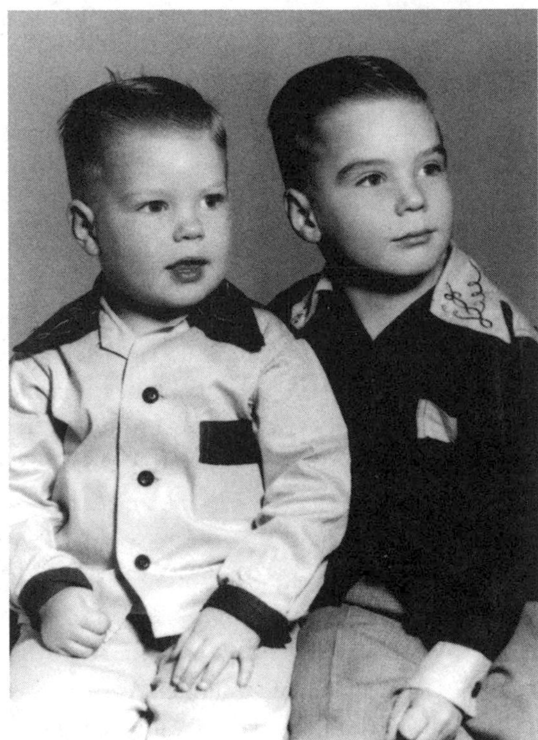

The Clark boys, Stephen (*left*) and Gary.

up. "I'll just get him," she said. She got down on the floor and lay quietly with her eyes closed. When Barney came in the front door, he called, "Honey?" She didn't respond. He walked into the bedroom. For a minute, he stood and looked at her. Then he stepped over her, went into the bathroom, and shut the door.

Outraged, she got up, opened the door, and said, "Well! So you didn't care if I had a heart attack or not?"

Barney deflated her: "I looked at you. You couldn't have fainted. Your cheeks were just as pink as they could be. Your breathing was even. I knew you were all right and decided you weren't going to fool me the way I fooled you."

After two years of premed courses, Barney and Una Loy went to Salt Lake City for his admission interview at the University of Utah School of Medicine. It was the first time he had been in the place. Realistically he gauged his chances. Competition was high. He was twenty-seven, four or five years older than most applicants who had not been in the military. He had no influential people endorsing his application. Probably the majority of candidates had better grades.

The interviewing doctor, following a routine, asked, "Mr. Clark, why do you want to be a doctor?"

Barney hesitated. The next voice he heard was Una Loy's. "He's got to do something for a living," she told the doctor. "He's got two babies to support."

Barney cleared his throat. Once he had thought it endearing when she piped up at any lull in the conversation. Now he was not so sure. The doctor went on to other questions. After the interview, Barney was cross. "You didn't help my chances any," he said.

"I thought somebody ought to say something," Una Loy replied.

"You made it seem like all I wanted was to make money."

"I'm sorry. I guess I should have said you only wanted to heal people." He said that would have been better. Still, the truth was that he did need to make money. With no explanation, the medical school turned him down. Barney was greatly disappointed.

Barney's Choice

Barney had a fallback position. For eighteen months, he had been a part-time distributor for Pepsi-Cola, Dad's Root Beer, and a grape drink. Now that he was graduating from BYU, he could work full time. As the outside man, Barney hustled his soda pop and made the deliveries. He liked the action and got a kick out of persuading stores that had never stocked his brands to agree to push them. When it heard about him, a major beer company asked him to be its distributor in much of Utah Valley.

He was debating the beer offer when he talked to Wes, who had left Provo in 1947 to attend the University of Washington's School of Dentistry in Seattle. "You ought to think about dental school," Wes urged.

"Oh, I don't know," said Barney. "I love it around here. Things are going pretty good, but I'll give it some thought." Barney talked it over with Una Loy. "If I take the beer job," he said, "I can start to make lots of money right away. If I go to school, it'll take me years to get anywhere."

"Do what you want to do," she said. When he did not respond, she went on, "The beer business might work, and it might not. If you go to dental school, you won't have to depend on anyone else for a job because you'll have a professional education."

She said this, although the idea of moving to Seattle scared her. Utah had always been her home, and she was near her family. Earlier in life, she had not even had the courage to go on a Mormon Church mission, unsure she could be away from home for two years.

Barney sent his application to the University of Washington. In April of 1949, he and Una Loy went to Seattle for his admissions interview and to check on housing. They left Gary with a neighbor but took young Stephen with them. Wes's wife, Linda, suggested they look for vacancies in Yesler Terrace, the rent-subsidized housing project where she and Wes lived. Leaving Una Loy with Stephen and the Browns' baby, Linda and Barney went to the manager's office. They were talking when suddenly the manager's desk began moving and slid clear across the room. The whole building was shaking. The manager screamed.

Having been in California, Barney knew what was going on. "It's an earthquake," he shouted at the woman. The extent of the shaking told him this was a major temblor. "Get in the doorway!" Linda obeyed, but the manager became hysterical. Barney slapped her to shock her and then put his arm around her to calm her. Leading her to the doorway, he held her until the tremors passed.

When the earthquake hit, Una Loy was on the toilet in the Browns' town house. She hastily pulled up her slacks, grabbed the two babies, and ran down the stairs to stand in the front-door jamb. When the shaking ended, she joined Yesler residents who had hurried into the street. She was waiting there when Barney arrived. The headline in the *Seattle Times* screamed, "Destructive, in Case You Didn't Know." On the Richter scale, the quake measured 7.1, a record for the Seattle area.

Washington's School of Dentistry accepted Barney. And long before any other students, his family got housing in Yesler. He believed comforting the manager during the quake had opened that door. Their Yesler town house had two bedrooms. Barney studied at an old desk in his and Una Loy's bedroom but usually only until 10:00 PM when the housing project's heat went down for the night.

When he came to bed, he told Una Loy, "The physiology and anatomy—they're great. I love them. It's like going to medical school." But as he moved on, he ran into trouble. "I've really got to struggle," he said. "I've got these big hands, and it's tough to carve dentures. Sometimes I don't think I'm any good."

A classmate, who had been a navy dental technician and had earned the nickname "golden hands," saw him struggling one day at a laboratory worktable. "Let me help you," he said. "I can do the plates for you."

Barney said no: "I've got to learn this. I'll stay here all night to get this right." Practice improved his dexterity. When Provo High classmate Frank Taylor came for a visit, Barney displayed some dentures. "How about these?" he said. "Took me a while, but I'm getting the hang of it."

The G.I. Bill paid his tuition and bought books, plus giving Barney seventy-five dollars a month for living expenses. "That will hardly cover us," Barney said.

He and a classmate went job hunting. The first four places turned them down. At the fifth, Associated Grocers, Inc., the employment man had lost a son in the Army Air Corps. He hired them to work all night Thursdays, using handcarts to load produce on big semitrailers for weekend distribution to stores. On Friday, Saturday, and Sunday nights, they took turns on watchman duty.

Una Loy was fairly happy in Seattle, despite the fears she had had about leaving Utah. She walked Gary and Stephen to the East Seattle day nursery in the morning, then went to a job as a searcher in a title company. One day the nursery director asked Una Loy, "Does Gary have a problem with his hearing?"

"I don't think so," Una Loy said.

"Well, do you have any trouble getting him to do what you ask?"

"Sometimes he can be rebellious. I tell him to do something, and he ignores me," Una Loy said.

"We noticed the same thing. But when we make very clear what we want, he's always surprised as if he hadn't heard us. As soon as he understands, he's very obedient."

The director gave Una Loy the name of Dr. Willard Goff. "He's a good ear, nose, and throat man," she said. "I've already talked with him. He'll see Gary."

The specialist discovered that Gary had a puzzling ear problem. Periodically his eardrum collapsed for no discernible reason. The doctor inserted a tube through Gary's nose that opened his ear with a puff of air.

His fee was fifty cents. "That won't cover your paperwork," said Barney.

"The center told me about you folks," said Goff. "I always have one patient that I charge this token fee. It makes me feel good to help the right people."

Dr. Goff gave Gary a number of treatments that year. When they did not achieve sustained results, he did surgery. Once again, his fee was half a dollar.

"That's not right," Barney said.

"Please," said Goff, "don't take my pleasure away from me."

As Gary's hearing improved, Una Loy and Barney realized he minded them better.

Friday dinner was manners night in the Clark home. Echoing Grandpa Mac and Uncle Vearl, Barney told his sons, "You come to the table scrubbed. No mud stains on your shoes. You're going to use napkins and the correct fork. No elbows on the table." He was firm but not harsh. "When you leave my house, I want you to know how to behave like gentlemen."

In 1952 when Stephen was not yet five, Barney had a man-to-man talk with him. "I hear you're picking fights and then getting Gary to finish them for you."

"But I like to watch Gary fight," Stephen said.

"I've taught you a little about boxing," Barney said, "but you shouldn't pick fights. And you sure shouldn't run away and let somebody else do your fighting." Barney didn't spank him; he just looked at him. When Stephen noticed his dad's raised eyebrows, he knew it was time to stop messing around.

At a birthday party, Gary blew on a horn. Then he wondered what it would sound like if he sucked in. The horn's whistle popped into his mouth, lodging in his throat. All of a sudden, he could not breathe. Another child yelled, "Gary's choking."

Barney came bounding up the steps, five at a time. With one hand, he clutched Gary's leg, then turned him upside down. With his other hand, he smacked his son's back, and the whistle shot across the room into the wall. Later, Gary said, "Gee, Stephen, Dad's sure strong."

Starting Out

Wes walked into the Clark's town house one Saturday afternoon. Not knowing what he was interrupting, he said, "Barn, let's go out for a cup of coffee."

"Oh no, you don't," Una Loy said. "I need him to replace the treads on the stairs."

"Oh, I can do it later," Barney said.

"Barney, I want you to do this right now," she said. "If you don't, you won't do it. Because when you come back, it'll be time to study, or work, or something else."

Wes began laughing. The more she fussed, the harder he laughed. "Aw, Una Loy," he said, "C'mon, sit down, have a cigarette and relax."

The notion that anyone would even kid her about smoking made her even madder, but before she could say anything, Barney said, "I'll see you later" and left with Wes. The next weekend Barney sued for peace by replacing the stair treads.

Having graduated, Wes was doing public-health work in Seattle. He said to his wife, "I go to work in the dark; I come home in the dark. Nobody smiles. And it's always raining." He wanted to go back to Utah. Then a dental practice opened up in Yakima, 150 miles east across the Cascade Mountains. After a trip there, Wes told Barney, "I like it. It's got four seasons, just like Utah. I'm making the move."

Barney could understand. He had to make a career decision himself. What was he going to do after graduation? He told Una Loy that he really wanted to become an oral surgeon. "But that wouldn't be fair to you and the boys. I'm thirty-two years old. I can't just keep going to school. I've got to get going," he said.

They had always assumed they would return to Provo. The dilemma was that they had only about fifteen hundred dollars in savings, hardly enough to open and equip a dental office. And Barney did not want to go into debt.

They were wrestling with what to do when Dale Mitchell dropped in. Another Utahn, he had become a friend of Barney's in dental school. He said he was going into the military and the job he held was open. It was in the office of Dr. Homer Lockett, who had an extraordinarily busy practice of two to three thousand patients in the nearby town of White Center, a bedroom community for many Boeing aerospace workers.

"You ought to talk with him," Dale suggested to Barney.

Lockett had an interesting proposition. He would provide office space and equipment, pay all expenses, and refer patients. Barney could keep from 30 to 40 percent of the fees he earned. Barney recognized the opportunity. He could get started in dentistry without any cash investment and learn the nuts and bolts of running a practice. Not many offices offered that.

Lockett liked Barney. Before hiring him, however, he asked several dental-school sources for an evaluation. "Homer," said his friends, "Clark's done well both academically and clinically—probably in the top quarter of his class. There's one thing you'll really appreciate. He's a nut like you. He's a workaholic." Lockett hired him.

On his first payday, Barney went to see Dr. Goff, the specialist who had operated on Gary. "I feel I must pay you for all you did for my son," he said.

"I won't take your money," Goff said, "but there is something you can do. In your practice, always have at least one family you're caring for free of charge. That will repay me."

"I promise you," said Barney, "that I always will."

Lockett came to work at 8:00 AM. Barney was already there. They tried to get out by 6:00 PM but often stayed to 8:30 or 9:00 PM, whatever the practice required. Lockett took just one week's vacation a year. He paid close attention to Barney's affable, low-key approach to patents. "You've got a good bedside manner," he told Barney. "They're comfortable with you."

After graduating, Barney used their fifteen-hundred-dollar savings for a down payment on a thirteen-thousand-dollar brick and cedar house. It had three tiny bedrooms upstairs and a huge basement playroom/den and was in the suburb of Burien, about five miles south of White Center. The subdivision was so new it had only three homes. Surrounded by trees, their place looked like a little house in a forest.

Being that isolated worried Una Loy. There was no telephone service yet, and she was pregnant again. As with all her pregnancies, the coming event inspired a dramatic announcement. Stephen begged her to come to his new school at lunchtime. He took her by the hand and introduced her to his teachers and the other kids. "This is my mother," he said. "She is going to have a baby."

After the delivery, the obstetrician told Barney, "You got your wish. It's a girl."

Although Una Loy would have been happy with half-a-dozen more babies, Barney told her, "Honey, that's it. Now we've got our family."

They took their daughter to church to be blessed and given a name, Karen Michelle Clark. One of the Mormon elders at the ceremony said, "How delighted you must be to have this cute little girl."

"Yeah," said nine-year-old Gary, "It is a good thing it was a girl because my dad said if it was another boy, he'd flush him down the toilet." Barney and Una Loy were deeply embarrassed.

Friends invited them to a buffet. Arriving home late to pick up Una Loy, Barney said, "I haven't had a chance to eat today. I'm really hungry." At the party, he had a couple of highballs. He began to feel light headed. He turned to Una Loy. "Honey, we're going home."

"We just got here. Maybe if you eat something."

"I'm not going to stick around for food. I'm in no condition." He thanked the host and hostess and said, "Una Loy, get your coat. We're leaving now!"

While checking on Karen and the boys after the babysitter had gone, Una Loy heard strange thumping and hoots of laughter from the living room. Rushing there, she saw Barney on the floor with his coat off and shirtsleeves pushed up. He was doing somersaults, engrossed in private hilarity. The noise woke Gary and Stephen. They came in and stared wide eyed at their laughing father. "What's wrong with Dad?"

"It's all right," Una Loy said, smiling, "Daddy's just having fun." His antics were so out of character that even she was amused.

With the pressure in the office, Barney drank lots of coffee and now smoked a pack of cigarettes a day. Instead of lunch, he snacked on glazed or sugar doughnuts in the Spudnut Shop below the office. Back in the office, he scrupulously brushed his teeth.

As soon as he had the money, Barney invested in four season tickets to the Washington Huskies' football games. The first time he, Una Loy, and two friends trooped into the end-zone stands he said, "We're halfway to heaven." He studied football plays through binoculars.

Una Loy was a hyperhollering fan. He chuckled every time she shouted, "C'mon you guys! Stop playing like a bunch of high-school kids."

Rx

One night in late June 1954, Barney washed up after working late and examined himself in the mirror. His eyes were very jaundiced. At home he said to Una Loy, "Look at my eyes."

"Why, they're all yellowy," she said. "What in the world is wrong with you? You're never sick."

"Last few days I've been a little nauseated."

"Why didn't you tell me, honey?"

"I didn't want to bother you. I'll go to a doctor tomorrow." During his examination, the doctor palpated Barney's abdomen. Barney winced when the doctor got to his liver. "It's a little tender," he said. The doctor wanted to know if he drank. "Couple beers a week, a highball every so often," Barney said. The doctor then asked about his work schedule. "Some days run pretty long," Barney admitted.

After more questions and probing, the doctor said, "You've got a hepatitis infection in your liver. You've been working too hard and gotten a little run down."

"What's the treatment?" Barney asked.

"Do as little as possible," the doctor replied. "Bed rest for at least six weeks and eat a lot of sugar—just suck on butterscotch balls."

Una Loy brought a garden chaise lounge into the living room so Barney could stretch out and watch television. Three or four times a day, he said, "Bring in Karen; let me play with her." Karen's hair was golden, and she had huge blue-green eyes. She was going to be tall. As he sat bouncing her, he said, "This is so wonderful. You know, she's the first one of our kids I've been able to enjoy as a baby."

Not working week after week galled Barney, as did having his teeth exposed to an unending sugar bath from the butterscotch balls the doctor had advised him to eat. He was always getting up to clean his teeth. He was so worried about tooth decay that he forbade Una Loy to pack Gary and Stephen's lunch boxes with peanut butter and jelly sandwiches. Still, he faithfully followed the doctor's orders.

Cooperation with his physician's suggestions did not extend further than worrying about his teeth. Barney continued to smoke heavily and eat a less-than-healthy diet that soothed his work pressures but did nothing for his hidden health problems. He was already making a gradual transition to serious future medical problems.

PART FOUR

13

The Gathering

You don't live in the world all alone. Your brothers are here, too.

—Albert Schweitzer on receiving the Nobel Prize

An Artificial Heart Ready for Humans?

As the 1970s drew to a close, some researchers, including those at the University of Utah, were convinced that the animal implants had proved the feasibility of artificial hearts. Animals, particularly calves, were surviving longer, usually until they simply outgrew the ability of their artificial hearts to meet their perfusion needs. Dozens of concerns regarding materials, design, and drive systems had been resolved. It seemed time to make the ultimate trial—in a human patient.

The mere prospect had many implications, and more years of work lay ahead before the first human implant. There were subtle changes in the animal research to answer important questions. Artificial hearts designed for a calf's chest would need to be slightly altered to fit a human being. A team of medical doctors familiar with treating heart disease and doing cardiopulmonary surgery would have to be assembled and trained to use the artificial heart and its support system. And the ethical debates sharpened.

When Pim Kolff had developed the artificial kidney in World War II Holland, he did not have to ask permission of anyone except his hospital superiors and his patients or their families. In 1970s America, government agencies, especially those that provided money to conduct research, had attached a gauntlet of oversight requirements to human experimentation by institutions. The Utah researchers conducted endless discussions about meeting those requirements and wording university applications to get a positive response. Aware of the media frenzy that had accompanied every new development in heart transplant surgery, they began also to think about ways to handle the inevitable media demands spawned by a human heart implant.

The Human Fit

At the top of the list of challenges were design decisions to modify artificial hearts for the human body. Robert Jarvik was in the artificial-heart lab in 1978 when the School of Medicine's Department of Pathology telephoned with news he had been awaiting. "We've got a cadaver: a young man, average size. He died from head injuries in a motorcycle accident. Might be just right to do the heart-fit trials you've been requesting. We have the necessary permissions." With the success of his Jarvik-5 (J-5) heart in animals, the young designer was contemplating his next big step—fabricating a heart specifically for the human body. How big should it be? He needed to be sure of the human chest's dimensions.

In the anatomy lab, the chest of the cadaver was already open for the autopsy. Jarvik looked at the pale pearl color of the skin and the grayish tan of the internal organs that had once flushed red with blood. He found that although it is easy to say a corpse is lifeless, it is hard to stare at one without thinking of what life had been like for this human being.

Sweeping away those thoughts, Jarvik teamed with a pathology aide to scissor out the incredibly light lungs. They injected quick-setting silicone rubber into the heart, leaving it rigid as stone and preventing it from collapsing when the chest cavity was filled with plaster of Paris. They slipped out the hardened plaster, cut it open, and removed the hardened heart. The researchers poured more plastic into the chest cavity to create a cast with the exact dimensions of the heart and its connections to the blood vessels.

Next they fashioned a mock ribcage of fiberglass. Placing the cast of the heart and its connectors inside gave them a three-dimensional view. Jarvik then designed a new heart model, the Jarvik-7 (J-7);[1] it was almost identical to the J-5, except smaller.

Animal Trials

Kolff and Don Olsen scheduled animal trials to test the J-7's performance, but they had few hopes the experiments would break any endurance records. Olsen summarized the reasons for the staff. "The J-7 was designed from the heart of a 150-pound man, but a calf can grow to 350 or 400 pounds. To sustain life in an animal that big, the J-5 pumps 155 cubic centimeters (cc) of blood with every stroke. The J-7's output is only 95 cc. Unless we make some special adjustments, the amount of blood pumped will be borderline for a calf."

"Those adjustments can be made," said Dr. Tagaaki Mochizuki, the visiting Japanese scientist who was appointed principal investigator for an implant into a three-month-old, 188-pound Holstein calf he named Fumi Joe. "We don't

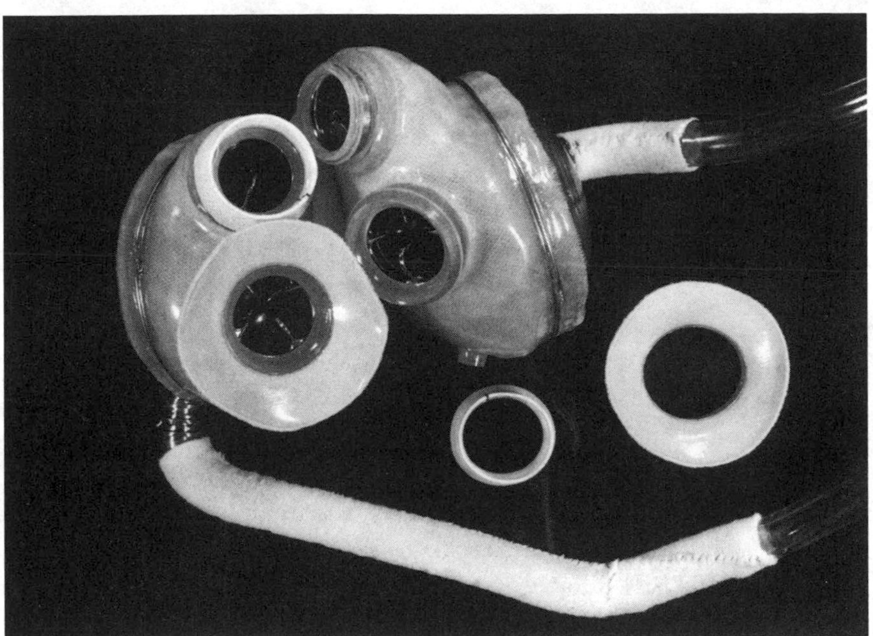

The components of the Jarvik-7 heart.

have to worry about the pumping volume of each beat. The crucial question is how much the heart pumps over a period of time. We can counteract low output per beat simply by increasing the number of beats per minute (BPM)." Fumi Joe's heart rate was turned up to 120 BPM. Even so, Mochizuki was concerned that the volume was inadequate. He pushed the pulse rate to 140, 150, and then 160 BPM.

That brought new worries. How could he be certain that this frantic rate would allow enough time in each pumping cycle for blood to enter and fill the heart? He could not do that without resorting to a technique Clifford Kwan-Gett, Kolff's former heart designer, had attempted a decade earlier. A high suction level was used to draw blood inside the pumping ventricles, which Kwan-Gett contended was unnecessary. He surmised that—with the right design—gravity took care of blood filling the heart. Subsequently, Olsen and other researchers had modified the technique, sometimes using just a touch of suction to discharge the compressed air used to create the previous blood pressure.

Fumi Joe's case was different. With the calf's heart pulsing 150 or more beats per minute, Mochizuki did not want to put all his faith in gravity filling the heart. He ordered suction at five to six times the usual amount. It was a dangerous decision. Suppose that this high vacuum pressure was so strong it collapsed the atrium, perhaps even sucked some of it into the ventricle. Death would follow in minutes. It was risky but under the circumstances unavoidable, Mochizuki felt.

The gamble paid off. For the first 125 days, Fumi Joe's J-7 heart kept up its rigorous pumping, filling and discharging without incident. The 126th day brought a hint of trouble—occasionally the heart's left ventricle was not filling on every beat. The Japanese investigator didn't think high suction was the cause. More likely, he guessed, some growth was beginning to obstruct the heart's inflow cuffs.

In the next month, the difficulties increased, and Fumi Joe weakened. Intestinal bleeding occurred, and there was edema. Blood spotted the urine. The heart failed to fill on eight of ten pumping cycles, so Mochizuki dropped the heart rate to 140, allowing more filling time. Drug therapy helped temporarily.

On the 178th day after Fumi Joe's surgery, it became impossible to fill the left heart at all. More intestinal bleeding occurred, but with treatment the calf survived until he passed the lab's previous endurance record of more than six months. Almost as if he knew his task was accomplished, Fumi Joe worsened dramatically. Edema puffed up his brisket (breast), and diuretics failed to shrink it. His red cell count dropped precipitously. What he desperately needed was a transfusion, but no compatible blood was available. On the 221st day, Fumi Joe died of hypovolemic shock—a shortage of circulating blood volume—typical of inadequate cardiac output.

The researchers' indispensable tool, the autopsy, explained the death. Around the heart's left inflow valve was a heavy layer of tissue that had rooted along the quick-connect cuff joining the left atrium to the heart. Olsen recognized it as pannus. The growth had spread until it cut off almost all blood flow in spite of the power of vacuum pressure. Regardless, Fumi Joe had fooled everybody. No one had thought he would live very long, yet the J-7 artificial heart designed for a human chest had kept this large animal alive for seven months—a new record for artificial hearts.

The Return of the Surgeon

In North Carolina, Dr. William DeVries was thinking it was time to move on. He had spent nine years in Duke University's medical center perfecting his surgery skills. By 1979 he had become a clinical instructor in cardiothoracic surgery. Throughout his Duke years, he had been in touch with the Utah program. Kolff dropped him occasional notes, and on a vacation trip to Utah, DeVries dropped in the lab. Sometimes he recalled that, when he had left Utah in 1970, he had been sure an artificial heart would be beating in a human chest within two or three years. Nearly a decade had gone by. DeVries was aware of the lab's problems and that, one by one, they were being overcome. "Must be pretty close now," he decided.

One day Kolff telephoned him. "There's a good opportunity for you back here. We need you."

"Thank you for saying that," DeVries responded. "But obviously I can't do anything without an appointment from the University of Utah School of Medicine." While Kolff could offer him a position in the artificial-heart program, he had no control over appointments to the faculty. However, there was a staff vacancy. The head of cardiothoracic surgery was leaving for private practice, and DeVries was invited to Utah for an interview.

When he returned to Duke, his redoubtable teacher and dean, Dr. David C. Sabiston, asked, "How did things go?"

"Well, there are some opportunities, but there are also problems, DeVries replied.

"I think you have to go there. I want you to go there."

"I think I would like to look at some other places, see what is available..." a cautious DeVries began.

"No, you are going to Utah," Sabiston declared. Few people, especially instructors, ever challenged the strong-minded Sabiston. DeVries knew the talk was over. He concluded that Kolff and Sabiston, who were friends, had talked about his career and that the dean had decided his student's best opportunity lay in Utah.

"He must believe it offers something valuable in the future," the young surgeon decided. "I know he's interested in fostering my career, not just for me but for society."

After an appropriate review, the Utah School of Medicine made a formal offer, and DeVries, his wife, and their seven children pulled up stakes to go west.

Kolff had his reasons for welcoming DeVries. Since 1957 in Cleveland, when they had seemed to take two steps forward and one back, Kolff and his team had clawed and scratched their way to unraveling the enigmas of the heart. Each time they achieved a new survival record, they came face to face with another problem. Now they were looking at the biggest challenge—putting the heart in a human chest.

This step was impossible without a clinical surgeon, one who believed in the artificial heart enough to dare to put it in a person. Kolff had once hoped his surgeon son, Jack, could win a faculty appointment at the University of Utah

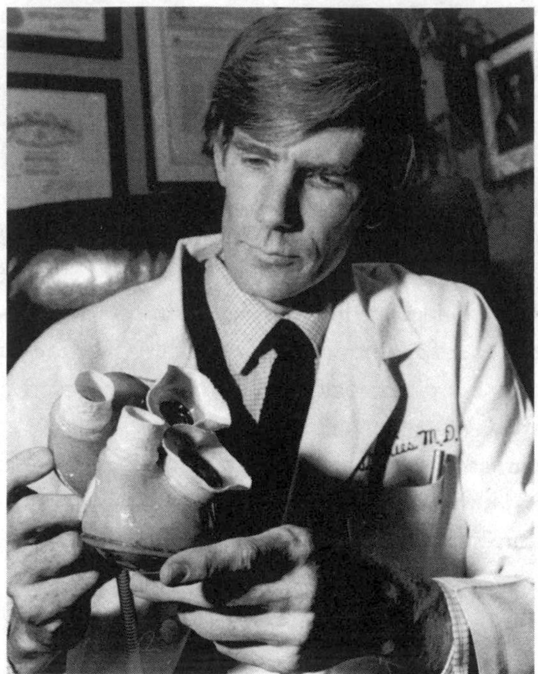

The return of William DeVries from medical training became the nucleus for the heart implant team.

School of Medicine. When that appointment never materialized, Kolff considered other candidates without finding anyone terribly interested.

As early as 1967, DeVries—then a medical student—had stood at surgeons' elbows, watching animal implants. Kolff was sure that under Sabiston's careful eye, DeVries had received the training he needed for the task. Furthermore, Kolff viewed DeVries as someone with the will and nerve to walk into the medical unknown.

In the summer of 1979, an international convention of artificial-heart researchers was held in Germany. Kolff took a delegation of his staff including Olsen, Jarvik, and Steven Nielsen. The Utah team made speeches, and the diverse European and Japanese researchers were impressed with their successes.

Kolff scheduled a staff meeting back in Utah and opened it to anyone who had an interest. A number of people wandered in to hear Kolff announce, "Dr. William C. DeVries has returned to the University of Utah from Duke University to join the medical center's clinical staff. Also he is in our Division of Artificial Organs. He will become the division's chief surgeon. To accommodate his schedule, we will change our implant day from Tuesday to Wednesday."

Olsen, who knew nothing about the Kolff/DeVries/Sabiston negotiations, felt his peers suddenly staring at him. For seven years, he had been chief surgeon and appreciated for his contributions. Without even a word of prior explanation, he was losing his title. Kolff was also rearranging the surgery schedule of the artificial-heart lab Olsen had run, again without consultation. However, a clinical surgeon was necessary. Kolff felt this was so obvious that he didn't have to explain it to Olsen or anyone else. Once he had recovered from his initial hurt, Olsen accepted the logic. That autumn he became DeVries's teacher in the Artificial Heart Research Laboratory.

"Obviously, you know surgery," he told DeVries. "What we do here is plumbing—taking out pumps and putting them in with new pipes. In this kind of surgery, we have to think three dimensionally. When we put in an artificial heart, we have to consider what it does to the vessels and organs behind and around it. We have to provide space for the heart, to see that the atria are not compromised and the aorta and great veins are not encumbered."

Unfortunately, DeVries also got a lesson in how hard it can be for a surgeon fresh out of residency to support himself and his family. His only dependable income was a pittance: a thousand dollars a year as an assistant (nontenured) professor in the university's School of Medicine. Any other income depended on what fees he could generate through surgeries, and he could not keep all of that. As is usual with teaching hospitals, the medical center allowed him to retain only a percentage. The rest went to the university. Devries estimated his share was about one-fourth what heart surgeons were making in private practice. In his first six months at Utah, his take-home pay was less than when he had left his training position at Duke.

He needed to increase his number of operations. Usually cardiologists refer patients to a surgeon, but despite nearly twenty years of trying, the University of Utah Medical Center had failed to establish an outstanding cardiothoracic surgery service. Many patients requiring heart operations were sent to other institutions, usually nearby LDS Hospital.

DeVries was reluctant to tell the university cardiologists and he wanted to build up the cardiothoracic surgery program. "They'll look at me and ask, 'Who's this guy?' They won't know me, know my training." So he went to Olsen. "Does the lab have any grant money I can draw a salary from?" he asked.

"I'm sorry, but we're strapped. I can't lay my hands on a single penny to pay you," Olsen replied.

DeVries then went across Foothill Boulevard to the VA Medical Center, which had been sending its cardiac surgery patients to other VA hospitals. He said he would like to become a part-time staff member and do at least some of the operations in the University of Utah Medical Center. The VA Hospital agreed. That brought in some money. At Duke he had trained in esophageal operations and procedures involving chest cancer. He could do those in Utah for extra income. Little by little he began getting referrals. That encouraged him to think that in time the university cardiologists would also send him patients.

In the artificial-heart lab, DeVries and Olsen developed a good rapport. Each Wednesday they stood across from each other, working as a team to implant hearts. After learning Olsen's way, DeVries introduced some suturing variations to build a comfortable technique. "Practice," DeVries said, "that's the goal: practice, practice, practice. Get so I know everything there is to know. I must be prepared no matter what happens."

Olsen and his staff were on the verge of solving what appeared to be their last major hurdle before human implants—combatting the strange growth called pannus that had killed Fumi Joe. Jarvik wanted a statistical count of how often it had occurred in the experimental animals. A review of the records documented that pannus had developed in the plastic quick-connects of more than 70 percent of the longer survivors.

Why did it form there, most often in the left heart's inflow path? What happened to generate pannus? In the literature, Olsen uncovered a report saying that when blood cells were damaged, they released a chemical that seemed to spur the growth of pannus-like tissue. That was a big clue. The Utah group set to work to determine where blood might be damaged in the quick-connects.

They studied devices that had never been looked at before to determine how they might bruise or rupture blood cells. They noted several areas with sharp angles and abrupt obstacles, notably where a ring protruded to hold the tilting metal valves. Like river rocks causing rapids, these were surely causing turbulence in the blood flow, a forerunner to damaged cells. It was a simple matter to redesign the quick-connects with a smooth, uninterrupted passageway for the blood.

Excited, they tested the new design in twenty-two calves. Autopsies found pannus in only six, and it was so slight it could not be considered life threatening. "It is clear that pannus formation has been virtually eliminated," Olsen and Jarvik concluded.

In animal after animal, DeVries kept honing his implantation techniques, trying to anticipate every emergency and ways to surmount it. In November 1979, he asked to talk privately with Kolff.

"We are ready for a human implant," the surgeon said. Kolff stared at him. For twenty-two years, he had been waiting to hear those words. Still, the only vestige of emotion was a slight narrowing of his eyes.

"If you say we are ready," he said after twenty or thirty seconds, "I will back you." He paused, "But we will have some troubles." Kolff was aware how much the situation had changed for experimenters since his early days. Before DeVries could attempt any human implant, he would have to convince what amounted to a jury that the procedure was both ethically proper and scientifically valid.

The Nuremberg Trial's Influence on Institutional Review Boards

The group charged with such decisions was the university's Committee for Research in Human Subjects, generally shortened to the institutional review board (IRB). At Utah the chair of the IRB Subcommittee for the Artificial Heart was German-born Dr. Ernst K. Eichwald, an internationally recognized pathologist credited with important discoveries in tissue transplantation. Other members included a psychiatrist, a philosopher, physicians, several nurses, a lawyer, neurologists, and a "citizen representative" from the community. The federal government mandated that every research hospital form such a committee and prescribed its membership.

The creation of these review boards in research institutions was a legacy of brutal Nazi experimentation on prisoners during World War II and the subsequent Nuremberg trials of 1946. Horror stories of human-skin lampshades and numerous other atrocities by Nazi doctors that were described as "medical experiments" had impelled a shocked international panel of judges to declare, "Never again!" As a statement of conscience, they drafted a code of medical ethics to guide experiments on human beings. "The voluntary consent of the human subject," the judges said, "is absolutely essential."

Unnecessary suffering was to be avoided, and the patient could choose to terminate the research. (In the unique circumstances at Utah, this requirement stimulated extensive discussion because an artificial-heart patient could not terminate the research without causing his own death.) Furthermore, the guidelines required that "only scientifically qualified persons" should do the experiments, and they had a "personal duty and responsibility" to protect the patients. In no case should the risk exceed "the humanitarian importance of the problem to be solved."

What emerged from the international debate initially was an honor code for researchers. They alone were left to decide if their work met the Nuremberg conditions with no outside review of their goals and tactics. As a result, the U.S. Public Health Service had no oversight of its own secret study on the impact of untreated syphilis in blacks at Tuscaloosa, Alabama. Long after effective therapy was available, the experiment continued, hidden from public scrutiny and in effect letting the subjects die so researchers could gauge the disease's progress.

In the late 1950s, some sixty-six American departments of medicine were asked if they had a formal set of guidelines to control what scientists did in human research. Only eight did, and just a few more than a third had—or favored the creation of—a committee to examine projects before they reached experimentation stage. A task force at the National Heart Institute said that investigators, universities, and research centers were not fulfilling their responsibility to research subjects with "sufficient care or universality." It was apparent an honor code was not enough.

Protection of patients and research subjects demanded that before scientists did human experimentation, they had to submit their projects for peer review. How to enforce that? In cases of federal financial support, obviously, the dollar was the weapon. Starting in 1966, the government ruled that to get federal funding, institutions had to have committees with power to veto any research proposal. Most institutions fell into line. More than 90 percent of them, however, appointed only physicians and scientists to sit in judgment on their friends and peers. Fearing that was too much of a buddy system, the government changed the rules. Committees had to be broad enough to include representation from lawyers, members of the clergy, and lay people.

By the time Utah's artificial heart had reached this level of debate, such committees had jurisdiction over all human research. But the artificial heart raised unusual questions. A 1973 task force of the National Heart, Lung and Blood Institute (NHLBI) noted that the device was unique because it was "the sine qua non of biological life" with implications not only for the recipient but also his or her family. The task force's conclusion stated that replacing the heart as part of

> fabricating man...poses problems beyond those usually found in the fields of medicine and medical ethics. Will its replacement by a mechanical pump and motor not merely place technology deep in man's bosom, but place man more deeply in the bosom of technology?
>
> Can we now envision the human brain linked to the computer? How much of the person can be supplanted by technology without loss of individuality, personality, humanness? Is it conceivable that the possessor of an artificial heart might believe himself less, or more, human?
>
> Might he not suffer the depression of the Tin Woodman in *The Wizard of Oz,* searching for a real heart, or confident of bearing a heart which can never fail, be deluded into a spurious sense of bodily immortality?

On the local scene, the questions reflected the concerns being voiced nationally and internationally. Just as he had promised, Kolff backed up DeVries with a letter to Eichwald:

> *Dear Ernst:*
>
> *As you know we have worked on the artificial heart for a very long time. Also, if we had wanted to, we could have had artificial hearts implanted via other surgeons in other locations. During the last two years we have been notified on several occasions that it was predictable that a patient whose body and mind otherwise were in good condition was going to die from irreparable heart failure. I have resisted every attempt to implant an artificial heart even in such cases as long as I felt that we were not quite ready.*
>
> *I believe that we are ready now but we should do it only when it is likely that we will restore the recipient to an (for him) acceptable and even an enjoyable existence.*
>
> *I feel that progress is fast now and that once life is sustained and health is maintained with the artificial heart alternative solutions for the patient may develop; either transplantation or a better artificial heart. Although I have worked on the artificial heart since 1957 I have not approached your committee for permission earlier. I feel that now is the time.*

The Protocol

Never before had anyone confronted the task that lay ahead for DeVries: shaping the precise language that would persuade an IRB to approve the implantation of an artificial heart in a human. The thirty-seven-year-old DeVries launched his June 1980 proposal audaciously, giving the implant a heroic context. He began with this passage from President Theodore Roosevelt: "Far better it is to dare mighty things, to win glorious triumphs, even though checkered by failure, than to rank with those poor spirits who neither enjoy nor suffer much, because they live in a gray twilight that knows neither victory nor defeat."[2]

Echoing Kolff's long-held philosophy, DeVries said use of the heart would be limited to "a patient who is surely going to die if not treated." He defined the pool of potential candidates in three categories:

1. The 140,000 Americans who go into cardiogenic shock after suffering severe and seemingly terminal heart attacks each year.
2. The 11,000 men and women who die annually from cardiomyopathy, the generally fatal disease that cripples the heart muscle.
3. The 5,000 or so patients whose natural hearts cannot be restarted after they have been on the heart-lung machine during bypass surgery for clogged arteries.

DeVries said those under seventeen and over sixty-five would be excluded. Also ruled out were those suffering from cancer, kidney and liver disease, and severe chronic obstructive pulmonary disease, as well as those lacking a "suitable social situation" to provide support. Nevertheless, he said that up to thirty thousand patients might benefit each year from the artificial heart. "There is little doubt as to the significance of the workable replacement to the diseased natural heart," he wrote. "There is also little doubt that we at the University of Utah currently possess the most successful artificial heart, driving system and surgical team available in the world."

To protect his choice against inappropriate candidates, DeVries said he would get a second opinion from Dr. Fred Anderson, a medical center cardiologist. The patient's lifestyle, family structure, and religious beliefs would be discussed before patient and family gave informed consent with the aid of a patient advocate drawn from the family physician, clergyman, lawyer, or someone appointed by the hospital.

DeVries anticipated that after the implant, the patient would not be hospital bound but could look forward either to returning home or going to Stanford University for a heart transplant, providing he or she met Stanford's rigid criteria, which included being under fifty and free of severe pulmonary vascular difficulties, diabetes, and infection.

But before the IRB could act on DeVries's application, the project faced a crisis from an unexpected source: the press became aware of the story, and the resulting publicity threatened to derail the plans to implant an artificial heart into a human recipient.

Reporters: Trust and Deceit

In the spring of 1980, Twila Van Leer, the soft-spoken medical writer for Salt Lake City's *Deseret News*, went to a Grand Rounds lecture in the University of Utah Medical Center. Most of it did not seem interesting for her readers, but buried deeply was a sentence that surprised her. Discussing clinical experimentation, the speaker said the University of Utah was planning to implant an artificial heart in a human being.

Back in her office, Van Leer telephoned one of her medical center sources. "I know about the animal experiments," she said. "Are you now ready for human implants?"

"Getting close," the surgeon answered. "But we don't want to release the story yet. If you can hold off, I'll make sure to contact you so you can have the story at the right time."

Van Leer—at forty-seven—was an experienced, prizewinning reporter. She wanted to be the first to break the news, but being a conscientious, noncompetitive person, she did not press for a story, especially since her source, who happened to be DeVries, said the medical center was not immediately ready to do any implants.

"You'll call me?" she asked.

"I will. And before we release the news, I'd like to talk with you about how it should be done. We're not terribly experienced in dealing with the press." That turned out to be a classic understatement.

Van Leer briefed her city editor: "This will be a big story. I'd like to go on special assignment for a couple of days to begin researching. We can have a series all ready when they release the news." Her boss agreed. What she failed to reckon with was the tongue-loosening powers of Neil Robinson's backyard barbeque.

Robinson was thirty-two and ambitious to be recognized as a writer. A midwesterner, he worked for United Press International (UPI) in Salt Lake City. In July 1980, he threw a party. Among the people he invited was a young woman who worked in the old St. Mark's Hospital building where the Kolff Artificial Heart Research Laboratory was located. "They're pretty excited in the lab," she said. "They're planning to take out somebody's natural heart and put in an artificial one."

"That's right," a young man who worked in the medical center chimed in, "it's just about set."

Though he knew nothing about the artificial heart, Robinson sensed this could be important news. The following Monday he looked for the UPI's file on the artificial heart. Though the animal work had been going on in Utah for thirteen years, he could find no stories about it or the potential for human implants.

"I know we've carried stuff on this," a UPI coworker told Robinson, "but damned if I can find the articles." Finally, they telephoned a staffer who had kept the files before being transferred to Los Angeles. Asked where the heart stories were, he answered, "Right where they should be—under calf hearts." Robinson grimaced at the logic, but he found the file. While it included accounts of animal implants, there was no mention of human experimentation.

Part of the reason was that—despite its critical importance—the IRB was largely unknown, even on the university campus. It did its business in closed meetings. Some members even wanted their identities to be secret. When DeVries's application went to the board, a choice confronted him, Kolff, and the university. They could make a public announcement and hope to control the news, revealing only what they wanted disclosed. That, however, flew in the face of the IRB tradition—no public announcements before it rendered a decision for fear publicity might pressure members.

Or they could say nothing, naively trusting they could keep news of the application under wraps. The formidable wall of secrecy shielding the IRB provided assurance there would be no leaks. But those university employees whose backyard barbeque chitchat brought UPI reporter Neil Robinson to the Artificial Heart Research Laboratory at old St. Mark's Hospital undid their confidence.

Thinking he was really onto something, Robinson telephoned Olsen and blurted out, "I understand you're seeking permission to put an artificial heart in a human being."

"I would be happy to talk with you about our animals," Olsen said. "I have nothing to do with clinical work on human beings." Robinson noted that Olsen had not denied a human implant was being planned. Maybe if he interviewed the veterinarian, he could confirm the report.

"Well, okay, but can I come to talk with you about the research work?" Robinson asked.

"Sure. Come ahead," Olsen responded.

Robinson first thought he had gone to the wrong office. The old St. Mark's building looked abandoned: an age-scarred structure left behind as people found happier homes elsewhere. He had to circle it to find the entrance into the animal barn. However, the bustle inside was astounding. Calves stood in cages with hoses connecting their implanted hearts to pneumatic drivers pulsing in an endless click-clack. Some calves placidly munched hay. One was stolidly walking on his treadmill exerciser. Smock-clad technicians monitored computers, checking minute by minute on the animals. It was all very high tech—with the definite smell of a dairy barn.

Robinson took the low-key approach reporters cultivate as an art—making the person being interviewed feel at ease. He was open, friendly, and interested. Olsen emphasized that he was a veterinarian, not a clinician, and that his expertise was limited to animal research. "Great," said Robinson. Walking the reporter around the lab, Olsen felt comfortable telling him about his work, even though he was conscious that Robinson periodically brought up the subject of human implants.

"Not my field," Olsen answered, citing the sensitivity around that subject. As the tour went on, however, he mentioned the human-implant application pending before the IRB. Robinson nodded without pressing the point.

The reporter also quizzed Jarvik, who showed him the J-7 heart he was working on, an electromechanical model that required only thin wires through the chest to an electrical source, instead of a bulky air compressor.

"Beautiful," said Robinson. Jarvik cautioned that as great as the possibilities appeared, the device was years away from full development. The calves' pneumatic units, however, were working now. Olsen and Jarvik also showed off an early model of a German-designed portable air-drive system no bigger than a woman's cosmetic case that was being tested. If successful, it would enable a patient to be untethered from the shopping-cart-sized heart driver for several hours.

Olsen mentioned that one possible use for the artificial heart was a prelude to a transplant, as Houston's Denton Cooley had done in 1969. As Robinson left, Olsen said congenially, "If you want an interview, and I am comfortable and am permitted to talk about it, I'll be glad to see you again."

Back in his office, Robinson began writing. The UPI's national desk in New York decided the story was important enough to carry on its A-wire transmission for the day's most significant news. The story it sent out on July 22, 1980, for release in the next morning's newspapers began,

> SALT LAKE CITY (UPI)—Doctors at the University of Utah say they are ready to implant a temporary mechanical heart in a human as a means of supporting life until a permanent transplant donor can be found.
>
> Dr. Donald B. Olsen, director of the university's Artificial Organs Laboratory, said Tuesday the school's human experimentation committee is considering an application by the surgeons to implant a polyurethane heart in a human. The patient has not been selected....

Arriving home at 8:00 PM that night, Olsen was stunned by the stack of telephone messages his wife, Joyce, had taken for him. Newspapers were calling from New York, San Francisco, Washington, Chicago, Los Angeles, and a dozen other cities, all asking for more details on the UPI story. Olsen called the UPI to talk with Robinson. He was gone for the day. "Then please read me the story," he asked. The first paragraph about the transplant potential relieved him. "At least he didn't mention the IRB," he told himself. When the reporter read the second paragraph, Olsen knew the roof had caved in. Aware of the IRB's determination to stay out of the media, he realized the gravity of what he had said. He desperately hoped that somehow it would not affect the application, but the anxiety would not go away.

When Van Leer came to work at 6:00 AM the following morning, the city-desk staff showed her the rival *Salt Lake Tribune*. The words "are ready" had been toned down to "are studying," but the *Tribune* had run the essence of the UPI dispatch on the top of its local news page. The usually mild-mannered Van

Leer had rarely been so angry. "How could the university do this?" she all but shouted. "I got zapped. I trusted them to call me."

An hour or so later, Jarvik phoned Van Leer. "I've seen the *Tribune*," he said. "Please, please, don't print that story." He knew the damage it could cause the heart application. That very afternoon the IRB subcommittee was convening for its first session on DeVries' latest proposal, and he was alarmed that the members would be annoyed by the publicity.

"You can't keep the lid on this anymore," Van Leer told Jarvik. She then wrote her own article. She reported, "The UPI account contained some errors." She also quoted a medical center spokesman as saying the story was premature.

That morning DeVries chastised Olsen for talking about the IRB. So did Jarvik. Kolff was gentler. From years of dealing with the media, he was well aware such things could happen. Nevertheless, the team's mood was glum as the members prepared to appear before the IRB. When they reached the conference room where the IRB subcommittee met, the frosty atmosphere chilled them. "This publicity is a precedent," said one member. "Never before have we had publicity about a proposal pending before us. Why did you do this? Were you trying to put pressure on us?"

Olsen asked to speak: "It was my fault; I take full blame. This reporter asked to talk about animal research. I revealed information I should not have. Because of the sensitive nature of the material, I thought my words were off the record. I had no intention of putting any pressure on you. I am indeed sorry."

Olsen felt sick. He prayed that his apology had softened some of the antagonism. For the rest of the meeting, the words just swirled around him. Committee member Dr. Ross Woolley reported that after the announcement in the press, the IRB had been hounded to open its meetings to the public. This seemed to be the only major problem that occurred after the premature announcement, and the university ignored it.

Witnessing the confrontation was Dr. Hiroshi Kuida, a professor of internal medicine and the medical center's chief of cardiology. Eichwald had great faith in him and had asked him to review the heart application. Kuida was curt. "I would approve the use of the device for only one class of patient," he said, specifying those who could not be weaned off the heart-lung machine. "You would have nothing to lose in using the artificial heart because the only other option is certain death." About DeVries's other two classifications, Kuida commented, "An implant is, in my view, not justified."

"What about using it temporarily in patients getting a transplant?" an IRB member asked.

"Ah," said Kuida, "There it would be reasonable to have it as an interim device for a patient who might otherwise die imminently. It could prolong life while a donor was being sought." Eichwald said it seemed to make sense to limit use of the heart to surgery patients. Others agreed. The consensus appeared to be that if DeVries insisted on his three-category pool of implant candidates, the application would be rejected.

Kolff saw the danger. "I remember that in Cleveland we had a research proposal that a committee was about to reject. I persuaded them to table our request so that it could be revised and brought back without the stigma of an earlier rejection. Can we table this application so Dr. DeVries can alter it?"

"We have no problem with that," said Eichwald. He appointed a small subcommittee to work with DeVries on making changes. Kolff left the room believing that they had made the best of a difficult situation.

He had more worries than the IRB, however. He was concerned the UPI story might poison the Washington wells he had been tapping for money from the NIH's NHLBI. Even though it funded much of the animal research, the institute had not been told of DeVries's application to the IRB because the university had no legal responsibility to do that. It seemed conceivable that bureaucrats could speculate that Kolff's team was doing an end run and diverting NIH money to experimental work on human implants.

An NIH Confrontation

Kolff had to mend fences. In June 1980, he had assured the IRB the heart was ready for implantation. Now a month later, he directed a letter to John T. Watson, the physiologist who headed the NHLBI's devices and technology department. Kolff wrote,

> *The unintentionally started publicity is mostly incorrect and regrettable. We are indeed talking with the Committee for Human Experimentation. We want [it] to take its time and advise us. We are not ready. NIH funds will not be used in any way. When the time comes, certainly not very soon, Kolff Associates, Inc., will donate the artificial heart and provide drive systems, etc. on loan.*[3]
>
> *We have no funds on any grant or contract for human experimentation. Of course we, and Kolff Associates, Inc., have benefited from previous and present NIH funding. Anything to be eventually used in human patients has been widely published and is available to the general public. It took me all day to quiet things down....*

He signed the letter, Pim.

Orchestrating the News

The press was like a pesky terrier nipping at the university's heels. "Is the story right?" national news and television reporters wanted to know. "What more can you tell us? When will the artificial heart be implanted?" It was clear that part of the drama was their amazement that such pioneering science was being done in Salt Lake City.

The university's first reaction was to stonewall the inquiries, downplaying the story and futilely hoping it would go away. Every day queries came to Pamela Fogle, who for several years had been the university science writer helping Kolff and his staff with public relations. She advised Kolff, "The longer we say 'no comment,' the more the interest will build. I think we have to call a press conference to clear the air."

The press had also been pestering the medical center's public-relations director, John Dwan, a Thurberish-looking ex-Marine. He agreed with Fogle that the press story had generated so much heat it would be impossible to avoid making some definite statements about the implant schedule. Kolff was not ready to do that. He arranged a meeting with Jarvik, Olsen, DeVries, and Fogle. Fogle again urged a press conference. Others disagreed. The discussion turned to brainstorming the questions the media was likely to ask and their possible answers.

Kolff said, "It would perhaps make a good impression on the press if we show off some of our hardware," meaning heart pumps and drivers. Several days later, he wrote Fogle, "I accept your suggestion for a press conference." He wanted, however, to orchestrate the responses to reporters and wrote a three-page scenario of questions and answers. Surgeons and their teams, for example, would not be identified. Why? He said they "would prefer to remain anonymous until well after the event to avoid pressure for publicity's sake." If anyone asked to interview the developer of the heart, the answer was that "we have many developers."

The answer to the question, "What kind of patient will get the heart?" should be, "He or she will be a person with an already failed or rapidly failing heart in an otherwise fairly healthy body. We shall not divulge the name of the patient. What the patient may choose to do after the event is, of course, his or her prerogative."

If questioned about the timing of a human implant, the reply should be, "First we must have [IRB] approval, and we cannot estimate when this will be, nor will we second-guess whether or not they will approve the proposal." Even after approval, the heart team had "many details" to work out prior to any surgery.

If reporters asked how long an implant patient would survive, the answer was, "This is a loaded question. On the basis of durability studies of our artificial heart, we can hope for one year. On the basis of animal studies, we can hope for six months. However, we cannot guarantee those numbers."

If asked, "Will the implant be temporary or permanent?" Kolff stated, "For a healthy person, survival of a few months to a year may seem a very short time. For the patient with imminent death as the only alternative, it may be a worthwhile venture that may allow him or her to settle affairs, to reconsider what his or her life was all about, and to set about enjoying life to the fullest."

As for the implant's impact on the patient's family, Kolff said that his experience with dialysis showed that "the family is always affected when one of its members has to live under more restricted conditions...in some [cases], the marriage broke up." Conversely, he indicated he knew that "some people testified that the years dependent on the artificial kidney were the happiest of their lives. Life is a precious gift, and not all of us realize it until we live on borrowed time; then we look at the world differently. It is our aim to prolong a life that will be enjoyable for the patient. A great deal will depend on us and a great deal on the patient. I think we shall each do our part."

Another milestone intervened, however, before the promised news conference materialized. In the late 1970s, a talented young engineer from Aachen, Germany—Horst Peter Heimes—had developed a portable heart driver. By 1980 it easily could maintain the driving pressures for a calf, but it did not yet have a redundant system. This was the driver that Jarvik had shown to UPI reporter Robinson.[4]

The Heimes driver was successful, at least on calves. On the sunshiny afternoon of August 12, 1980, a calf named Lawson made a brilliant, theatrical debut. He walked across the lawn outside the artificial-heart lab at the St. Mark's building with a number of fascinated newspeople attentively watching. By that time, Lawson had lived 104 days with an artificial heart. What excited the television cameramen and still photographers was that Lawson required no heavy air compressor to take his stroll.

"Impressive" was the review from the *Salt Lake Tribune* medical writer. And in truth it was a spectacular backdrop for the press conference Fogle had set up to satisfy the media's curiosity. Lawson was Exhibit A for the effect Kolff wanted to produce in the reporters, which he established by declaring, "We want to create happiness."

"When will the heart be ready for humans?" he was asked. Kolff said that was up to the IRB. That was not good enough for the reporters, who pressed him for

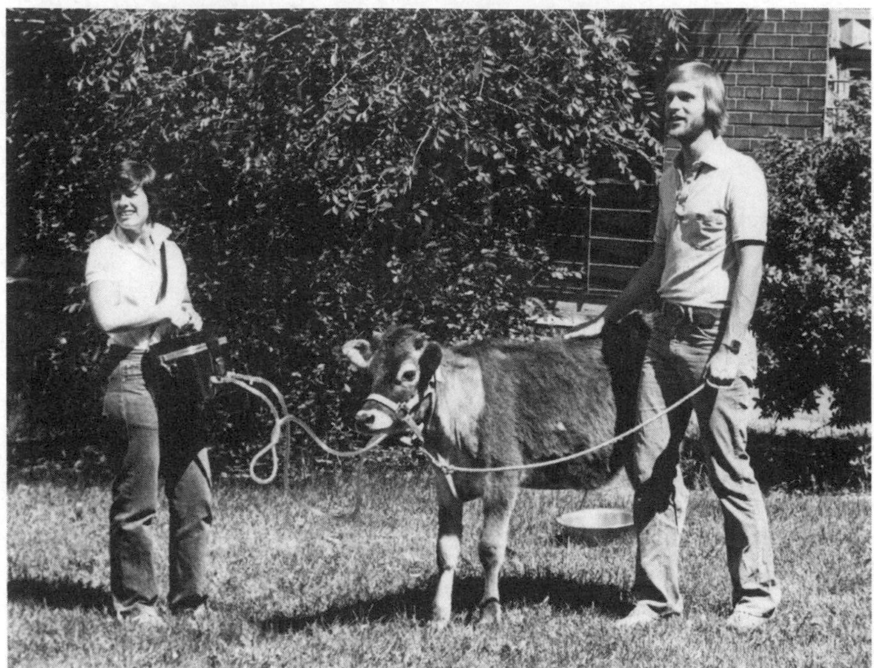

The calf Lawson with the portable driver invented by Peter Heimes.

more details. "A heart will not be ready tomorrow," he said, adding he would not be surprised if a human implant took place within a year.

Placating the Research Team

On the evening of the press conference, before any stories appeared, Kolff sat down to think of what the coming implant would mean to the staff whose long dedication had helped to make the operation possible. Concerned for them, he wrote the following:

> When the artificial heart will be implanted into a human recipient, the principal surgeon in charge is the one who takes the greatest risk to his career, the greatest part of the blame when things go wrong, but also the greatest publicity. It is this last part that I want you to ponder long before the time of the actual implantation.
>
> It may be very difficult for those of us who have worked so very long on the total artificial heart to accept that total publicity will be handled by the surgeon. His name will be flashed on the TV screens and over the news media. If some of us are mentioned it will be due to the surgeon's generosity of thinking of us at that moment.

> As you know, I have traveled very extensively during the last few years. If I enter a dialysis unit, which may treat 100 patients, part of them may still be treated with the type of coils (with minor modifications) that we ourselves devised. When I give my name to the head nurse, any of the technicians or any of the younger physicians, you can be quite certain nobody has the vaguest idea that I had something to do with the artificial kidney when they were still in the cradle.
>
> What I want to warn you about is that you may not like the way the publicity is going to be handled. Some of this may be inevitable, some of this may be unjust and none of it is done with any particular design towards hurting you. Our main reward must be to know that we have done our best and that in time patients will be saved who are now doomed and they will be saved through our efforts. Think about this, discuss it with me if you want to and let us bear our fate with understanding.

Despite the many problems he had experienced getting the artificial heart to the point of human use, Kolff was satisfied that it would be a success and his years of hard work and persistence were coming to fruition.

The IRB Makes a Decision

The IRB subcommittee accepted only the pool of five thousand patients DeVries had identified in his third group, limiting him to postsurgery patients who could not be weaned from the heart-lung machine. On September 10, 1981, the FDA approved the Utah application and authorized implant of the artificial heart in seven patients.

Several patients in University Hospital agreed and signed the consent form before undergoing heart surgery. But from November 1981 through April 1982, all cardiac-surgery patients who signed the consent form survived surgery, and their natural hearts were started after the procedure. In April 1982, the IRB received an addendum requesting that the team be allowed to expand the protocol to include patients with end-stage cardiomyopathy.

Coincidently, a flurry of media reports on the board's activities was spurred by the appeal of a thirty-eight-year-old Florida man who wished to be the first patient to receive the artificial heart. He was represented by a flamboyant attorney who had ready access to the media. He made considerable demands on the university in general and the IRB specifically. After all the hoopla, the sick man did not meet the university's requirements, and the search went on.[5]

Notes

1. In between, Jarvik had designed a J-6 heart, but it was very rough, so only one model was made, and then the heart was abandoned.
2. Theodore Roosevelt, "Strenuous Life," speech given to the Hamilton Club, Chicago, Illinois, April 10, 1899.
3. Over the years, Kolff occasionally formed small companies with the permission of the university to market some of the products developed in his lab. Kolff Associates, Inc., dealt with the artificial heart.
4. By 1984 the portable Heimes driver was successfully used with the second patient implanted after Barney Clark—William Schroeder.
5. There were, of course, detractors all along the way. On October 19, 1982, nearly two months before Barney Clark's surgery, the then-president of the Utah State Medical Association, Dr. Robert G. Wilson, criticized Dr. John Bosso, the chair of the Utah IRB, in a letter:

    Dear Dr. Bosso:

    As President of the Utah State Medical Association, I hear voiced by increasing numbers of physicians grave concern over the implantation of an artificial heart in a human. Also, I have deep personal reservations and have for some time wished to speak out on this issue.

    I realize that the procedure to be done has gone through what you feel to be an exhaustive examination by members of your Review Board, surgeons and others at the University of Utah Medical Center and even ethicists. However, I feel for many reasons that the conclusions, which were reached, were wrong.

    The implications of costs have not been properly addressed. Looking back on renal dialysis, were we able to turn back the clock and stop dialysis before it was ever thrust upon the public, we would not be in the dilemma of having to make the unpleasant decisions that may be made in the very near future. Certainly the impact of an artificial heart and the directions it will lead us will have even greater consequences upon society and its ability to pay for all the medical care it thinks it deserves. My point simply is this: if we don't speak up now, it will be too late to speak up after the first procedure has been done....

    Sincerely yours

    Robert G. Wilson, M.D., President

14

Exploring the Backgrounds of Key People

The summer before the Kolffs came to Utah, I loaded trucks on the swing shift. That was real hard work, but it was kind of interesting because I met lots of people. I remember one man who was an intelligent guy. I asked him what he was going to do when he graduated from school.

He said, "I have a nice job, a nice car, a nice apartment, a nice girlfriend. What else is there in life?"

I was quite shocked. Before then I had never been so aware of my ambitions. It surprised me to see, all of a sudden, that I was a bit different than the average guy. I have a little more drive than the average guy. I have been that way all my life.

—William DeVries

Creating a team to implant the first artificial heart in a human being posed particular challenges for Dr. Kolff. The people chosen had to have not only exceptional medical and technical talents but also believe in the experiment.

The Heart Surgeon

A rawboned, twenty-three-year-old freshman named Bill DeVries was just months into his first year at the University of Utah's School of Medicine when his anatomy instructor, noting his aptitude, said, "You should think about going into academic, rather than clinical, surgery."

DeVries was aware that university doctors not only cared for patients but also taught and did research. "That's a good idea," he said. Later in the year, the instructor repeated his suggestion. "I have kind of got it in the back of my mind to do that," DeVries answered.

However, telling a medical-school senior about the conversation, DeVries asked, "How do you go about doing that?" The senior counseled him to hook himself to a star: "Associate yourself with somebody famous in the medical school who can help you. Work really hard for him. A strong letter of recommendation is invaluable."

DeVries wondered where he could find someone who met those criteria. Picking up a copy of the student newspaper, his senior friend pointed to a story about the noted Dr. Willem J. Kolff speaking that afternoon to medical students. "This guy has come to Utah. Why don't you go talk with him?" he suggested.

DeVries went to Kolff's talk and was fascinated by his report on artificial organs. Afterward he told Kolff, "I am a medical student here. I would like to work for you."

"What's your name?"

"DeVries."

"That's a good Dutch name. You're hired," Kolff said.

DeVries was surprised. He did not know that before the lecture, a professor had told Kolff, "We have a freshman named DeVries. Excellent student. He'd make you a good summer worker."

Some twenty-five years earlier, DeVries's father, Henry, had emigrated with his family from Holland to Grand Rapids, Michigan. He was fifteen, tall, and had a clump of sandy hair. Henry was one of eight children. "We can afford for only the young ones to go to school," his father said. "To help support us, you and your older sister have to work." Though he knew only Dutch, French, German, and Flemish, Henry got a job in a print shop, where he learned English setting type.

Henry's quiet demeanor hid fierce ambition. Determined to become a surgeon, he graduated from college and then got his medical degree from the University of Michigan. He did his internship at Salt Lake City's LDS Hospital, where he met a nurse named Cathryn Castle. A tall, California redhead, she had a friendly personality that bubbled with an Irish sense of humor. Known as Kay, she liked to think of herself as fun loving and independent. She thought Henry DeVries was sober and serious—and he was eleven years older. He was a Baptist; she was a Mormon.

In March 1942, they married. "Why?" a friend asked.

"Because," she answered, "I never met anyone with his kind of dedication." Their son, William Castle DeVries, was born on December 19, 1943, in the hospital for the Brooklyn Navy Yard. Henry's enlistment in the military had taken the couple to Brooklyn. Henry saw his son through the nursery glass only once before he shipped out to the South Pacific aboard the destroyer *USS Kalk*. On June 12, 1944, off New Guinea, a Japanese bomber dropped out of the sky to make a direct hit on the *Kalk*'s torpedo tubes. Twenty-two enlisted men and four officers were killed, including Lt. Henry DeVries. That night, as the *Kalk* limped to port, DeVries's father was buried at sea.

During his first three years in Salt Lake City, young Bill grew up among women—his mother, his widowed grandmother, and a young aunt. "It's terrible," his mother told them. "He's got no father, no grandfather—just a lot of us."

"I know a wonderful man for you," a babysitter told her. "He's a widower and has this nice little girl he's raising."

"Not interested," Kay said. "I've too much to do." She was getting a teaching degree at the university. But later on, she changed her mind. The man was Donald Nuttall, manager of a large supermarket and a Mormon. The two of them had the same sense of humor, shared the same interests. A date was taking his daughter and her son to the zoo or to play tennis in Liberty Park. When he saw Nuttall, little Bill always ran to hold onto his leg.

After Kay and Donald were married, the family moved to Preston, Idaho, where Bill entered school. He was the tallest in his class and probably the shyest. "I'm concerned, Mrs. Nuttall," his first-grade teacher said. "I know Bill reads very well, but he won't read in the group. I can't get two words out of him."

So the class was flabbergasted during a "sharing time" when Bill held up his hand to talk. Pointing across the street to a hospital, he said, "My mother's over there having a baby. When I left home, her pains were five minutes apart. That means she was contracting. The baby will be born sometime today. We hope it is a girl. And my father is coming over to tell me when the baby is born." After that unexpected start, Bill participated in class talks every day.

When he was a third-grader, another teacher called. "Bill has a little bit of a problem," she said. "His name is DeVries, and yours is Nuttall. The kids ask why, and he can't come up with an explanation. Do you have anything of his father's that he can bring to school and talk about?"

Kay dug out an old scrapbook, which Bill took to school. He explained, "This is a picture of my father. His name was DeVries, and he was a doctor, and he was killed." He showed the children a picture of the destroyer *Kalk* and his father's Purple Heart. They never asked about his name again.

Kay and Donald talked about his adopting Bill and even consulted a lawyer. However, adoption meant they would have to forgo the small federal pension that Kay had been putting into a trust fund for her son. Besides, she said, "The DeVries family loves and adores Bill. I can't take the name away from him. I'll accept the little social inconveniences—like people calling him Bill Nuttall and me Kay DeVries."

When people asked Bill what he wanted to do, he had no doubts: "Be a doctor." Kay told him that his father had practiced to be a surgeon by wrapping thread around his thigh and tying and untying knots, so Bill sat in the kitchen manipulating knots as his father had done to make his fingers nimble. He was still only eight or nine when the family dog and parakeet became his patients. Pretending they had leg wounds, he strapped on bandages over and over.

Bill liked to work with his hands. Planting himself on the floor, he used a razor blade to slice balsam wood for model airplanes. Tired of the blueprints he left strewn about, his mother told him, "If you don't pick them up now, I'm putting them in the wastebasket and taking them to the dump." He refused and went out to play.

When he came home, the floor was clean. "Where are my drawings?" he asked. Told they were at the town dump, he walked three miles to root among the trash until he found most of them.

"He's determined," Kay told Donald. "If he gets something in his mind, right or wrong, he's going to do it."

After the family moved to Ogden, Bill announced he was "running away"—but not too far. He pitched his tent in the nearby hills, picking a spot where his mother could see him every time she glanced out the kitchen window. Kay sensed that he imagined slights from others and then brooded about them.

He definitely had his own sense of morality. When Bill was in junior high school, he needed only one more merit badge to become an Eagle Scout. A friend told him he had earned his badge by lying. Bill decided, "I'm not going to do this. I'm not going to finish." His attitude was, "If you can get something by cheating, who wants it?"

After a week, his mother said, "You're only hurting yourself by quitting. It's inconceivable that you'd work this hard for this long and not finish."

Bill went to talk to his Mormon bishop. Returning, he told his mother, "I'm going to do it."

He built ten birdhouses of various sizes, strung them in the hills, put out seed, and tracked birds for a week. He became an Eagle Scout and was proud of his achievement.

Bill was not one to follow the leader. He did not have a big gang of friends. Rather, he had two or three close pals, and he was the leader. He was not an outstanding student but did well in science. He loved sports. In a field near his home, he dug a pit, persuaded Donald to fill it with sawdust, then added standards and a crossbar—a practice run for high jumping. He could set his own goals and break his own records.

His high-school coaches concentrated on sprinters, so Bill bought a book to teach himself to jump. Every morning at 6:00 AM, he was on the field running and jumping. He had a gangly grace. When he uncoiled from his usual slump, he was six feet, three inches tall and growing. One year the track team voted him the "most improved athlete," and the next, "the most outstanding." He won the Utah state championship with jumps that set a record for that season's high-school track competitors.

Bill's athletic skill won him a scholarship to the University of Utah. He thought about playing basketball, but the coaches did not think he was aggressive enough, and he recognized that he did not have "the killer instinct." He used the trust fund his mother had saved to pay the rest of his college expenses, including joining a fraternity. During his first year, he gave his books no more than a passing glance. His C grades reflected his nonchalance.

Anne Karen Olsen was in his chemistry class. She was ambitious and studious and tall like Bill; they both had eyes as blue green as the sea. Through the year, he kept hanging around her, and they began dating. Pointing downtown to the Mormon Temple one night, he announced, "One day we'll be married there."

Karen laughed, but then Bill did something that really impressed her: he changed from a mediocre student to a superior one. That indicated he had qualities she had not suspected. They were married on June 12, 1966, during their senior year of college. Later, they were sealed in the temple, just as he had predicted.

The professor interviewing DeVries for admission to the University of Utah's School of Medicine asked what he would do if he was not chosen. "Be a basketball player," he said. The professor was startled. DeVries could afford to be flippant because the prestigious George Washington School of Medicine in Washington, DC, had already accepted him. But when Utah accepted him, he decided to stay. He was western born and bred and would feel more at home among the mountains.

DeVries commented after the Barney Clark surgery:

> If I were to die right now, I would say, 'Sure, it's been hard, but I am doing what I like to do. . . .' I have a great deal of drive to get things done right, and I have a lot of goals I have not reached, but I see them on the horizon. . . . [My goals are] to build this practice up, to get a fantastic teaching

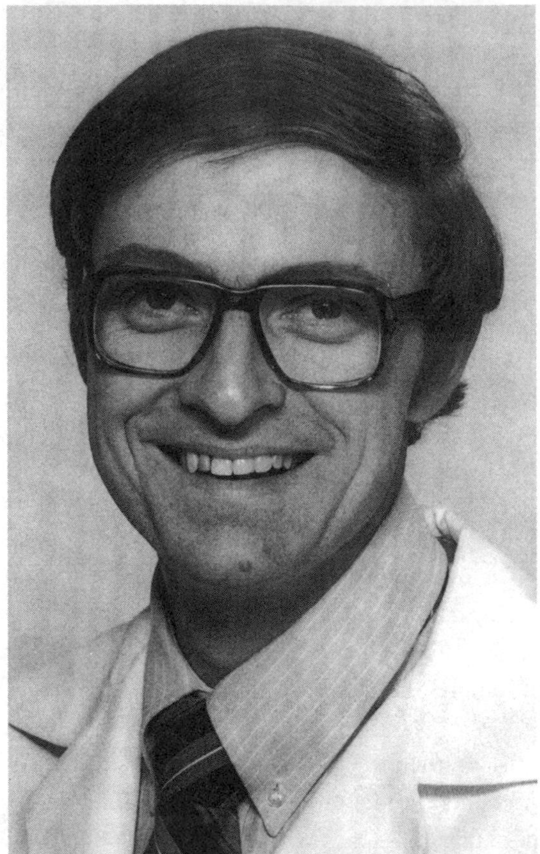

Before he came to Utah, Dr. Lyle Joyce was convinced that artificial hearts were not feasible.

> [position] to do research here, and have people come into the hospital and really rely on being treated better than anywhere in the world; and to walk into a room and have a patient say 'I am glad you are my doctor; you are going to take care of me. I have no question in my mind that you will do the best.'[1]

The New Surgical Faculty Member

In 1980 a new faculty member joined DeVries on the staff at the University of Utah Medical Center. Dr. Lyle Joyce had brown hair and large brown eyes, wore horn-rimmed glasses, and stood five feet, ten inches tall. With his pleasant, open manner, he made friends quickly. Patients found it easy to confide in him. He had a keen sense of how to organize himself and reach his goals. Step-by-step, he was advancing to a dream he had nourished for most of his life.

Joyce grew up on a farm near the small town of Plainview tucked into Nebraska's northeastern corner. As a youth, he heard radio reports about the heart-surgery feats of Houston's Dr. Michael DeBakey. The thought that doctors could put scalpels and needles into the human heart excited him. "That is what I want to do," he decided. Typically he did not waste time fantasizing about his new ambition. It was something he was going to do. He simply had to get ready to do it.

In Plainview High School, Joyce was the all-American boy: clean-cut, the best student in his class, and a pole-vaulter. He loved the farm, especially because it revolved around livestock. His father was often his own veterinarian, and Joyce learned much about medicine from helping him treat animal illnesses and do autopsies. His practical outlook and mechanical skills served him well when he later got involved with the artificial heart.

His family depended on each member working on the farm, but his parents encouraged him to explore other options. Leaving the farm would break a family tradition that extended all the way back to England, but in the fall of his senior year in high school, Joyce told the superintendent, Eugene Lavender, that he wanted to be a surgeon. Lavender advised the boy to look for the far horizon: to "go for the gold." "Lyle, you've got only one limit—your own ambition and your willingness to sacrifice to achieve it. What you want to do, you can do," he told his student.

Joyce told Lavender that he had been thinking about going to the University of Nebraska in Lincoln.

"You've been telling me about Dr. DeBakey's program in Texas," said Lavender. "If you're serious about going into cardiac surgery, why not go to an area nearby to train? How about DeBakey's school, Baylor University?"

"My family could never afford it," Joyce responded.

"There are ways to get around that, but first you should take a look, see if you like it," Lavender said.

That Christmas Eve, in the middle of a blizzard that piled three feet of snow on the roads, Joyce, his mother, and his sister started off on the nine-hundred-mile drive to Baylor University in Waco, Texas. After battling snowdrifts, Joyce was incredulous to discover shirtsleeve weather. "I don't care what kind of a study program they've got here," he said to his mother. "This climate is for me."

Baylor had a special program for its best and brightest students—the top 1 percent—and it accepted the Nebraska farm boy into this elite class. With a scholarship, he could attend Baylor for less money than he would pay at the University of Nebraska. In his premed program, he concentrated on science, always focusing on being a heart surgeon. In the summer between his junior and senior years, he got an extraordinary opportunity to work in DeBakey's experimental lab at the Baylor College of Medicine in Houston.

That was his introduction to artificial-heart research, and it was disappointing. As an operating-room (OR) orderly, he assisted surgeons Michael DeBakey and Domingo Liotta as they implanted artificial hearts and ventricular-assist devices in calves. Often he stayed up all night babysitting the animals. He felt discouraged that nearly all of the calves died soon after the implants. Joyce went back to Waco that fall, full of doubts that artificial-heart technology would ever reach the stage of human implantation. He forgot about that while he concentrated on finishing his undergraduate work.

That year he met Tina Farr, a pretty, dark-haired Baylor coed, who often had prayed that "God will take me to the right person." In Joyce she found someone with whom she could share her innermost thoughts. Slowly but surely, she decided that "Lyle is the one."

Joyce was a Methodist. He told Tina, "I'll become a Baptist like you if you become a Republican like me." They were married in 1970. Even before Joyce received his medical degree, the couple agreed that they wanted to help others. They spent a summer in Bangalore, India, running a clinic and helping build a new hospital. Joyce completed a residency and earned a PhD in surgery at the University of Minnesota, a school noted for its innovative cardiac operations. That spurred hope that he, too, would someday be part of trailblazing surgery.

When it came time for his cardiovascular residency, Joyce was particular. He was looking for a place with a heavy surgery schedule. He called and asked residents in various medical centers around the country how many coronary bypasses and valve replacements they did in a year. To his surprise, the University of Utah reported three to four times more than the others. When Joyce was skeptical, his contact explained that Salt Lake's major hospitals cooperated to give cardiothoracic residents work in three facilities with many different doctors. Joyce decided Salt Lake City was the place for him. He reported to DeVries, who told him of the weekly animal surgeries. "I'd like to see those," Joyce said.

In the St. Mark's Hospital building, Joyce was surprised by the sophisticated technique the Utah group had pioneered for implantations and the way the calves were cared for after surgery. This was much better than his experience in the Baylor lab. He saw numerous calves that were surviving, some even exercising on a treadmill. As he looked at the survival records, he realized his earlier conclusions about using artificial hearts in human beings had been wrong. With renewed enthusiasm, he became convinced that human implantation was imminent. He kept working with DeVries and Olsen on animal surgeries, sharpening his skills, knowing he wanted to be around when the artificial heart went into a human chest.

It was clear by 1981 that the team at Utah was ready for the first human implant. DeVries was the only surgeon at the university trained to do such an implant. He clearly needed an associate to share the workload to accomplish such a remarkable feat. Joyce turned down offers from several other programs in the country to join DeVries on staff.

The Joyces had three children by the time they arrived in Utah, and Tina was pregnant with their fourth during the Barney Clark implant. Their lives were about to change.

The Heart Innovator

In the fall of 1971, a surgical-supply-company executive telephoned Kolff. "I've got this very bright young researcher. I think you can use him in your lab. If you hire him, we'll pay ten thousand dollars toward his salary."

"Not interested," Kolff told the executive.

The young researcher was astounded. It was unthinkable that anyone would reject that kind of an offer. Curious and a little irritated, he called Kolff directly. "Do you remember who I am?" he asked.

Kolff replied, "Yes, I remember you, and I think you should go back to Italy and finish medical school."

"I don't want to do that. I want to work for you."

"Well, tell me more about yourself. Do you have a car?"

"Yes."

"Well, what kind is it?"

That seemed a strange line of questioning, but the researcher answered, "A Volvo."

That was also Kolff's car, but he only replied, "Oh?" After a pause, he said, "Just a minute. I see my administrator through the window." The young man was encouraged, but Kolff was actually discussing something else with his administrator.

Returning to the phone, Kolff inquired, "What's the lowest amount you think you can live on?"

"One hundred a week" was the reply.

"Fine. Come to Salt Lake." The figure suited Kolff nicely. It was about half of what the company executive had offered. The remaining five thousand dollars could be applied to general lab expenses.

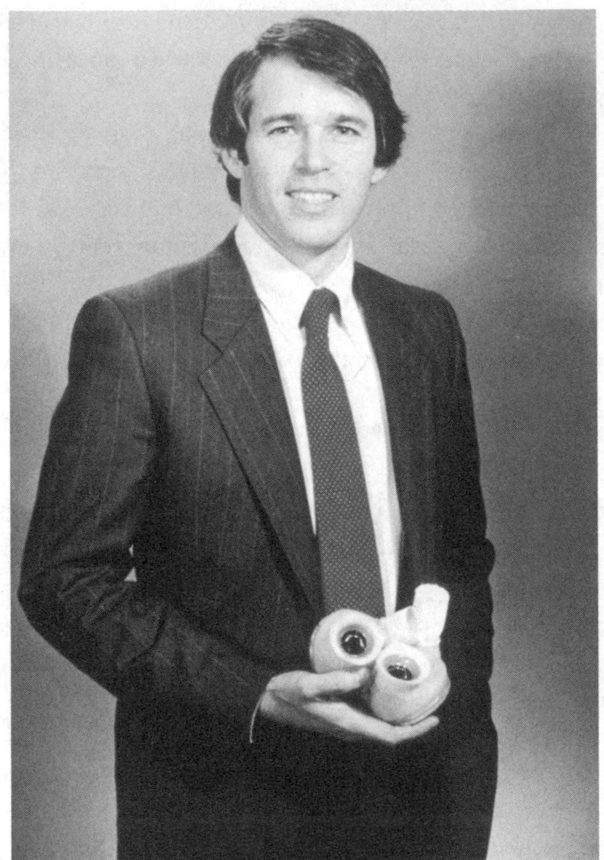

Robert Jarvik helped overcome numerous technical challenges to design a heart that could be used in a human patient.

However, things did not work out that way. After the researcher was hired and already working, Kolff heard again from the executive. "I'm sorry. The board will not pay the young man's salary," he said. "I'm afraid you'll have to cover it." This was Kolff's introduction to Robert K. Jarvik.

Jarvik was twenty-five and thin with arresting blue eyes. His diction was unmistakably New England. He liked to play the role of the challenger, someone who had to be convinced. Before Jarvik accepted an idea, he wrestled with it. He asked, "Who says that's right? Why should I believe it?"

Jarvik was born in Michigan and grew up in a comfortable Connecticut home, the third and youngest child of a successful physician. In preschool he was something of a loner. As a preteen, he thought most of the family talk focused on his siblings. He hung out with his brother's friends and felt older than he was.

Some days he was aware he had few friends of his own. That bothered him, but he comforted himself by saying, "I'm just like my brother's friends."

When the family sailed in his father's boat to the restored whaling village at Mystic, Connecticut, Jarvik wandered among the craft shops, watching men use lathes to build model ships. He was intrigued that one man spent three years carving a model from a beef bone. He saved his money to buy a lathe to shape a "Jarvik ship."

Periodically he went to the local hospital to watch his father operate. He noticed how repetitive it was to clamp tissue and sew one stitch at a time. He thought, "There must be a better way." His answer was a stapling gun, and he began sketching one.

Jarvik was interested in art and began studying architecture at Syracuse University. After a time, he switched to premed. He received poor marks because he did poorly in the final exam. He was irritated he received no credit for his innovative work. In his junior year, he went back to art. He wanted to take a course in making jewelry but lacked the prerequisites, so he rigged the class computer cards to qualify. He excused himself by declaring, "The prerequisites aren't cricket, either."

At Syracuse Jarvik met Elaine Levin, the daughter of a government economist and a middle-level Pentagon supervisor. A vivacious brunette, Elaine had one date with him and no interest in another. Eighteen months later, while she was waiting for a bus, a student with the saddest possible excuse for a beard approached her. "Remember me?" he asked. He prompted, "Rob Jarvik." For some reason, the wistful attempt at a beard made him more attractive.

When Jarvik and Elaine became engaged, it was not enough for him just to give her a ring. On a trip to Alaska, he panned for gold nuggets. He engraved his name, not hers, on the ring, explaining, "That's the Italian custom."

When Jarvik was a senior, he began applying to medical schools. He found one that would admit him in Bologna, Italy. The day after their marriage in 1968, the couple flew off on their Italian adventure. Bologna, a famous medical school, had a tradition dating back for centuries: class attendance was not required. At the term's end, the faculty quizzed each student in Italian while classmates sat listening. The only grades were pass or fail. Although he did not attend class very often, Jarvik passed.

Jarvik actually was concerned by his lack of concentration in studying. At one point, he built a device that locked him in his chair so he could not get up until Elaine released him. About the only result, she decided, was that "as long as he was in the chair, I had to wait on him." To help him remember medical terms, they composed songs to stamp the elusive words in his brain.

Because they could always tap their families, the young Jarviks were not church-mouse poor. They did, however, try to live within a meager budget. Jarvik made uncomfortable furniture from orange crates, padding, and vinyl. Splitting a fifty-lira candy bar was a big event.

Jarvik was technically enrolled at Bologna in 1970 though in fact he was in New York, still hopeful an American medical school would accept him. In two years, he was turned down twenty-five times, including a rejection from the University of Utah. However, he learned that the U.S. Public Health Service was offering fellowships in biomechanical engineering. "I can do that," he told Elaine. He was right. Fellowship in hand, he enrolled at New York University.

He devoted hours to designing the surgical stapling tool he had envisioned years earlier. He navigated the red tape of patenting it and began to think he might have a career creating surgical instruments. He took his stapler to a surgical-supply house, hoping to market it. The device did not fit the firm's products, but Jarvik connected with the executive to whom he talked. He had gone through similar frustrations before finally being admitted to medical school.

"Applying to schools as an out-of-state student hurts your chances because the lion's share of admissions goes to local students," he told Jarvik. "Think about moving. Maybe go to Utah. There's a fellow out there that I know. Once you're there, you can apply as a resident to the medical school." He then made the telephone call that resulted in Kolff hiring Jarvik.

In their first meeting, Kolff outlined some of the problems the lab was going through, showing Jarvik various heart designs. Jarvik looked at the dome shape of the Kwan-Gett heart and was puzzled. "Who says an artificial heart has to be round?" he asked.

The Veterinarian

Don Bert Olsen was accused of having tunnel vision when he focused solely on a dairy-cattle practice when he was in veterinary school at Colorado State University. Dr. Rue Jensen, who taught pathology and later became the dean, advised him that research was far more fulfilling than veterinary practice. Olsen was not convinced.

Olsen was born on April 2, 1930, the first child of Bert Hansen Olsen, who had been born in Manti, Utah, on July 1, 1907. The senior Olsen became an underground miner in Bingham, Utah. He married Doris Bodell on May 28, 1929. The Great Depression became so severe that all the mines closed, so with three children, the couple moved onto a farm with Bert's parents in Axtell, Utah.

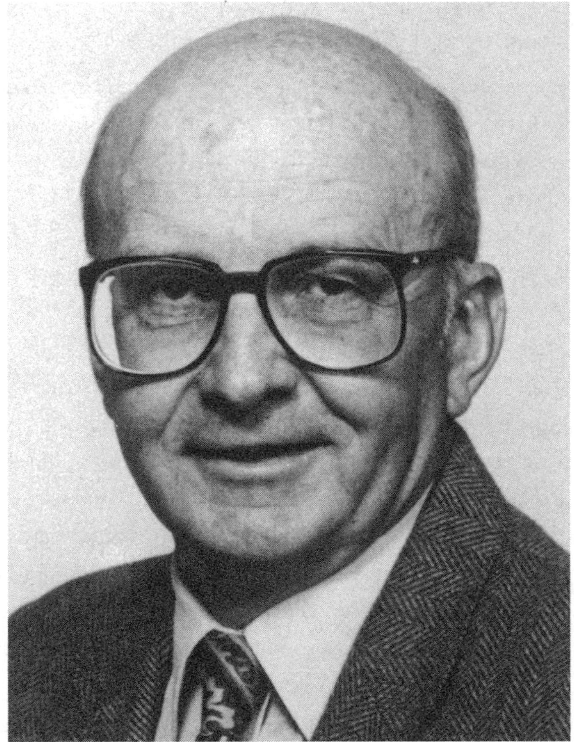

Adding Dr. Don Olsen, a veterinarian, to the Utah team was a great boost to the extensive animal experimentation.

There they could raise a garden and some pigs, chickens, and cows to feed their family. After the Depression ended, Bert returned to the mines.

Don was in the third grade when his father contracted silicosis, known as miner's lung. Bert was informed that he should get out of the mines permanently or face dying a miserable death. The Olsens and their children—now four—moved to another farm in Axtell in 1938. Trying to survive on a small, irrigated farm on the fringe of the Great American Desert presented many challenges, including limited water for irrigation, no culinary water, and no electricity.

At that time, all farm work was done with horses. Bert was clearly prouder of Don when his son learned to drive farm equipment with four head of horses than when he later received his first degree from Utah State Agricultural College. Even though he missed a great deal of school, Don was the first boy from Axtell to graduate from Gunnison High School in seven years, excelling in agriculture classes; most of the Axtell students dropped out of school to work.

For three years, Don tested the milk from all the family cows (as many as twenty-five, all milked by hand) for butterfat. For his diligence, the Future Farmers of America awarded a purebred, registered heifer calf and a state farmer's degree to Don. He also judged dairy cattle in competitions with other students from rural schools at county fairs, the Utah State Fair in Salt Lake City, and Utah State Agricultural College in Logan.

Bert offered to help his son purchase a neighbor's farm so they could share farm equipment and build a grade-A milking barn, but Don preferred to attend college. His high-school vocational-agriculture teacher applied for a scholarship sponsored by Sears, Roebuck & Company to Utah State Agricultural College.

It was a bashful farm boy who boarded the bus for Logan. Registration day was terrifying. So many people scurried from one line to another that he was completely lost. Olsen had decided years before that he wanted to become a veterinarian, so he searched for the Veterinary Science building just beyond Professor Caine's dairy herd. He approached Dr. Wayne Binns and asked for help. Binns recognized a farm boy who was completely out of his element and helped Olsen select the appropriate courses. Later, Binns served as his advisor. The least traumatic step for Olsen was paying his tuition with the letter from Sears Roebuck.

Olsen had never studied so much and so hard. In high school, assignments had boundaries within which one learned, but in college there were no boundaries. Assignments were open-ended, and the entire subject had to be studied. He learned in bacteriology that there were many types and they could produce a wide variety of diseases. That made him wonder how the Olsen family, dipping water from an untreated irrigation ditch twenty miles downstream from a reservoir, had survived.

Olsen married vivacious, blonde Joyce Cronquist on June 30, 1950. Joyce was the daughter of the owner of a large dairy farm in Cache Valley. His grades went up nearly a point after their wedding in the Logan Temple of The Church of Jesus Christ of Latter-day Saints.

After graduation from veterinary school in June 1956, Olsen set up a practice specializing in dairy cattle, but after five years, he remembered the advice of Dr. Jensen, his former dean, about going into research because it was much more rewarding. He made a decision that would transform his future in ways he could not imagine.

In 1962 Olsen moved on to a more challenging career in research at the University of Nevada, Reno, where he studied diseases that impacted Nevada's sheep and cattle industries. He was on a team with Dr. George Smith, a pathologist, and Lester McKay, an engineer; they received a large grant from the Fleischmann Foundation to establish a laboratory for environmental pathophysiology. The lab received subsequent research grants from both the American Heart Association and the NIH.

The major equipment in the laboratory was a cinefluoroscopy X-ray unit that was used by some of the doctors at Washoe Medical Center. Human patients were bundled up and brought on a gurney through the rose garden and into the animal laboratory in the morning before animal experiments began. The local hospital had no cinefluoroscopy equipment for those patients.

Olsen had some interesting adventures at the University of Nevada. Dr. James Anderson, a practicing cardiologist and chair of the University of Nevada's Board of Regents, and Smith, Olsen's research partner, were anxious to initiate a two-year medical school at the university. To promote the school, Anderson, Smith, and Olsen were invited to the Desert Inn in Las Vegas, where they visited the offices of eccentric multimillionaire Howard Hughes. Noah Dietrich, Hughes's executive administrator, came in, exchanged a few pleasantries, and then exited. After a short time, he returned and presented the group with a twenty-five-million-dollar check signed by Hughes!

Hughes had a motive for donating such a large sum for a two-year medical school on the Reno campus. The previous owners of the Desert Inn had wanted Hughes to move out of his suite on the top floor of the hotel so they could rent it to high-rolling gamblers. To solve the problem, Hughes purchased the hotel. As the new owner, he had to obtain a Nevada gaming license. Never in the history of the state had the gambling commissioners issued a gaming license without the applicant appearing personally for extensive interviews. For Hughes an appearance was out of the question since he had become severely reclusive. After his magnificent donation to the University of Nevada, Hughes received several licenses for his many casinos without once having to appear before the gambling commission.

Kolff employed Olsen as a consultant in 1967 to solve the problem of sheep dying on the OR table while being implanted with artificial hearts. He offered to hire Olsen full time, but Olsen had an NIH postdoctoral fellowship at the University of Colorado School of Medicine. He then planned to return to the University of Nevada as a vice president for research. However, this first foray into the Utah artificial-heart program seemed to portend that he would become, peripherally at least, part of the bellwether implant team.

Surgery at the University of Utah

Their consultation arrangement continued for four years until Olsen joined Kolff's team full time in 1972. He was given an appointment as an assistant professor in the Department of Surgery in the University of Utah's School of Medicine. His first assignment was to act as a scribe during animal implants, recording data for each step of the procedure. He was responsible for the postoperative management of the artificial-heart recipients, animals that up to that point had rarely survived more than a few hours, and also conducted autopsies on all the animals.

One day in 1973, Kolff invited Olsen to lunch. He announced that his current Dutch surgeon, Dr. Jay Volder, would be returning to Holland and Olsen was to become the implant surgeon. Olsen argued that he was neither a medical doctor nor a cardiothoracic surgeon, but Kolff refused to listen to him, stating that Olsen had implanted one artificial heart successfully and that the Utah team believed he would succeed. Olsen became the implant surgeon at the University of Utah in the fall of 1973.

The Founding of Kolff Associates, Inc.

When Kolff was invited to Utah, the university's president told him that if he wanted to start small companies, the university would be happy to help him. In 1976 Kolff wanted to begin an artificial-heart company called Kolff Associates, Inc., and he called a meeting in Building 518 after work to announce his plan to all of the artificial-heart workers. As he canvassed the room, the comments were very positive in favor of a new, for-profit company.

Olsen, however, reminded the group that the Jarvik artificial heart was not theirs to sell. He remembered signing an employment agreement stating that any and all inventions were assigned to the university as the sole owner. He stated that Kolff Associates would have to license or obtain permission or rights from the University of Utah to market the heart and other equipment.

Kolff was upset. "Of course it is our heart and heart driver," he protested. "We built them with money from grants from the NIH and other contributions. Of course they are ours to market." Olsen's objection resulted in his being offered many fewer shares of the one-penny stock than others in the group.

The Utah-developed artificial heart and pneumatic driver were sold to laboratories around the world. Olsen was the chief salesperson and deliveryman, and he trained research teams to implant the hearts and operate the equipment. The Kolff Associates' Board of Directors was appointed with Kolff as chair. Other board members included Dr. Jack Kolff, Lee Smith, Robert Jarvik, Clifford Kwan-Gett, and Olsen.

Years later, in April 1982, Jarvik set up meetings with potential investors. The name of the company was changed to Kolff Medical, Inc. Jarvik felt the new name would facilitate fund-raising through stock sales. Prior to investing, company representatives came to Utah to complete due-diligence studies. The group met with board members and announced that Kolff Medical did not own the artificial heart and related equipment that it had been selling over the years—exactly what Olsen had told Kolff Associates. Kolff Medical licensed the technology from the university, and Jarvik and Kolff met with the due-diligence team for many hours.

Jarvik later met with Olsen and reported that the due-diligence team felt that Olsen did not have adequate founders' stock and stock options. They recommended that he be given much more stock to ensure he remained a member of Kolff Medical. He received several thousand additional shares before the investors agreed to participate. However, Olsen informed Jarvik that the additional shares did not necessarily buy his support for Jarvik's plans.

The first investors were the Humana Audubon Hospital in Louisville, Kentucky; Hospital Corporation of America (HCA) in Nashville, Tennessee; and a medical group from Miami, Florida. Warburg Pincus, represented by Rodman Moorhead, was the only nonmedical corporate investor.

A few weeks later, Jarvik announced that the financial security of the laboratory was established. He had sold three contracts for a million dollars each to train surgical teams from the three investing hospitals to implant the Utah artificial heart in human patients. The three teams would come to train in the laboratory each month over the course of a year.

The training arrangement created additional animosity between Olsen and Jarvik. Olsen was furious and accused Jarvik of completely destroying the future of Kolff Medical. He argued that only a small handful of hospitals could commit their surgical teams to a year's training, and who else could pay the one-million-dollar costs? Furthermore, Olsen said the FDA would then consider a full year's training as the standard requirement for all human artificial-heart implants.

A loud argument ensued, and Jarvik asked Olsen how many calf implants it would take for training. Olsen replied that the physicians who were coming were all trained, experienced surgeons. They all had experience in cardiac transplant surgery where the heart is removed prior to implanting an artificial heart. He insisted that he could teach them with a lecture and implant the artificial heart into one calf, and the next day do a second calf implant and remove the artificial heart from the first calf in preparation for a cardiac transplant. Only training in the technical differences between implanting an artificial heart and a natural heart was necessary.

Jarvik believed Olsen had made everything too simple, but the teams from the three investing hospitals welcomed the abbreviated training time. The FDA readily adopted the training program of three surgeries on two calves, and many additional surgical teams welcomed this more realistic and affordable schedule.

Kolff scheduled a meeting of the Kolff Medical Board of Directors at 5:00 PM one afternoon. Before the meeting, he came to Olsen's office and announced that he was going to nominate Robert Jarvik as president of Kolff Medical. Kolff and Jarvik had a father-son relationship, but they did not always get along well, so Kolff's announcement came as a complete surprise to Olsen. He urged Kolff to cast a wider net to see what might be available. Kolff said he had thought the matter out: he felt Jarvik was aggressive and would make the shareholders a lot of money.

Olsen protested, "But Dr. Kolff, you and Rob rarely agree on anything; you fight all the time, and you have even taken him to a psychiatrist to try to resolve the animosity."

Kolff then said he did not need Olsen's vote anyway because he had already talked to all of the other board members and they were in agreement. When Olsen's vote was the only negative one at the meeting, it did nothing to improve the relationship between Olsen and Jarvik.

Outside Funding for Kolff Medical

After the early difficulties in establishing a base of funding for the artificial heart, the early venture capitalists infused a great deal of money into its development and marketing. On March 25, 1983, the *Deseret News* printed an Associated Press article by Robert Burns, indicating,

> Investors—including some of the nation's largest medical companies—poured more than $5 million into Kolff Medical, the tiny company which developed the Jarvik-7 heart... Kolff Medical had been selling the artificial hearts to research institutions since 1978, and in 1980 the revenue from such sales topped $100,000 for the first time....
>
> In Kolff's absence the board of directors adopted an incentive stock-option plan that awarded them more stock than it gave him. Jarvik was awarded the most. He declined to say exactly how many shares he received, but the major non-investor shareholders received 90,000 to 100,000 shares each. Olsen received 60,000 shares and the other penny-per-share investors received fewer. Dr. Kolff was limited to 10,000 shares. With an exercise price of one dollar per share, these options would become extremely valuable if the company prospered.
>
> Rodman Moorhead found three additional investors that filled the company's requirements, precisely: Hospital Corporation of American, Humana and American Hospital Supply, a $3 billion-a-year firm that distributed healthcare products. Each was to invest $1 million and

Warburg Pincus put in a similar additional amount. Rounding out the $5 million target includes two venture-capital firms, Southwest Venture Partners and General American Investors and a small amount by Ed Massey and two other board members.

On February 16, 1983 the Kolff Associates partnership gave way to a new privately held corporation called Kolff Medical Inc. Despite the magnitude of outside financing, the original shareholders retained nearly 64 percent of the equity in the partnership. New investors were paying $12.38 per share of Kolff Medical stock at the time.

Note

1. Earl Selby, interview with William DeVries, May 28, 1983.

15

The Importance of a Calf

I profess both to learn and to teach anatomy,
not from books... but from the fabric of nature.

—William Harvey

The Poet and the Calf

He stood a little more than three feet tall and weighed close to two hundred pounds. He was a rich brown and had huge dark eyes and ears he could wiggle. His name was Alfred, Lord Tennyson, and he was a Jersey calf with an artificial heart. Tennyson was the unquestioned king of the barn by New Year's Day of 1981.

His cage was right in the middle of the first row of animals so that everyone saw him first. Tennyson had a habit of staring at visitors and using his mobile ears to ask them to pay court to him. He then raised his head so that arms could encircle his neck and hands could scratch his forehead. He was so appealing that it was impossible not to like him. His barn records described him as "frisky, bouncy, and sociable."

Except for the air-driver leads protruding from his right chest, it was hard to believe Tennyson had an artificial heart. He was one of the better treadmill exercisers the lab ever had. He mooed loudly, had no physical problems, and ate with gusto—including an occasional slice of pizza. In every way, Tennyson was the irresistible showcase for the quality of life possible with a man-made heart. Jerseys grow more slowly than the Holsteins commonly used in research, so they survived longer, and Tennyson carried high hopes. He was an important bridge between calf experiments and a human implant.

Tennyson's principal investigator (PI) was William Lawrence (Larry) Hastings, a twenty-eight-year-old who was like his calf. His twinkling eyes and ready laugh showed he, too, enjoyed life. As a Quaker, he espoused nonviolence. Between him and the calf grew a bond that transcended research—he loved Tennyson.

It was pure accident that Hastings was in the artificial-heart program, although the work was in his heritage. At nine he had crept down the basement stairs to watch his father, Dr. Frank Hastings (later to head the National Heart Institute's artificial-heart unit), design an artificial heart. Despite his medical background, however, he finished high school more interested in Victorian poetry.

At a friend's suggestion, he visited Utah State University and enrolled as an English major. His Quaker philosophy attracted him to the antiwar activism then sweeping campuses. He had a dream the world really could be changed, so he switched his major to prelaw. But law bored him, and he switched again—to biology. His father had died, so he told his mother, "I'm thinking about going into medicine."

With other premed students from Utah State, he traveled to Salt Lake City in 1975 to visit Kolff's Artificial Heart Research Laboratory. The research ignited no fires in him, and when he graduated the next year, he still was not sure medicine was right for him. "I'd like to see what it's like from the inside," he told his wife, whose name, ironically, was Victoria.

For a year and a half, he was a hospital surgical orderly in Reno, Nevada, his wife's hometown. He concluded, "The medical profession is like any other organization—disorganized, good, and bad." Nevertheless, he decided to be a doctor, and when Victoria got a Forest Service job in Spanish Fork, Utah, he applied to the University of Utah School of Medicine, but he guessed he would not be accepted when his recitation of the way he chose medicine almost put his interviewer to sleep.

Then he remembered that one day in his father's Washington office, he had met Dr. Kolff, who had extended an invitation for any of the four Hastings boys to visit him. "Wouldn't hurt to see him," Hastings thought.

When he walked into Kolff's office, he got a warm welcome and a strange question, "Do you have a car?"

"That's how I got here."

"Good. Then take me to St. Mark's." En route Kolff asked, "What are you doing?"

"Nothing much; just looking for work."

Kolff considered that. "I'll give you a job," he finally said. "But I must warn you that I will pay you as little as I can get away with." At the research lab at

St. Mark's Hospital, Hastings saw what the job was—being a calf sitter. Dr. Don Olsen even had an organizational chart for this group of workers: calf-sitter trainee, second calf sitter, first calf sitter, senior calf sitter, and supervisor. Their schedules went around the clock seven days a week so that there was always a crew to monitor vital signs, administer drugs, keep records, and clean up.

"It's entry level," Hastings decided. "About as low entry as it can get." Twenty-four hours later, he signed on as a trainee for $2.70 an hour. His task was to stand like a sentry behind the animals—broom and dustpan at the ready—to sweep up their droppings.

It just happened that a group of Kolff's peers was in the lab that week, determining whether to recommend that NIH research grant funds be renewed. Discovering the diligent sweeper's identity, one of the review party asked, "You're Frank Hastings's boy? I knew your father well. Splendid man. Glad to see you're here." At first Hastings wondered why he had been assigned when the committee came through. He could not quite believe Kolff had planned it, "but on the other hand, my father did have a lot of friends. Dr. Kolff doesn't miss a trick."

Hastings moved up quickly. Within six months, he was offered a promotion to supervise the thirty calf sitters. He was the only calf sitter not in school during the day, so he was the logical choice. "It's a terrible job," warned a young woman who had done it before. "You're always on call. When somebody bugs out sick, you're on the hook to find a replacement or come in yourself. It's your responsibility to see that everything is done on time and right. You'll have more headaches than you ever thought possible."

Hastings smiled, thanked her, and took the job. His next ambition was to become a PI, the person who ran postsurgery. The job was to follow protocol and make decisions, under Olsen's direction, about an animal's care. He asked endless questions of established PIs to learn the required skills. By then the Kolff team was the only one in the world that had maintained life in an animal with an implanted artificial heart for more than two hundred days, but a full year passed before the calf Fumi Joe set a new record. Hastings set his own goal—survival approaching a year.

Holsteins gained weight so quickly that they outgrew the ability of their mechanical hearts to support them. Hastings decided to get a smaller breed. Olsen suggested he consider Jerseys, and Hastings, who did the lab's animal purchases, went to a dairy farm specializing in them. "Might have one for you," the farmer said. "About four months old now. You can get it down in the meadow."

Hastings headed for the calf. It did seem smaller than a Holstein. "He'll never outgrow the heart," Hastings decided. He moved cautiously toward it. The calf did not stir, not even when he put a rope around its neck. "Come on, boy, we're going home," he coaxed the calf.

That was May 11, 1980. Hastings trucked the calf back to the lab, where he was carefully examined. The calf appeared to be in magnificent condition so an implant was scheduled. On May 17, Hastings brought in water pails, brushes, and soap and carefully scrubbed the calf from head to hooves. The next day he did it again. Then he ordered the sitters to withhold both feed and water. He administered an antibiotic to quell possible gas production from any food that remained in the calf's four stomachs. "Okay," said Hastings, "he's ready for the heart."

Center Stage for Tennyson

At 6:00 AM the next morning, Hastings was in the lab to take the calf to the OR. Anesthesia was administered, and the calf was prepared for surgery. DeVries was the lead surgeon, Olsen his assistant.

Despite the success of the J-7 artificial heart in Fumi Joe, the surgeons had decided to use the larger J-5 model, believing its superior pumping volume would increase survival time. In addition, in the surgical technique Olsen had developed, they used special ventricles, each with one man-made valve to let blood into the heart. The calf's natural valves to route blood into the pulmonary artery and aorta were retained.

The surgery went smoothly until DeVries suddenly realized that blood was leaking from the natural aortic valve, which had somehow been nicked. The surgeons had rarely faced such an emergency. Their only option was to substitute a new left ventricle, one with two mechanical valves, one for the inflow and one for the aorta. That left the calf with one natural valve and three artificial ones. "Quite unique," said Olsen.

The tubes carrying air to pump the heart had a new type of apron flange called a skin button that was intended to promote better healing and bonding with the skin. Since skin buttons had never been used before, DeVries could only make an educated guess about how far to separate their entry incisions. The surgery took four hours—not bad, considering the valve crisis.

Before leaving the lab, Olsen warned Hastings to be prepared for a rough time. "Typically," he said, "Jerseys have a longer reaction to anesthesia." Hastings nodded.

Knowing that a PI had the right to name his calf, one of the sitters asked Hastings what the calf would be called. "Much too early for that," he answered. "You never name one until you're sure it will live. If it dies, you are wasting a good name."

The calf came out of anesthesia very groggy. Not until 10:00 PM that night could Hastings and the others transport it to a cage in the barn. At 4:00 AM the next morning, Hastings saw the calf struggle to its feet, but its legs were wobbly, and in a few minutes, it sank back on its chest. Hastings examined the animal's eyes. Bad. They were glazed—the sign of how sick the calf was—and could not follow moving objects around the room. Hastings offered some feed, but the calf could not eat. Miserable, it just kept grinding its teeth.

The following day the calf's temperature skyrocketed to 104 degrees (normal is 101). "Infection," said Hastings. "He may not last." He ordered an antibiotic, but the fever stayed up. He switched to another drug. No results. Finally, he called in one of the lab's heavy hitters, a powerful, high-risk antibiotic reserved for emergencies. It, too, failed.

When the calf reached eight days after implant, Hastings still was not sure it would live, but he could no longer delay giving it a name. He had been planning on Rossetti after his favorite pre-Raphaelite English poet. "Too good to waste on a doubtful animal," he decided. He also liked the poet Tennyson, so he told the calf sitters, "We'll call him Alfred, Lord Tennyson."

By the thirteenth day, Tennyson was extremely listless and eating very little. The fever hovered around 103 or 104. Hastings, who thought no experiment was worth an animal suffering, went to Olsen. "I'd like you to help me make a decision," he said. "I don't want to prolong this if it is not going to get us anywhere. Tennyson is very sick."

"Give him a few more days," Olsen advised. "Let him have a chance to fight it through."

"All right. I'll put off the decision on terminating until the twenty-first day," Hastings said.

He secretly and poetically decided that somehow Tennyson became privy to his conversation because—on the next day—the fever subsided. Apparently the calf's own immune system had kicked in to fight the infection, and Tennyson started eating. On the twenty-first day, there was no decision to make. The blood-cell count was almost normal, and the temperature was only slightly elevated. Best of all, the calf's bright eyes had lost their glaze.

When Hastings came into the lab, Tennyson kept moving his head to stare at him no matter where he walked. "Tennyson, Tennyson," said Hastings, "you've earned a treat." He opened his hand to extend a sugar cube. Tennyson lapped it up, then looked at Hastings as if he expected another.

For the first thirty days, the calf had been caged in a corner of the barn.

"He's better than that," Hastings told the calf sitters. Pulling a little bit of rank, he moved Tennyson to center stage—right in the middle of the floor where he would attract attention.

Generally, it takes at least two weeks to a month for a calf to recover fully from the assaults of the implant and begin to assert its own personality. One calf named Elizabeth Barrett Browning was aloof, spurning every effort to win her friendship. Others, like Oscar Wilde, were rambunctious and rattled their cages. Tennyson, however, was genuinely sweet to everybody. People coming to work at the Institute for Biomedical Engineering that shared the building started detouring through the barn so they could say, "Hi, Tennyson!" He picked up his head to let them rub it. His long tongue went out to lick any hands in sight. When his admirers turned their backs, he swiped playfully at wallets, combs, or anything else protruding from their pockets.

A Special Birthday

On the 88th day, Hastings noticed a splotch of white pus in Tennyson's skin between the two air drivelines. Where had this infection come from? Suddenly, Hastings was afraid Tennyson was going to die. "What is it?" he asked Olsen.

"We put the drivelines too close together," the veterinarian said. "Instead of bonding to healthy skin, the buttons on the lines bumped against each other and killed the tissue."

Both men recognized the peril. Situated at the entry points for the drivelines, the infection seemed to have a clear channel to invade the entire body. "The special skin button was meant to keep any infection localized," said Olsen. "That's our only hope."

Hastings cleaned the area with Betadine antiseptic, but it was too strong. Quickly he switched to a nitrogen compound that attacked the infection but also permitted new skin to develop. There was no evidence of fever, which would have indicated that the infection was spreading.

This was good news in the lab because ultimately Tennyson became the longest living animal with an implant. He inherited this title from Lawson, the calf that had won such good press by strolling across a lawn with only a small portable driver. On October 5, 1980, Lawson succumbed to infection and blood clotting after surviving a little more than 158 days.

When Tennyson remained fever free for the next two months, Hastings said, "If we can check the infection this long, there's a chance that Tennyson can break the record." It was the first time he felt confident, and he wrote in the animal's chart, "200 days and going strong."

At 209 days, however, Tennyson's cheerful personality disappeared. His eyes glazed, and his abdomen bloated, possibly due to bad hay. The bloating was not dangerous, but it could press on the diaphragm and inhibit breathing.

Hastings got the calf to swallow a tube, and he squeezed on the puffed-up belly. Out came a cloud of a horrible-smelling gas. People in the lab ran for cover, gasping at the smell, but the bloat subsided. At 3:00 AM the next morning, the night shift woke Hastings at home. "He's bloated again," the calf sitter said. "What should we do?"

"Don't do anything. I'm on my way."

Hastings drove to the lab, where he found Tennyson's belly so tight that hitting it was like banging a drum. Again he debloated him. Unknowingly echoing what Kolff had said about a calf in Kampen forty years earlier, Hastings joked, "We could keep the lights burning in Salt Lake for some time with all this gas." Over the next eight days, Hastings made four postmidnight runs to the barn. "I know you could do this," he told the calf sitters, "but it's my calf, my responsibility, and I think I should do it."

On the 217th day, Hastings came back from lunch to find his calf stretched out in his cage. In Tennyson's side was a trocar tube into the first stomach. Panicked, he rushed to Olsen, exclaiming, "What have you done to my animal?"

"Relax," said Olsen. "While you were gone, Tennyson bloated so badly his eyes were bulging out. He almost stopped breathing. Puncturing his rumen was all I could do to save his life."

Hastings was still livid. "There's got to be a better way," he said.

It was the Christmas season, and Hastings had promised Victoria he would go with her to visit her folks in Reno. Did he dare to leave Tennyson? Reluctantly he went, but he told her, "My heart is not in Reno." On Christmas day—as early as he could conveniently leave—he flew back to Salt Lake. He was relieved that Tennyson's abdominal incision was healing with no sign of infection.

December 27, 1980, was important for the once-sickly calf that had battled his way through infection, fever, and bloating. On this day, he became the world's longest-surviving animal with an artificial heart. "We're having a party," Hastings announced. When others asked who would buy the cake, he was offended. "Buy?" he asked. "For Tennyson I'm baking the cake." He did—a chocolate layer cake inscribed, "Tennyson 222+ Days, Happy Birthday."

Tennyson liked the cake. He was, however, not too keen on the champagne that Hastings provided for the guests, including the thirty or so calf sitters, heart-maker Tom Kessler, and several visiting Japanese scientists. They cheered as a calf sitter put a sign on Tennyson's cage reading, "The Champ." Olsen,

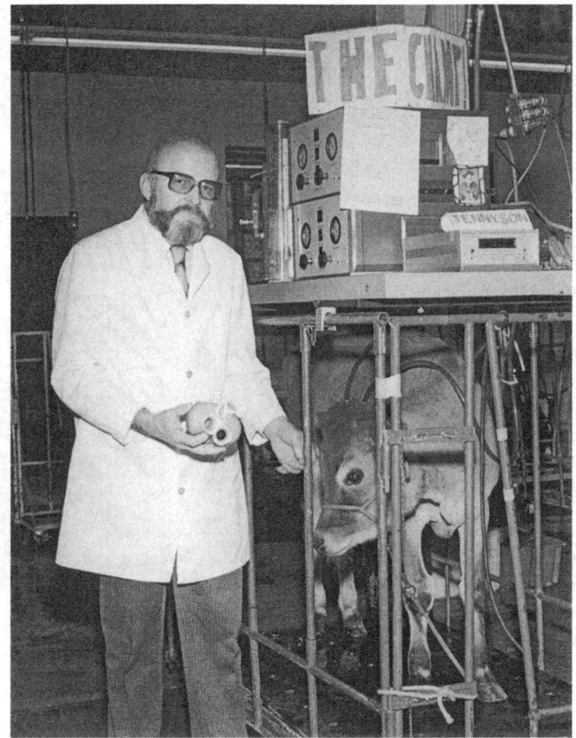

Tennyson, here with Don Olsen, was a lab favorite.

visiting family in Montana, telephoned his congratulations. Then Kolff called. "Did he make it?" he asked.

A trifle cocky, Hastings replied, "Of course."

Later, he and a dozen others went to a café to continue the celebration. In about an hour, a waiter asked, "Is there a Dr. Hastings? There's a call for him." Feeling so good he did not bother to correct his title, Hastings took the call.

On the line was a UPI reporter. "The lab said I could catch you here. What about Tennyson? Did he set the record?" he asked

"You bet," said Hastings, and for the next fifteen minutes, he talked about his calf's triumph. It was his first interview.

Triumph

For the next twenty-six days, Tennyson was the talk of the lab, especially because he seemed to be in such marvelous condition—alert, full of personality, his driveline infection under control, eating well, and bolting down every sugar cube in sight. It didn't last. On day 248, Hastings did not like what he saw. For

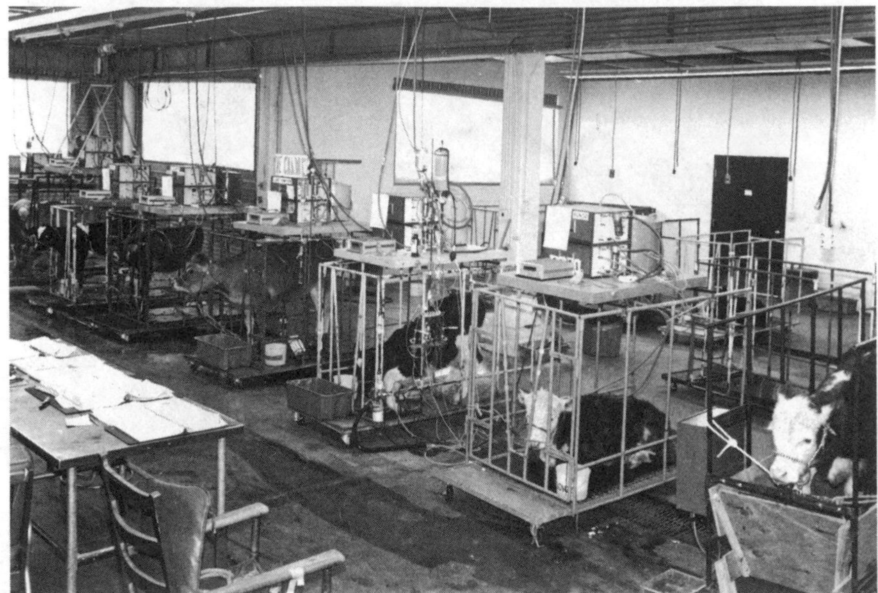

The St. Mark's barn often had two sheep and fourteen calves.

the third time, Tennyson's eyes were becoming glazed, and the jugular vein in his neck was much distended. That could indicate that blood was backing up. After all this time, it appeared his artificial heart was failing.

With Olsen's approval, Hastings took his calf to the OR. The tentative diagnosis was that the heart had developed occlusions, possibly pannus in the inflow valve and a blockage in the outflow. Olsen said they could operate and either clean out the clogs or replace the ventricle, but the risk of mortality was high.

The lab team held a meeting, and Hastings said he would rather try medicine. "We've still got infection around the drivelines," he said.

Olsen added, "There is also the chance strong adhesions have developed between the heart and the surrounding tissue—very difficult to sever. His chances of survival aren't good. I say, let's take him back to the barn."

Tennyson was brought back to his cage, where antibiotics and a diuretic were administered. The therapy had a temporary success, but by day 260, it was obvious that the calf was dying. His temperature spiked to 105 degrees. His constant movement to get comfortable betrayed his suffering. Hastings was giving him painkillers three times a day with little effect.

On day 267, Hastings called Olsen. "I think we had better put an end to this," he said. "I can't let him suffer. As much as I hate to say it, I think we have to terminate him."

Olsen thought a minute. "I agree," he said.

"I'll do it tomorrow," Hastings said. That night he said to his wife, "It'll be the hardest thing I have ever had to do. I feel like his father."

At 2:00 PM the next afternoon, Hastings walked into the barn. The hematology aid, who had taken so many blood samples from Tennyson, was there in tears. So were a surgical scrub nurse and the calf sitters. This was not just a scientific experiment—Tennyson was their beloved friend.

Normally a two-gram vial of sodium pentothal will put an animal of Tennyson's size to sleep. Hastings doubled the dose to be sure. He walked to Tennyson, who looked up at him and then raised his head so Hastings could put his arm around his neck. "He knows it's time," Hastings said. He injected the Pentothal. A minute went by. At two minutes, Tennyson's eyes closed, and he sank to his knees. Hastings sat down with him. For ten minutes, the two old friends stayed there. At last Hastings rose and—with two quick clicks—turned off the heart driver. Then he lay down beside his calf.

Hastings did not meet his goal of a one-year survival for Tennyson. Yet he knew that if the IRB reviewing DeVries's application to do a human implant questioned whether the artificial heart could sustain life long term, the committee had only to look at the triumph of the brave calf Tennyson.

Calves Versus Sheep for Implant Research

Although human use was always the primary objective for the artificial heart, it was critical to find the best animal models. Several decades of trial and error taught researchers a lot. The common replies to the question, "Why were both calves and sheep used in the artificial-heart experiments?" were resiliency and fit. Calves were preferred because they have fewer complications during lengthy bypass surgery and respond very quickly afterward, standing and eating hay. They have the preferred weight of 170 to 220 pounds and the ideal chest size for implanting the artificial heart that would fit best in humans.

Calves are not problem free, however. They are still very young and have delicate lungs like human infants. Young calves also have fetal hemoglobin circulating in their red blood cells. These cells are fragile and rupture easily, releasing the hemoglobin, even at the low stress level created by the artificial heart. When the Utah lab became more successful in keeping calves alive longer, the difficult problem of size surfaced. A healthy calf could grow about two pounds a day, so by three months, it doubled its weight and needed much more blood flow. Since the heart remained its initial size, the pulse rate had to be increased to meet the additional demand.

Implanted calves eventually outgrew their artificial hearts. When their body weight doubled, they experienced congestive heart failure and had to be

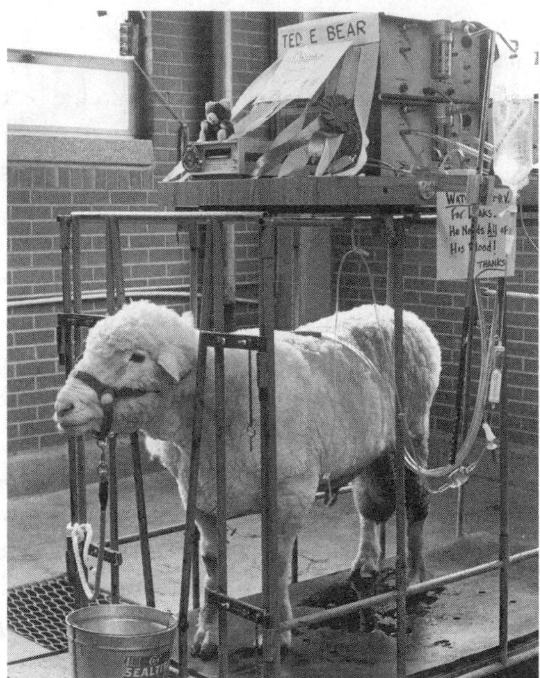

Ted E. Bear was one of a number of sheep that received an artificial heart.

terminated. Olsen switched to Jersey cattle, which grew more slowly than Holsteins to address the problem. The change—as we've seen—produced Tennyson, one of the lab's notable successes.

Sheep were initially more difficult to keep alive on the artificial heart than calves. Their responses to anticoagulation were different, and they needed special postoperative care because they were not as resilient as young calves. The adult sheep, however, maintained a steady body weight on a maintenance diet. Calves frequently battled infections at the exit site of the air drivelines as they grew. This was never a problem with adult sheep since the lanolin on their skin was bacteriostatic and rarely became infected. The sheep Ted E. Bear lived nearly a year, setting a record at that time for an animal with an artificial heart.

Using Artificial Hearts as a Bridge to Cardiac Transplants

As early as 1978, Olsen had concluded that if the artificial heart ever came into widespread use, it would be as a temporary bridge to a cardiac transplant. Raised on a dairy farm, he knew twin calves were unique. In veterinary school, he learned that the blood vessels in their placentas were connected so all hormones, proteins, and stem cells were exchanged in utero. Later, when he studied immunology, he learned that the tissues exchanged between embryos tolerated an organ transplant. A few medical publications about skin transplants in twin calves supported that theory, but the tolerance was not considered permanent.

Olsen submitted a research proposal to NIH to implant the artificial heart in one calf and after six to ten weeks remove it and transplant the natural heart from its twin. The project was funded in 1979 for three years and renewed through 1985.[1] Since no one on the Utah research team had experience with cardiac transplants, Olsen contacted the Stanford cardiac-transplant team. Dr. Bruce Reitz came to Utah for the first explant-transplant surgery. The Utah team did all of the subsequent surgeries successfully.

Because of Olsen's research, the Utah Artificial Heart Research Laboratory was frequently highlighted in the news after Tennyson. Shortly after Olsen received funding for experiments with twin calves, the media were invited back to the lab to make the acquaintance of a new celebrity, Fernando, a Hereford calf. Fernando was three months old when Olsen replaced his natural heart with an artificial one. The device was removed after Fernando had thrived on the artificial heart for forty-four days and was replaced by a heart transplanted from his twin, Roberto. Since the twin calf's tissue short-circuited rejection problems, Fernando was in his ninety-fourth day with his third heart when the press came calling. Mostly ignoring them, Fernando walked around the barn, stealing hay from the calves whose air drivelines kept them confined to their cages. His experiment was terminated after six months, and all his organs were still normal.

Charlie the Holstein Bull

Charlie had the most unusual story of any calf implanted with an artificial heart and later transplanted. In 1982—after the successes of Tennyson and Fernando—Olsen purchased black-and-white Holstein twin calves. They were named Charles, affectionately called Charlie, and Diana after the newly married British royals. Charlie received an artificial heart. For seventy-four days—excluding a two-week recovery period following the implant—every test on Charlie produced the same test results as those on Diana. He grew to a healthy, nearly four-hundred-pound bull calf. He was then taken back to surgery, his artificial heart was removed, and Diana's heart was transplanted into him.

The Utah State Fair took place about three months after Charlie's heart transplant. Olsen asked if the calf sitters would be interested in entering Charlie in the dairy-cattle exhibit. They enthusiastically agreed, and Charlie went to the

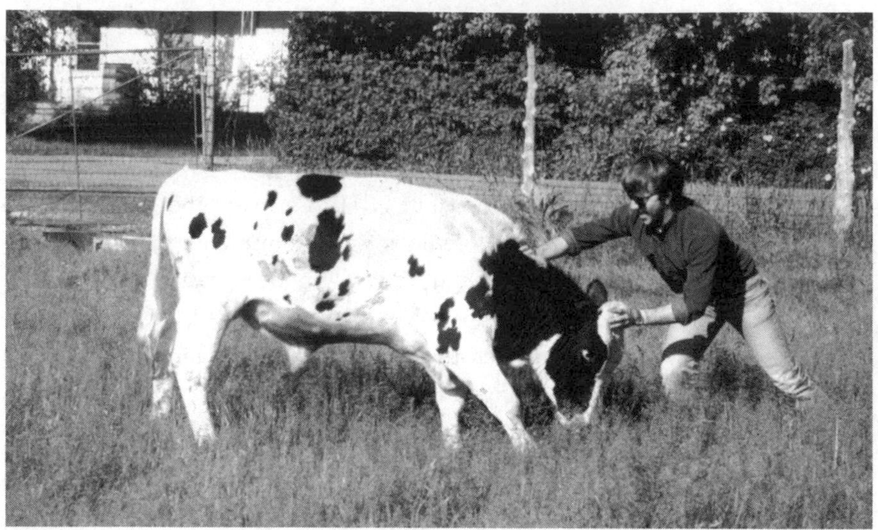

Charlie was a very popular exhibit at the Utah State Fair.

Utah State Fair. A large sign over Charlie's stall read, "The University of Utah. The calf that had three hearts." To intrigue fairgoers even more, an artificial heart similar to Charlie's was attached to a water pump to demonstrate the way a machine could function as a heart.

Fairgoers liked the exhibit, and the calf sitters were kept busy explaining Charlie's unusual medical history. This friendly young bull was a great ambassador, and his exhibit was so popular that the fair board presented Charlie with a special Grand Champion Ribbon. Artificial-heart research got a shot in the arm.

The protocol of Olsen's research program called for termination of the calves after about six months so that their organs could be studied for changes or abnormalities. When the time came for Charlie's demise, the calf sitters were distressed. They had grown to love Charlie, who by then was a coddled and affectionate lab pet. They pleaded for Charlie's life. Olsen agreed to save the calf, but he knew that Charlie would soon outgrow the laboratory. He called a friend in the dairy business and asked him to take Charlie as a herd sire. Though an imposingly large, nearly adult bull, Charlie was as gentle as a puppy and had unusual affection and tolerance for humans.

Three years and three months after Diana's heart had been transplanted into Charlie, the dairyman called to report that he must get rid of the bull. He now had daughters old enough to breed so he must be removed—a rule to ensure healthy offspring. Charlie was sent to slaughter. At the time, he weighed 1,750 pounds.

The tiny heart from Diana had grown in perfect harmony with Charlie's body, clearly demonstrating that cardiac transplants could be safely done in infants. Charlie established another world record in addition to his body size and survival time—he had sired fifty-five healthy calves!

These successes in Utah artificial-heart development eventually resulted in approval to implant an artificial heart in a human. However, more detours were on the way, and the IRB was only one of the roadblocks on the journey.

Note

1. Don. B. Olsen, principal investigator, "Artificial Heart Implant, Later Cardiac Transplantation," NIH grant R01 HL24419 (1979 to 1982) and R01 HL24412 (1982 to 1985).

16

Preparing for the Ultimate Test

Man is but a reed, the weakest in nature.
But he is a thinking reed.
—Blaise Pascal

A Sleepless Night

Beth Ann Cole woke with a start. She did not know what time it was, but she was instantly aware of what had roused her—the agonizing thought that another human being's life might lie in her hands. It was a thought that kept bothering her. As a new member of the medical center's IRB, she was among the thirteen men and women who would pass judgment on William DeVries's application to implant the artificial heart in a patient.

Cole took her appointment very seriously, conscious that her mission was to protect both patients and the university from ill-advised experimentation. Was the artificial heart ill advised? If the IRB permitted implanting in a person, was it signing the patient's death warrant?

In late fall of 1980, Cole was thirty-seven, married to a plastic surgeon, and the mother of two children. A professor in the University of Utah's College of Nursing and also director of its graduate program in psychosocial nursing, she had migrated to Utah because that seemed logical after her conversion to Mormonism. She tended to think before speaking, though sometimes her words came in a rush of emotion. She was well educated: a bachelor's degree in science from the University of Cincinnati, a master's degree in child psychiatric nursing from Boston University, and a PhD in family studies from Brigham Young University (BYU).

By nature optimistic and convinced that people can generally achieve most of their goals with hard work, she thought how rewarding it would be if the artificial heart extended life. But as she lay awake, she was struck with the enormity of what DeVries was proposing. She prayed for guidance, but she knew that she alone would have to make her decision. She felt that God accepts human imperfections, and people just have to do their best. In that spirit, she would make her choice.

As a nurse, she thought first of the patient who would receive the heart. Since a male cadaver had sized the J-7 heart, she assumed the first recipient would be a man. Where would DeVries find a reasonable candidate? Would that person be informed enough to give rational consent? What about his motives? Obviously, one would be a chance to extend life. But what if a patient wanted fame, his name in medical history books?

Cole's work in family studies told her that an implant involves more people than the patient. He would need a support system to help him transition to a radically different lifestyle. His wife would have to make as big a commitment as he did. She would be the one to take him home from the hospital, if possible, and devote a major portion of her waking hours to him. For her and all involved family members, there would be an emotional price to pay.

And what was the likelihood the device would work in a human chest? No one on the IRB's subcommittee was a cardiothoracic surgeon. Cole had not even seen an animal implant. By what standards could she decide if success was a reasonable expectation? However, she knew that—while her knowledge was limited—she could rely on the board's collective conclusion. The members were hardly rubber stamps. They had already grilled DeVries aggressively, making him describe in painstaking detail the animal experiments that had convinced him the heart was feasible. No question was glossed over, and discussion continued until the answers were satisfactory.

DeVries was willing to make certain compromises, but the revised application he submitted in October 1980 still clung to the hope of using the heart with patients who had suffered heart attacks or had irreversibly diseased hearts. Cole felt that both types posed problems. Since a patient in shock from a heart attack obviously could not give informed consent, would it be ethical to allow an implant? Cole wondered how she would feel if she woke after a heart attack to find herself tethered by six-foot lines to an artificial heart's 375-pound air driver, especially when consent for the implant had been given by family members. Was that maintaining life at any cost? Would death be preferable?

And what of the patients whose diseased hearts had simply lost their pumping power? It appeared death was closing in, but who could know that for certain? Was it morally right to take out a heart whose lifespan could not be predicted? Cole sighed. There were no easy answers.

Behind the IRB Curtain

Ernst Eichwald, the IRB subcommittee's sixty-six-year-old chair, looked like a rumpled, spry Einstein with a head of gray hair, bright, inquisitive eyes, soft speech, and a hearing aid he didn't bother to conceal. He loved to prowl art galleries and search out restaurants with the best German food. He was also still an avid skier. For seventeen years, he was editor of the international scientific publication *Transplantation*, a tribute to his distinguished work in helping overcome tissue rejection in organ transplants. With medical degrees from both Germany and Utah, he had recently completed a term as chair of the School of Medicine's Department of Pathology.

In 1974 he was in a Salt Lake City restaurant when another patron—knowing he was from the university—belligerently asked, "What are you fellows doing up there? I hear you're putting artificial eyes in blind people. What kind of business is that for a university?" Eichwald said he knew nothing about that, but back on campus, he investigated, and that was how he found out there was an IRB.

He went before the board and asked the members if what he had heard was correct. "Absolutely not," he was told. Fascinated by the IRB's role in judging whether an experiment's potential benefits outweighed the risks, Eichwald gladly accepted an appointment to the committee. Within a year, he was appointed chair of the newly formed Subcommittee for the Artificial Heart by John A. Bosso, the chair of the IRB. By the time DeVries's application came in, Eichwald estimated that the IRB had reviewed three thousand bids to start or continue research on human subjects.

Eichwald liked DeVries. Recalling the young surgeon as one of his pathology students in the late 1960s, Eichwald thought him "very charming." Nevertheless, that did not soften the way he treated DeVries before the IRB subcommittee. He and the members took exception to the surgeon quoting Teddy Roosevelt's words about daring mighty things in his application. What if something went wrong in the surgery? Would people think the quote indicated that the university was more interested in its staff's "glorious triumphs" than in the best interests of its patients? Consequently, DeVries removed the quote from his revised application.

The subcommittee also criticized Kolff's letter of support for the implant. Some members thought that his saying the implant should only be done when it would restore the patient to an "enjoyable existence" possibly promised more than the artificial heart could deliver.

The IRB subcommittee very carefully reviewed the many requirements mandated in the FDA-approved Patient Consent Form. A major item that confounded the members was the "freedom to withdraw" clause. Consent forms historically include a statement that the patient is free to withdraw at any time during the procedure and will receive continued care. For artificial-heart recipients, this statement might imply a sanction of suicide because if the patient removed him or herself from the drive system, death would result.

Kolff described for the IRB the key on the front panel of the heart driver. Reporters had written a great deal about Kolff and that key. When it was turned, the heart driver would immediately stop, and the implanted animal or human would die. Could that be considered murder? The key was removed from the driver and sequestered where only DeVries and Joyce had access to it.

Given the unique challenges of the artificial-heart proposal, the IRB included a limited right-to-withdraw statement, which said that although patients might put themselves at considerable risk by not following advice, they did have the right to continue to live or die with or without the pump. The patient could not stop the heart but was allowed to refuse further instructions—or even demands—from medical personnel.

The IRB wanted more documentation on the criteria DeVries proposed for patient selection, specifically about financial status. Members worried the cost might be so astronomical the implant would only be accessible to the rich, which was alien to the medical center's philosophy of medical care. They even debated about how an implant patient targeted for a transplant would get to Stanford for the surgery. What proof did DeVries have that the artificial heart would function in an airplane cruising at thirty-five or forty thousand feet?

DeVries called an airline. "What's the cabin pressure in flight?" he asked. The answer was that—regardless of the altitude—most cabins are set to an atmospheric pressure of about eight thousand feet above sea level. Olsen then arranged for a sheep with an artificial heart to be trucked to Snowbird, a Utah ski resort 7,760 feet up in the mountains, where the animal spent several uneventful hours. DeVries sent photographs to the subcommittee and told its members they proved the artificial heart would survive pressurized airplane cabins.

The most germane question remained whether use of the artificial heart was justified. Was something less permanent—a left ventricular-assist device to bolster the natural heart, for instance—more feasible? Kolff and DeVries insisted that ventricular-assist devices had not yet achieved a high level of success. Their worry was that while the assist unit was in place, the patient's heart and body would further deteriorate, diminishing the possibility of an artificial heart succeeding. As the inquiry dragged on, DeVries heard that his proposal was "sure to be approved at the next meeting," but that meeting only generated more questions.

Even so, decisions were being made. Eichwald had decided he would vote no on DeVries's application, although not from any fears the heart was unworkable. The long-term survival of Tennyson and Fumi Joe seemed to indicate that it could sustain life. However, like Dr. Hiroshi Kuida, the cardiologist he had called as a consultant, Eichwald wanted to limit the device to patients whose hearts could not be restarted after cardiac surgery. Others on the board were just as vehemently in favor of giving DeVries wide latitude in choosing his heart candidates. "We are at an impasse," said Eichwald.

Another member figured out a way to cut this Gordian knot. "We have two basic categories of patients: the surgical—those in heart operations—and the nonsurgical—those with heart disease. These two are clearly distinct, so why not separate them? Suppose we limit the use to surgical cases? If that succeeds, we can reconsider the nonsurgical ones." Eichwald could vote for that. So could Cole and the others.

Accepting that severe a limitation on patient selection was a hard concession for DeVries. He wanted the protocol to include heart-attack patients. Except for a bad heart, which he would replace, the patients' vital organs would likely be in good condition, boosting hopes for long-term survival. He also saw the artificial heart as worthwhile for cardiomyopathy victims, even though their condition might have damaged liver, kidneys, or lungs. Even then the heart could be the only alternative to death.

Nevertheless, holding out for the other two categories would surely doom his entire proposal. Swallowing his disappointment, he said he would agree to use the heart only with surgical patients who had nonfunctioning hearts. However, his compromise did not end the IRB discussions; there were still more questions. Disturbed by the apparent never-ending impasse, Dr. Leonard Jarcho, a neurologist, said, "I have been against this proposal, and I am not sure I am for it still, but I think we owe Dr. DeVries a vote. If everybody is against it, there is no reason to continue. If people are for it, then we can say that." A vote was taken and was overwhelmingly in DeVries's favor.

On January 27, 1981, Eichwald appeared before a press conference to announce the IRB had cleared the artificial heart for experimental use in a human being, limiting it to heart-surgery patients who faced certain death. Because of that, he added, there was no risk or danger from the device. He stated that he would be "elated" if an implant patient survived two or three weeks. For a recipient to survive two or three months would be "a tremendous success." The subcommittee, however, had severely shrunk DeVries's pool of potential implant patients from a possible annual total of thirty thousand to only about a tenth of that.

Reporters wanted to know what his fee for the surgery would be. "Nothing," DeVries said, disclosing that professional fees would be waived. However, he said the heart would cost $5,000, as would the heart driver, with another $3,000 to $4,000 in estimated bills for what he guessed would be a ten-day hospital stay. It could also cost up to $30,000 to equip the patient's home with ramps, air compressors, and special electrical connections and cover air fares. All in all, costs would total perhaps $50,000, not an alarming amount.

Kolff predicted that thousands of otherwise-dying patients would eventually benefit from the heart. He was asked if more patients would be helped by the artificial heart than the artificial kidney. Unhesitatingly, he replied, "The artificial heart will be far more important than the artificial kidney."

At the press conference, the clear implication was that the IRB subcommittee had approved an implant, and so it had—but only conditionally. Final approval was dependent on DeVries and a subcommittee appointed by Eichwald agreeing on a protocol defining exactly what the surgeon could do to whom. The subcommittee members analyzed almost every phrase in the surgeon's proposal before shaping a protocol everyone could accept.

His description of the Utah heart group as the world's "most successful surgical team" was changed to say it had "a great deal of experience" with the artificial heart. The maximum age for an implant patient was shaved from sixty-five to sixty. The surgeon thought one cardiologist would be sufficient for a second opinion, but the IRB raised that to two. DeVries said the plan was for the patient to live at home. The IRB specified that home had to be within forty-five minutes of the medical center to facilitate postsurgery checkups.

Above all, the IRB wanted to be sure an implant patient had enough information to make an intelligent decision about volunteering for the surgery. Before signing an informed-consent form, the patient—as DeVries had suggested—should consult family and other advisors. The IRB added that the patient had to be told that "his lifestyle would be significantly different with an artificial heart" because of being tethered to the heart driver. The IRB also stated a patient had to have a history of medical compliance and a willingness to follow doctors' orders. He had to be mentally competent to handle the driver, able to deal with "his illness with stable psychological mechanisms," and be free of alcohol or drug problems. Furthermore, he had to demonstrate a "stable home situation with spouse, sibling, or reliable person."

After everything was explained, the patient would be asked to sign forms permitting surgery on his diseased heart, plus an implant and possibly a transplant. In addition, there were forms permitting the medical center to release information to the media. The patient was to be told that after his diseased heart was repaired, it might not restart. Then DeVries would try to activate it with drugs and possibly an intra-aortic balloon pump like the one developed in Kolff's Cleveland lab. Only after exhausting all possible therapies would DeVries do the implant.

And what could the patient expect with an artificial heart? He would not be bedridden and could move from room to room. Short automobile rides would be possible with a portable driver, along with most normal life functions, such as using the toilet, eating, reading, and deskwork. "Does that include sex?" a reporter asked DeVries.

He replied, "We hope that goes okay."

At Home in the Headlines

In February 1981, the university held an open house for the media to observe an actual animal implant in the Artificial Heart Research Laboratory. Present for this operation were reporters, including a *Newsweek* correspondent, photographers, and television crews with lights and cameras. The Utah heart was now at home in the headlines, undeniably national news. The *New York Times* sent its widely respected science/medical writer, Harold M. Schmeck Jr., to write a story that took up two-thirds of a page in its "Science Times" section. The *Chicago Tribune* headlined another long story, "Artificial Heart May Save 60,000 Lives Every Year."

Time magazine said the Utah surgery was even more spectacular than a heart transplant. The heart's cachet as a hot ticket in the media peaked when an emissary for Harry Reasoner of *Sixty Minutes* came out to argue, unsuccessfully, that his man should have the exclusive rights to interview the first implant patient before the surgery.

ABC's *Good Morning America* featured DeVries. His hometown newspaper, the *Ogden Standard Examiner*, said, "This man's journey has taken him to the 'heart of life'" and reported that DeVries kept a motto from Alan Ashley-Pitt in his office. It read, "The man who follows the crowd will usually get no further than the crowd; the man who walks alone is likely to find himself in places no one has ever been."

With eye-catching visuals like that, the news of Utah's progress spread overseas. Heart patients in Japan, England, and South America called DeVries, pleading for implants. "I'm sorry," DeVries had to answer. "We cannot yet accept anyone to receive the artificial heart." Before he could implant the heart, there was one more hurdle—running the gauntlet of Washington's bureaucrats, and that, he feared, might be the toughest obstacle of all.

The NHLBI's Efforts to Block the Utah Implant

The news that the Utah IRB had approved the heart did not go unnoticed in Washington and especially in the university setting in Bethesda, Maryland, where the NIH's NHLBI was headquartered. The NHLBI was shocked. It was mandated by Congress to oversee development of heart devices, and it had to learn from newspapers that DeVries had received his IRB's sanction for a human implant!

For more than a decade, the NHLBI had opposed giving the artificial heart priority over left ventricular-assist devices. Some years earlier, when he had headed the National Heart Institute, Dr. Donald Frederickson had been asked for his reaction if a total heart replacement became available. In her book, *Heartbeat,* Natalie Davis Spingarn quoted him as saying he would not "exactly cry out with joy. It is a very costly, temporary solution to heart disease and not an appropriate piece of technology for today."[1]

But what if DeVries's implantation was successful? It took no brains to envision the ensuing public furor. Would Congress then begin asking why the NHLBI had put most of its eggs in the ventricular-assist-device basket? Would the NHLBI be left in the bureaucrats' worst possible posture—with its flanks and perhaps even more exposed? Suppose the treatment failed. Would that not be a setback for all heart research, one that could scuttle much of the NHLBI's funding? It almost seemed that going ahead with the implant would put NHLBI in a no-win situation—damned if it was a success, damned if it was not.

How to escape this trap? The NHLBI first wanted to be sure that the Utah IRB had given approval. Kolff and DeVries confirmed that. "Had a copy of the protocol been sent to the institute?" No. "Would one be?" Yes. No statute said DeVries had to clear his plans with the NHLBI. In fact, a new law said another federal agency, the FDA, now had control over medical devices intended for human use. Utah was going strictly by the book in asking the FDA for permission to implant the artificial heart. Only the FDA had the authority to grant exemptions from the law so that new devices with high risk could be tried experimentally, providing there was proper patient consent and local IRB approval.

For most of the twentieth century, manufacturers could make medical devices without any government clearance. If the government objected, it could seek to block sale or distribution of the devices, but it had to prove its case. A 1976 law put the shoe on the other foot by declaring the creators had to prove their devices were both safe and effective. It was easy to document safety with the artificial heart, but what about effectiveness? Heart failure in animals was not similar to chronic heart failure in humans. No reliably acceptable way to prove effectiveness existed.

A tug-of-war was on. Even before the FDA received the Utah application, the NHLBI was gearing up its program to derail the proposal. Frederickson, who had so vigorously condemned the artificial heart, had by this time risen to head the entire NIH. He personally directed that the NHLBI's Civilian Advisory Council be asked to "examine issues raised by the Utah plans." Just a year earlier, this same council had said the NHLBI was right in giving assist devices top billing over an artificial heart. Then Frederickson told the NHLBI to carry the case against the Utah application directly to the FDA.

The NHLBI point man for the issue was Dr. Peter Frommer, the agency's deputy director. A veteran bureaucrat with a bristly crew cut, Frommer met with the FDA and also sent a long letter urging extreme caution in considering the Utah heart proposal. Acknowledging that the right to rule on the heart lay with the FDA, Frommer said, "We do not seek to change this," but the NHLBI wanted to share its "technical and clinical investigative expertise." He wrote, "Almost certainly, the NHLBI and NIH will be affected by public reaction. Since this will be clinical research in its most newsworthy, dramatic and emotionally charged form, it can very plausibly impact on clinical investigation in general."

Although somewhat handicapped in his comments by not having yet received the Utah proposal, Frommer said the NHLBI had questions about the artificial heart's safety and effectiveness. He also asked whether "alternate experimental devices," meaning ventricular-assist pumps, would not be preferable to the artificial heart. He pointed out the NHLBI had funded research about using these assist devices to help restart hearts after operations, precisely the situation where DeVries wanted to use the artificial heart. In the fifteen most recent cases, Frommer said, four patients had recovered and survived from seven to thirty-three months. "We recognize," he added, "the other eleven died," but he ascribed the deaths to complications unrelated to the devices.

Noting the tethering necessitated by the replacement heart, he said that even if patients survived the surgery, "they would still face an unfavorable prognosis and serious limitations in the quality of life. Their care would incur substantial expenses and other resources. These prospects raise a whole host of societal issues."

Glenn A. Rahmoeller, the earnest young director of the FDA's Division of Cardiovascular Devices, wrote Frommer, "Socioeconomic factors are not generally a critical part of making a determination of whether or not to approve a study. The fundamental decision is based on whether we believe that . . . the risks to the subjects are outweighed by the anticipated benefits to the subjects and the importance of the knowledge to be gained." Rahmoeller reminded Frommer that FDA regulations made local IRBs, not federal agencies, responsible for patient protection because the boards expressed "local community attitudes and ethical standards." He also pointed out that the congressional committee spearheading the medical-device law had declared it was usually better to let IRBs, rather than government officials, supervise clinical testing of the devices. "But," added Rahmoeller, "within the limits of the law, the FDA would be glad to receive whatever assistance NIH would like to provide."

Warning Flags

Back in Utah, misgivings about the heart project were building. Kolff summoned DeVries one day to ask, "What about the J-7? Are you sure it will fit in the human chest?"

"Of course it will," DeVries reassured him. Kolff then pulled out letters he had received from overseas researchers, including an extremely close friend in East Germany, who had been sent models of the J-7 heart. They said they could not get it to fit. On top of that, Dr. Jack Kolff, the scientist's son who had started a cardiovascular service in Philadelphia's Temple University Hospital, said that his attempts to fit a cadaver had also been unsuccessful.

"Let me show you," DeVries told Kolff, taking him to the nearby VA Hospital where he had fit cadavers. Picking up the left half of an artificial heart, he put it in the chest, explaining, "You have to put this ventricle way over on the left side as far as it can go. Then the right ventricle goes on top of it, and the chest can be closed."

Kolff studied what DeVries had done. "It fits," he agreed.

Olsen had also made several trips to Rostock, at that time part of East Germany, to assist Dr. Horst Klinkmann, the clinic director of the Department of Internal Medicine in the University of Rostock. Klinkmann's group was establishing an Artificial Heart Research Laboratory and also designing an artificial heart. On some of his trips, Olsen carried the J-7 for trials. Olsen indicated to the German researchers during these visits that the inlet and outlet of the left ventricle had to be more divergent to improve blood flow. He demonstrated that the left ventricle fit better without compressing the pliable left atrium if the pericardial sac was opened into the left hemithorax. After putting that ventricle in place and suturing the aorta, the right ventricle was positioned in the chest and held in place by Velcro and the air-driving tubing's exit sites. Then the chest was closed.

Olsen then clamped or tied off the aorta and pulmonary arteries and the superior and inferior venae cavae. With the diaphragms removed, the ventricles were injected with a rubbery material to fill the atria, venae cave, and pulmonary artery. After the material solidified, it was removed and evaluated by its shape. If the ventricles did not fit correctly, the thin-walled atria and superior vena cava appeared compressed, disturbing or limiting the blood flow. This "casting in place" was the best way to assess fit with the chest closed.

A Gift from the Neurologically Dead

In Philadelphia Kolff's son, Jack, who was still doing cadaver experiments, was not altogether sure about the DeVries-Olsen technique for putting the artificial heart's two ventricles in the left chest. He thought perhaps it would be better to separate the ventricles and put one in each side of the chest, but could he prove that? Because of anatomical differences in humans, he could not test his theory on animals. He needed to try his idea in a human with functioning blood circulation. That would require FDA authorization, which he did not have.

In May 1981, a brain aneurysm (blood-vessel blister) ruptured in a woman patient at Temple University Hospital. Although her body was otherwise intact, she was declared neurologically dead. Here was Jack Kolff's opportunity. The family agreed to let him implant the artificial heart, and because the patient had legally died, there was no need for FDA approval.

Subsequently Jack Kolff's team did more implants in brain-dead patients, including one that ran on a pump for seventy-two hours—the longest an artificial heart had ever beaten in a human chest. The experiment ended when the family requested the body for the funeral.

Dealing with the Media and Objections from the NHLBI

In the University of Utah's School of Medicine, Dean Dr. G. Richard Lee was also thinking about the implant. He could foresee the firestorm of publicity it would generate, which made him wrinkle his nose in distaste. He did not believe in conducting science amid headlines. Since a media blitz was inevitable, he thought he should prepare for it. "I'd like to talk to your staff," he told Kolff. Meeting them in the lab at St. Mark's, Lee asked each one's opinion of going ahead with the human implant. There were some reservations. Perfectionists in the group worried whether they had anticipated every possible problem. But Kolff was in favor, and so was Olsen.

Then Jarvik spoke up. "We are not ready," he declared.

Kolff was enraged. "That is wrong," he said. "The implant should go ahead."

That made Lee think. In his mind, Kolff was the authority. He recalled that Kolff and others had told him Jarvik was not the sole designer of the artificial heart. "He is only one in a long line of people who have made their contributions," Kolff had informed the dean.

Later, however, Lee asked DeVries, "What's going on? Rob Jarvik has reservations."

DeVries was embarrassed. "I have never doubted for a minute that the heart will work," he said. Lee nodded, convinced that DeVries was correct. The official sponsor for the heart application that had reached the FDA on February 27, 1981, was Kolff Associates, Inc. The application listed DeVries as the principal investigator, the only one who could do the implant surgery. Under the law, the proposal was deemed approved unless the FDA said no within thirty days.

On March 18, 1981, Kolff had an unannounced visitor, John Watson, boss of the NHLBI's Division of Cardiovascular Devices. Ostensibly on a scheduled trip to review the progress of federally funded programs in the Artificial Heart Research Laboratory, Watson asked for a list of everyone involved in the planned human implant. Kolff foresaw that this list would enable the NHLBI to determine whether anyone was being paid from its grants. If any were, the NHLBI could cut off the funding because its money was earmarked for animal research. Some eight months earlier, Kolff had written Watson assuring him no NHLBI funds would be used for work on human heart implants. Therefore, he thought Watson's request for the list was intimidation.

"I suggest you see Jim Brophy," Kolff said, referring to the university's vice president for research and a wily negotiator in dealing with federal agencies. Brophy shrewdly told Watson he would be glad to furnish the list as soon as he received a formal written request. Even under the rubric of assuring that funds were being properly used, such a letter would be undeniable proof the NHLBI was dipping its oar into a pond reserved for the FDA. The NHLBI chose not to send the letter.

However, Watson did go to see DeVries in his office with its cramped cubbyholes spilling over with research papers, books, and scientific publications. "What federal grants are funding your work?" Watson asked.

"None," was DeVries's terse reply. Watson queried if there were some channels by which federal aid was funneled to him. "None," said DeVries. It was true that he did implants for the federally funded animal experiments at St. Mark's, but he donated his time. The surgeon suddenly thought of the odd way serendipity works. A couple of years earlier he had asked Olsen for support money from his government funding for the animal implants. Now that rejection was emerging as a blessing. DeVries thought, "He's got no control over me because I don't get any of his money."

"Do you know what you are doing? Have you ever done anything in heart research?" Watson asked. DeVries concluded Watson knew nothing of his background: that he had worked in the heart program as far back as 1967. He thought, "He probably thinks I'm some young kid just out of his residency, someone Kolff hired to come in and do this."

"This [the implant] cannot do any good," Watson said, "only harm."

"What if it is successful?" DeVries asked.

"It will not do any good at all. Won't help us with funding," Watson stated.

DeVries thought that Watson was genuinely frightened. He became disturbed as the bureaucrat continued, "There are people like Bill Pierce.[2] They have spent all their lives working on the artificial heart. You may put one of these things in and kill the patient, and everything he has done will be destroyed. Kolff will be destroyed as well. You will have ruined the reputation that these people developed over the years..."

That struck DeVries. "It's not just me who's going to the line in this. It is all the people who preceded me. He's right about that. And that's frightening," he thought. He gained new insight into Watson's job that wiped out any resentment. He thought, "Under the system, his job is to be honest, to see that the funds are allocated correctly and conservatively." Nevertheless, DeVries was not going to back down.

After the Clark surgery, Earl Selby asked DeVries about the incident. "The NIH—after the first Cooley implant—got frightened to death that their whole program was going down the drain," he suggested.

DeVries replied,

> Watson said, 'You don't know what you are letting yourself in for. You are a young person, and you don't understand what is going on. This could literally slam the door on all artificial-heart research in the future.'...I said, 'If it is a dismal failure, that is what will happen.' But I also said, 'If it is a success, it is going to be fantastic.' [Watson] said, 'Success won't do anything if it's a failure. You can't win. You can only lose.' He was frightened...that a failure...like Cooley's would change things forever, that he would never be able to generate another penny for anybody.

Late the afternoon of Watson's visit, Kolff drove him to the airport. The bureaucrat said, "We are just deadly afraid that an unsuccessful experiment will set us all back."

"I do not anticipate failure," Kolff assured him.

In Washington a reporter asked the NHLBI's Frommer to comment on Utah's FDA application. "Haven't seen it," Frommer said. To his surprise, the reporter handed him a packet of fifty-eight photocopied pages, saying that the university had described it as the FDA proposal. "I'll read it," said Frommer.

The document offered his first reliable insight into the Utah plans. He discovered that far from ignoring the heart-assist devices favored by the NHLBI, DeVries had cited the work of at least fourteen investigators and concluded their clinical results "have been generally disappointing." Said DeVries, "Within the past five years, well over 200 patients have been supported with [assist pumps].... Only approximately 40 have been able to be weaned from their devices and fewer than 20 are reported to have left the hospital and even fewer were long-term survivors."

After reading this, Frommer wrote yet another letter to the FDA. This time he did not merely urge caution; he said flatly that the risks of using the artificial heart outweighed any possible benefits. This was a significant statement. If it was true, the FDA was legally bound to reject the heart application because its regulations forbade approval of any project with a negative risks-to-benefit ratio.

Frommer's letter went on to say that the Utah team:

> Failed to understand that with assist pumps, benefits were superior to the risk.
> Claimed the assist units were plagued by complications of hemorrhaging, infection, and multiorgan failure but was silent about how the artificial heart could avoid these.
> Was vague about average survival times and causes of death in its animal experiments, and
> Gave only a "brief and broad-brushed" description of its artificial-heart system.

Although he said the NHLBI supported local IRBs, Frommer took a swipe at the Utah board's competence in approving the artificial heart. He stated, "I am not familiar with the... expertise of the [IRB] and I do not know what material they had to review, but these sections [about the artificial heart] would be grossly inadequate to form a favorable technical assessment in the judgment of an NIH scientific review group."

In late March of 1981, the FDA had an answer for Utah: it was, "No—but..." While the application "was not approvable in its present form," the agency said it "would be happy to receive a revised application." In many respects, the FDA's letter to Utah seemed designed to respond to the behind-the-scenes complaints of Frommer and the NHLBI.

The FDA, for example, wanted more data to show that benefits outweighed risks. It wondered why DeVries had not given greater consideration to assist pumps. It declared the patient's informed-consent form did not adequately describe possible complications, and it sought more information about the length of survival and the quality of life that a heart recipient could expect.

DeVries, Kolff, and Lee Smith, the biomedical engineer who was president of Kolff Associates, Inc., regarded these comments as routine. "Happens all the time with the FDA," said Smith, who had undergone a briefing on the agency's procedures. Accordingly—after getting the agency's letter—he convened a meeting of thirteen scientists from the company and the university to discuss what was needed and form task forces to supply answers.

Infighting in Washington: Round Two

With the network of Washington contacts he had built over three decades, it was inevitable that Kolff would sooner or later learn of the NHLBI's efforts to block Utah's human implant. One even passed him a copy of Frommer's second letter to the FDA. Kolff sent copies to DeVries, Jarvik, Olsen, and Eichwald. His accompanying note on May 1, 1981, said, "The enclosed is an obvious subversive attempt to intimidate the FDA and to stop us from applying the artificial heart."

On the copy, he scrawled notes contradicting Frommer's comments. Reacting to the NHLBI official's challenge of the competence of the Utah IRB, he said, "Members of the IRB have visited our animals and our experimental facility. Dr. Frommer, as far as I can remember, has not." He also said that of 5,000 patients who die each year because their hearts cannot be restarted after cardiac surgery, "23 received [assist pumps]. That leaves 4,977 patients who die under the present state of the art. We propose to take one of those patients..."

As he had done every year since he served as its first president, Kolff went that May to the American Society for Artificial Internal Organs (ASAIO) meeting. There he met Robert Kennedy, associate director for the FDA's device-evaluation office. Kolff found him extremely friendly and encouraging. Kennedy voiced hope that Utah would ultimately get permission for the human implant. Kolff said that Kennedy was "very much annoyed" because Frommer had written not only to the FDA but also to U.S. Health and Human Services Secretary Richard S. Schweiker, to whom both the FDA and the NIH reported.

After returning to Utah, Kolff wrote a letter to Chase Peterson, University of Utah vice president for health sciences. According to Kolff, Kennedy had talked for ninety minutes at the meeting with DeVries and Jarvik. Kolff said they had learned that Schweiker had met with top officials from both the FDA and the

NIH about "the Utah problem" to determine which agency would make the decision on the heart proposal.

Kolff reported to Peterson,

> After having heard from all parties, the Secretary of Health decided there would be no deviation from the usual procedure—that is, the FDA is to handle this case. I will not try to guess at the motive of the National Heart Institute [NHLBI] for the actions that they have taken, but want to state they are unusual, unethical, uncalled for and a clear attempt to prejudice the court. Therefore, I suggest we restrict our communications with the National Heart and Lung Institute [NHLBI] to the bare minimum; that we do nothing to antagonize them, delay any response as long as it is humanly possible to any request or any action that the National Heart Institute [NHLBI] takes.

Assured that the FDA was making "the Utah decision," Kolff told his wife, Janke, "We have played the permission game from the FDA, exclusively according to the rules. The Heart Institute [NHLBI] has tried to break the rules. They lost on all points. They have not been enough sportsmen to send me a little note congratulating me."

But the NHLBI was not done fighting. It was playing hardball with new ammunition. A report from its advisory council concluded that the institute was right on all counts, and the University of Utah and its IRB should reconsider human implants.

The council particularly pointed out that the media were attracted to the implant story. Within seven pages, it said Utah's plans had been "much publicized" and "widely publicized." On top of that, the plans had drawn "extensive publicity." Without supplying details, it cited the "possible emotional trauma from extensive publicity" and "the hazards from excessive publicity."

In that spirit, the NHLBI's Frommer said, when he sent the report to Utah, that the implant plan had been "widely announced." The report said there was "potential bias" in having the same doctor be both the "treating surgeon and the investigating surgeon," an apparent reference to DeVries being the principal investigator and also the implant surgeon. The Utah researchers wondered if the same separation had been enforced in the assist-pump experiments. The council report did not address this question.

To avoid any suggestion that the advisory council was totally against artificial hearts, the report stated that artificial hearts could be used when there was no other means to maintain life for a year. The members did not explain how they had arrived at that time period, or whether the same criteria were applied to assist devices. In forwarding the report to Utah's Vice President Peterson, Frommer said that it could be considered an outside review of Utah's plans. As he acknowledged, it might be considered "unsolicited advice." The IRB subcommittee did not reconsider its approval for the implant.

Cooley... Again

In Holland a bus driver named Willebrordus A. Meuffels was not even thirty-five. He was short of breath and racked by angina pectoris. With his family history (a heart attack had killed his father at fifty-six), doctors sent him to Denton Cooley's Texas Heart Institute in Houston. The opinion was not to operate. Meuffels was put on a regimen of drugs and a low-fat diet and sent home. The chest pains became sharper and more frequent, forcing him to quit work. His Dutch physicians sent him back to Houston.

When he arrived on July 20, 1981, Meuffels was anxious but not in acute distress. His blood pressure was 110 over 80, his pulse 78 and normal. An electrocardiogram showed nothing abnormal. However, an arteriogram of his coronary arteries disclosed that his heart muscle was starved for blood. Three arteries were partially blocked, two so severely they allowed only a quarter of the normal blood flow. The diagnosis was atherosclerosis or deposits of plaque from build-ups of cholesterol and other chemicals. Cooley did what he had done thousands of times—by his count more often than anybody else in the world—a triple bypass, taking bits of a vein from one of Meuffels's legs and suturing them to divert blood around the clogged arteries.

All went smoothly until the surgeons tried to take their patient off the heart-lung machine. Stubbornly the heart refused to start pumping. After intensive therapy, it gradually revived. Within ninety-five minutes, it was beating strongly enough to disconnect the heart-lung machine and transfer Meuffels to the Intensive Care Unit (ICU). Three hours later his blood pressure fell alarmingly.

Fearing a heart attack, doctors massaged Meuffels's chest. When that brought no response, they cut open the incision from his bypass surgery and began to compress the heart by hand. Feebly it began pumping. They called for heart-whipping drugs such as Lidocaine. They failed. So did repeated electric shocks. Their only hope was to get Meuffels back on the heart-lung machine. With doctors literally at his side—reaching into his open chest to squeeze his heart into beating—he was wheeled through the halls to the OR.

In forty-five minutes, he was on bypass. Except for that, Meuffels was "dead on the table," the classic description of the patient DeVries had envisioned to implant an artificial heart. Waiting outside the OR was Meuffels's wife. Cooley sent one of his assistants to explain what they were facing. They could let her husband die, or they could try to sustain him by implanting an artificial heart on a temporary basis until they found a donor heart for a transplant. Amid tears she gave both oral and written consent for the implant.

Cooley had an artificial heart available, one developed by Dr. Tetsuzo Akutsu, the same surgeon/researcher who had built the first artificial heart in Kolff's Cleveland lab. Akutsu had worked since the late 1970s on ventricular-assist pumps and artificial hearts in Cooley's cardiovascular research center. Because of Meuffels's obviously poor chances of recovery, Akutsu was reluctant to see his heart wasted on this patient. This design had been finished only two weeks earlier and had not even been tested on any animals. Cooley had never bothered with calf experiments. He once said to *Life* magazine, "Why should I spend my time sewing it [the heart] into a cow? You don't even need a medical degree for that."

On July 23, 1981, the media carried the news that Cooley had put Akutsu's artificial heart into Meuffels and was hunting for a donor heart to transplant. That was fine with Kolff. He was looking to a permanent lifesaver with his artificial heart. He telegraphed Cooley, "Congratulations. Well done. Save the patient's life while you are blazing the trail. Best wishes for your patient, my fellow Dutchman and for you from all of us in Utah."

Jarvik was hosting a small party in his home the night of the Houston implant. DeVries called to tell him about Cooley's surgery. Jarvik was nonchalant: "That is probably the most interesting thing I have heard all day."

Meuffels's implant experienced problems almost from the beginning, starting with diffuse bleeding that was difficult to control. Because of that, the Cooley team decided not to sew the sternum closed so they had access to the chest. Only the skin and the subcutaneous tissue along the incision were stitched. Within eight hours, Meuffels's left lung became congested, and signs indicated possible fluid in the right lung. What Cooley described as "mechanical obstruction" became evident in both a pulmonary vein and artery, possibly from being squashed by the heart. The next day the amount of blood oxygen sank precipitously while carbon dioxide—the poison that lungs normally siphon off—rose. Cooley ordered an oxygenator to be connected to provide more oxygen.

It was now imperative that the Texas team locate a heart for a transplant. Miraculously they found one in Tennessee, where a thirty-year-old man had died after a motorcycle crash. His body was flown to Houston so his heart could be transferred to Meuffels. However, at 8:00 AM on August 2, 1981, Meuffels died of multiorgan failure. He had lived thirty-six years with a natural heart, fifty-six hours with an artificial heart, and seven and a half days with a transplanted heart.

Meufflels's story did not end there. The FDA complained that by law it had to approve the clinical implant of medical devices. Cooley had implanted his artificial heart without even a word to the federal agency, contending his patient's emergency had dictated his actions. The agency did some thinking before it wrote, "We fully appreciate the emergency confronting Dr. Cooley and we have no reason to question the circumstances surrounding implantation." It added that if Cooley had any plans to put in another heart, he should "please submit [an application for a device exemption] to the FDA." A Washington newsletter called that "a wrist slap."

The FDA Approves Seven Patients in Utah

Three days after Meuffels's death, the secretaries at Kolff Associates, Inc., finished the mammoth job of copying and collating the new application seeking FDA permission to implant an artificial heart. To answer the agency's questions had taken four months, and the size of the document had nearly tripled to 225 pages. The new application included patients with chronic heart failure in the pool of potential candidates.

The FDA gave the application a line-by-line reading. It also sent copies to various consultants, seeing what holes they could poke. Several worried the heart might be implanted in a minor. Another faulted switching to backup units if the heart driver failed. A third said he thought it would be exceedingly rare if a natural heart could not be revived after surgery, so why would the artificial device ever be needed? Were any caveats serious enough to block approval? The FDA officials decided no. On September 10, 1981 they announced that they were giving DeVries approval to do not one but a series of seven implants.

Kolff permitted himself to smile. He had worked a quarter of a century for this moment. Of all the researchers who had labored on the artificial heart, he was the one who had persevered the longest and now had received the first government sanction to implant the device.

The following day news stories about the FDA announcement blossomed around the country in the *New York Times,* the *Washington Post,* the *Chicago Tribune,* and the *Los Angeles Times.* The story also made its way into the *Seattle Times.* Among the latter's subscribers was Barney Clark. At the time—with his own heart condition not yet critical—he believed the news was irrelevant.

The FDA, however, still was not completely satisfied. It wanted some further fine tuning on the language proposed by DeVries for the informed-consent form. Once the refinements were made, it took seven pages to include everything the agency thought necessary. The form said the recipient had to be so sick he or she would die unless the natural heart was removed and an artificial one implanted. Also, according to the form, DeVries thought that the left ventricular-assist pumps advocated by the NHLBI possessed more complications than benefits.

But accompanying the artificial heart—the form pointed out in blunt terms—could be a gallery of horrors. The heart could spawn deadly blood clots, could mechanically fail, could lead to infection, hemorrhaging, pneumothorax, and blood-cell damage. Once the heart was in, more surgery might be inevitable to correct problems. An implant, said the form, was "highly experimental." A recipient could "anticipate pain, discomfort, inconvenience." No promises could be made about success, possible length of life, or the quality of that life. Cooley's two temporary implants were mentioned; the form said they had resulted in survivals of only "several hours." Moreover, the patient had to assume all the risks, including picking up "considerable" costs due to extended hospitalization.

The FDA wanted to give patients ample chance to pull out. It specified the consent form had to be signed twice with at least a twenty-four-hour gap in between to allow plenty of time to reconsider. When DeVries pondered the consent form, he wondered where he would find a patient whose condition justified the heart and who also had the grit to face all the medical uncertainties.

DeVries did not know that—years before in Minneapolis—when Walter Lillehei had performed the first successful cross-circulation procedure from parent to child to repair a ventricular septal defect in Gregory Glidden, the parents had signed a consent form consisting of one simple sentence: "I, the undersigned, hereby grant permission for an operation or any procedure the university staff deems necessary upon my son, Gregory Glidden."

Time and bureaucracy had now complicated human research. The simple straightforward permission granted by the Gliddens had all but disappeared under the mountains of paperwork and hours of debate required of the Utah artificial-heart team. But with the resolution of the FDA's final questions, the University of Utah entered a new phase—waiting for the right patient.

Notes

1. Natalie Davis Spingarn, *Heartbeat: The Politics of Health Research* (Washington, DC: Robert B. Luce, 1976).
2. Dr. William Pierce of Pennsylvania State University's Milton S. Hershey Medical Center was a noted experimenter on devices both to assist and replace the natural heart.

PART FIVE

17

Ready for Surgery

Thoughts
Relief: No awkward decisions.
What to do with a man incapacitated.
And a "heart that keeps on pumping,"
And the whole world's attention
Is on us.

—Barney and Una Loy Clark

Barney Clark Flies to Salt Lake City

By late 1982, Barney was familiar with the Utah artificial-heart program, and his medical condition appeared to meet the criteria that had been hammered out for IRB and FDA approvals.

The Friday following Thanksgiving (November 25, 1982), William DeVries received a telephone call from Barney and his Seattle cardiologist, Dr. Jeff Block. Barney was not dying, but he was confined to his home, and his condition was deteriorating. Block thought his patient might have less than a week to live. Barney said that if he was going to do something about his situation, now was the time to do it. DeVries suggested that he fly to Salt Lake City by air ambulance to reduce the risk of dying en route. Barney didn't think that was necessary and flew to Salt Lake City on a commercial plane, arriving at 5:00 PM. Western Airlines had a long concourse to the baggage-claim area, which worried flight nurse Donna Weeks. To protect Barney from the press stationed at the airport, he and Una Loy were flown by helicopter directly to University Hospital.

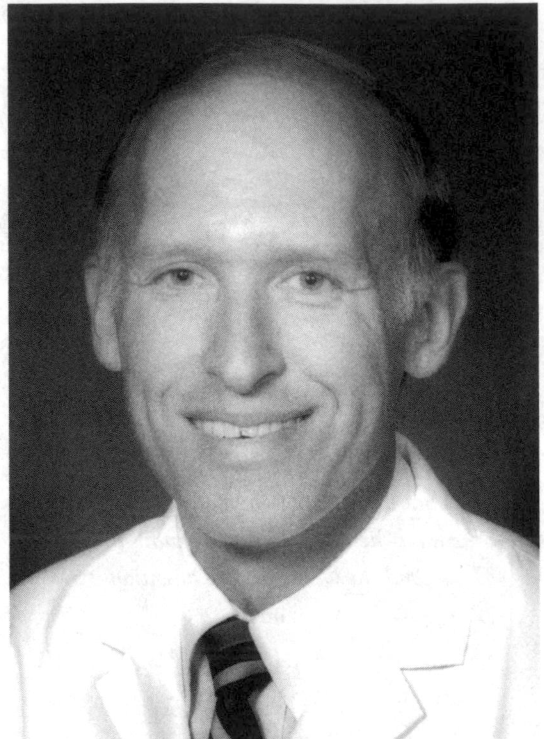

University of Utah cardiologist Dr. Fred Anderson.

Barney Is Admitted to the University of Utah Medical Center

Cardiologist Dr. Fred Anderson officially admitted Barney into the University of Utah Medical Center on Monday, November 29, 1982. Anesthesiologist Dr. Ted Stanley went to Barney's room to discuss his pending anesthesia and the informed-consent requirements. "Barney was very, very sick," Stanley said. "He has a disease which has slowly progressed to the point that it's like having two feet in the coffin, not just one." Stanley and Dr. Nathan Pace discussed how they could do the things that were necessary to get Barney safely under anesthesia and keep him stable until he could be connected to the heart-lung machine.

Barney's extremities were blue, his arms and legs were cold, and his abdomen was distended, indicating ascites, an accumulation of fluids. He had moderate peripheral edema. All were symptoms of profound cardiac failure. The paradox with which the IRB had wrestled was coming to the OR. While surgeons did not want to cut the heart out until the patient was nearly dead, that created the worst possible scenario for anesthesiologists. To get the patient anesthetized while keeping the natural heart from deteriorating or stopping until the heart-lung machine is connected and functioning is a challenge in any open-heart surgery; Barney's poor condition made it even worse.

Barney remarked, "The last year and a half I have lived because of the pills they gave me. Somebody had to test them first, and I am trying to do something similar." But he also felt very strongly that he was going to die. "In my death, as in my life, if I can help the next person to do a little bit better, that is something I want to do." He bravely went on, "I know that I am going to die. I accept that, but I want to know that someone later on is helped."

Barney could not walk and had an erratic heart rate. He was experiencing brief ventricular tachycardia (rapid, uncontrolled heartbeats) that could be fatal. He also had moderate renal impairment.

DeVries was asked if he had done a physical examination on Barney. He said, "He did not come to me for a physical. He came to me for information about the artificial heart. Others have given him physicals, and he came with a detailed medical history."

DeVries told Barney's family members that all costs would be donated except the hospital expense, which might run from ten to fifteen thousand dollars. It was even possible that those costs would be donated. Kolff Associates, Inc., was donating the artificial heart and the use of the driver and other equipment.

Dr. Lyle Joyce had been significantly involved with animal experimentation and had also worked with DeVries for two years in the hospital, where he had received accolades for his sensitivity to surgical patients' families. He had limited opportunity to visit with the Clarks immediately before the surgery, however, because so many hospital personnel were interviewing them. When Joyce finally approached this patient, he felt the difference. Joyce thought, "He knows he is dying, and he's about to enter an uncharted experiment."

The cardiologist's primary measurement to determine how nonfunctional a heart may be is the ejection fraction—the percentage of blood being pushed from the ventricle with each beat. Barney's cardiac ejection fraction was 7 to 9 percent (the normal heart's is 65 percent). His heart was in severe failure, and his body automatically shunted blood away from the kidneys, skeletal muscles, and liver to preserve the brain and the heart. However, Barney was still lucid, and his memory was astonishing. Calmly Joyce commented on this presurgical situation. "If Barney were going to die, now would be that time."

Two cardiologists named Anderson also played key roles. Jeff Anderson, who had originally referred Barney to DeVries, had assured Barney's son, Stephen, that he was 90-plus percent sure that his father would meet the IRB's criteria to receive the artificial heart.

Fred Anderson was a member of the university's evaluating team. His assignment was to collect and evaluate all necessary medical data to determine the patient's prognosis. The cardiologists had to ensure that the patient had the specific medical profile spelled out by the FDA and the IRB. The patient had to be in the New York Heart Association class-four heart-failure classification. According to those requirements, the patient had to have

A ventricle ejection fraction of less than 18 percent;

A cardiac index of less than 1.5 liters of blood pumped each minute per section of body surface area squared;

No active inflammatory disease, dismissing possible recoverable heart failure; and no significant surgically correctable lesions.

"The patient shows significant cardiac failure symptoms at bed rest," Fred Anderson concluded. He remembered Barney had been much sharper during his visit in October. On December 1 at 7:30 AM, Anderson wrote in his journal, "Visited with patient; examined him. Essentially unchanged; talked about dental school, numbers of dentists in practice in Seattle, etc.; seemed relaxed and didn't talk about the heart."

Normal blood-clotting time is twelve minutes, and the higher the number, the more likelihood of bleeding during surgery. The level needed to be twenty-five to thirty-five minutes for good anticoagulation. Barney was taking Coumadin to prevent blood clots from forming in his poorly beating heart. These clots could break free, travel to the brain, and potentially kill him. However, it was also necessary for his blood to clot after surgery.

Making the Decision to Operate Earlier

At 5:00 PM, the Cardiac Intensive Care Unit (CICU) called Fred Anderson to report that Barney had experienced a thirty-second run of ventricular tachycardia (V-tach) arrhythmia that had stopped spontaneously; he then appeared okay, but patients with heart disease frequently die from arrhythmia. With DeVries and Dr. Ross Woolley (a member of the IRB), Anderson reviewed the recorded ECG strips; they showed clear-cut V-tach for about thirty seconds with another briefer run. The V-tach seemed to be related to stimuli. Barney had been about to have his blood drawn when the arrhythmia had started. There were also short periods of premature ventricular contractions (PVCs), a serious further sign of possible cardiac arrest and death.

The intra-aortic balloon pump was brought close to Barney's room to support his circulation if needed. The question was whether to wait until morning, or do the surgery that night when Joyce finished his present case and the larger OR and patient-monitoring equipment would be available. The consensus among DeVries, Woolley, and Anderson seemed to be that it was hard to know whether Barney would die that night if they did not operate, but it seemed very likely.

At 6:00 PM, Anderson went with DeVries and Woolley to speak with Una Loy and Barney's daughter and son-in-law about performing the surgery earlier than planned. "We don't think your husband is going to live until morning; I want to go ahead with the surgery early," DeVries told Una Loy.

She replied, "Yes, I saw it on television."

Local radio and television news had already reported that the surgery was going to occur that night, rather than the next morning. With so many people and facilities involved, the news had leaked out quickly. These persistent information leaks about the pending surgery—mostly incorrect—were hard on the family and most annoying to the team.

Barney told DeVries, "I wish we could go ahead and do it now."

DeVries said, "Your wish has come true."

Barney's last words before being anesthetized went to Una Loy: "If I don't see you again, you have been a darn good wife."

DeVries recognized the comment as another proof of what a close couple they were. "I knew it even before that," he said later. "I knew it in October when they were here. They were asking questions as though they came out of one mouth."

DeVries also asked the assembled team members their opinions about doing the surgery that night, even though it was up to him to make the final decision. If Barney's heart continued to fail during the night, his brain could be permanently damaged.

Some of the hospital personnel caring for Barney advised the team that they had "better go early. He has deteriorated in appearance and in cardiac rhythm during the day." Barney just did not look as well to them.

Because Joyce was already doing a case in the largest OR, Anderson noted, "All the necessary people are in the OR already for the case going on, and none of them wants to go home, leaving in such a snowstorm."

Final Preparations

Anderson requested the use of a physiologic recorder during the surgery. He wanted to be able to read on a screen what the pressures were at any specific time and also have a permanent paper recording of those pressures that could be reviewed later. This would help the doctors understand the patient's response to drugs and the effectiveness of the heart-lung machine. The blood pressures he was interested in were the aortic and the pulmonary artery. Another very important pressure was the left atrial, which would tell exactly how the artificial heart was working. Based on the readings, the pneumatic controller could adjust the pressures. Pace and Anderson also asked that the "electronics for medicine/patient-monitoring equipment that provides a paper readout and permanent record of all the measured parameters be made available."

That evening Don Olsen had attended a Kolff Associates, Inc., board meeting where Kolff announced Barney's surgery would occur the next morning. Olsen found himself driving home in a heavy snowstorm over snow-packed roads lined with deepening drifts. Since he lived on a steep hillside, Olsen decided to park his car facing downhill so he could leave early the following morning for the surgery. His wife, Joyce, met him at the door with the news, "Bill has called twice and wants you to hurry to the hospital."

Olsen immediately waded back through the snow to his car, grateful he had had the foresight to park on the street. He started the snowy journey along slippery Foothill Boulevard back to the University of Utah Medical Center. At the hospital, he quickly changed into surgical scrubs about 8:30 PM.

Anderson changed into green hospital scrubs and stayed near the nursing station watching Barney's EKG. The screen showed an increase in PVCs and a decreasing heart rate, both bad signs.

Joyce finished his cardiac case about 9:00 PM, which freed up the larger OR. The orderlies, nurses, and attendants hurried to clean and prepare it for Barney's surgery. The requested electronic-monitoring equipment was also calibrated.

Pace and his residents were taking a break in the lounge and watching television as John Dwan, the medical center's public-relations director, announced that Barney was in the OR. One of the local 10:00 PM news programs reported, "Patient stable now. The family is with him for a few minutes, and the surgery will be done tonight."

Pace got up and remarked wryly, "If Barney is in the OR, then we'd better take him there."

Ready, Set, Go

All hospitals are alike—a confounding maze of hallways bathed in bright fluorescent lights and lined with countless doors leading to places with warning signs that read "Do Not Enter" or "Hospital Personnel Only." These expanses of terrazzo flooring echo either the purposeful steps of those who know where they are going, or the uncertain meandering of those who do not. University

Hospital was no different on this snowy December night, except for one special hallway, the one connecting the CICU with the OR suites. Clattering down this passageway was a cumbersome bed with its occupant, his head propped high on a pile of crumpled pillows.

Following the bed was an unusually large parade of personnel. Each was dressed in the familiar green outfit of the hospital staff, some cloaked with unbuttoned white coats, which billowed like the sails of a ship providing the group with its forward momentum. And forward they went. There was no turning back from the decision to embark on one of the most historic medical adventures of the twentieth century.

The task was to successfully traverse the unmeasured distance from the safe confines of the CICU, with its monitoring equipment, to the equally safe OR. This hallway was a no-man's-land in medical care. All hospitals teem with stories of patients who developed life-threatening medical problems while in hallways, elevators, or other inhospitable dead zones—the outcomes were hardly ever positive.

This knowledge was on everyone's mind as the members of the staff closest to Barney quizzed him with the question asked of all patients headed to the OR: "How ya doin'?" Instead of a realistic response, such as, "If I wasn't on my way to the OR to have my failing heart removed and replaced by a plastic heart never before used in a human being, I'd be fine," he murmured, "I'm okay," between labored breaths.

That was Barney, a man who was to become loved and respected by everyone who got to know him during the next unknown number of days. He was a man who faced the uncertainty of this event with a stoicism and resolve that made him a hero—a man of valor—and the perfect patient. He was the type of man of whom the eighteenth-century dramatist and poet Conte Vittorio Alfieri had said, "Often the test of courage is not to die, but to live."

At that moment, however, the goal was simple—to reach the OR safely. Despite all of the unanswered questions regarding the J-7 heart, everyone present that eventful evening in Salt Lake City believed that it was now the only possible way to prolong Barney's life. It simply had to work, or death was inevitable.

Entering the cardiac-surgery OR immediately lessened the anxiety of the transport team as well as the patient. The undersized monitor propped precariously at the foot of the bed with its equally small display of heart rate and blood pressure was exchanged for the large overhead displays. And the tackle box of emergency medications transported with Barney was replaced by the standalone medication cart of the anesthesiologist. This environment provided as

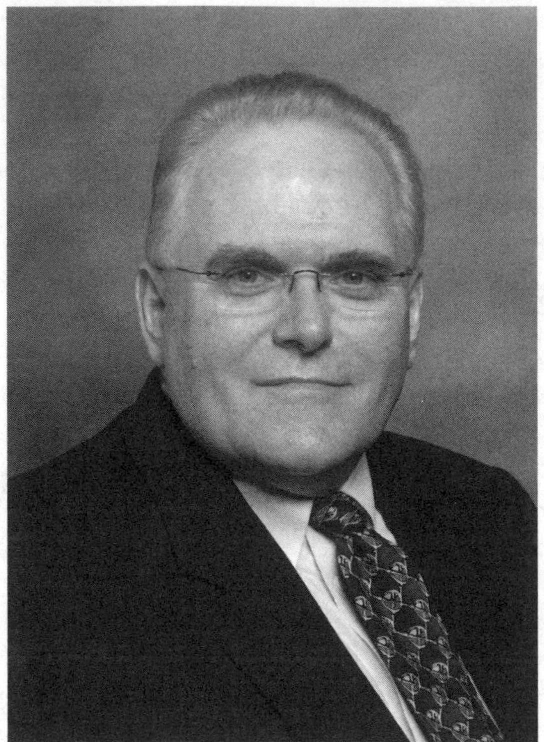

Anesthesiologist Dr. Nathan Pace.

much safety for the patient as a hospital could offer. Television and the movies tell us that the surgeon rules the OR. That is a falsehood; the OR is a shared venue, and the physician who shares it with the surgeon is the anesthesiologist. On this night, that was Dr. Nathan Pace.

Ode to Nathan Pace

Pace knew that nearly all patients facing heart surgery are very frightened, and most people want to be knocked out. He had already told Barney about the possible impact of anesthesia on his failing heart. The anesthesiologist understood Barney could not withstand the usual pre-anesthesia procedures and that remaining relaxed would help the anesthesia process. Most patients would never have tolerated that, but Barney's blood pressure revealed he was calm.

As Barney struggled to slide himself from the hospital bed onto the operating table, Pace took charge of his care. He knew that the key to the next phase of Barney's care was going to be the tricky task of placing him safely asleep under general anesthesia. It would take all his skill.

Normally patients arriving in the OR have already received intravenous sedation to prepare them for the operation. The severity of Barney's heart disease, however, made administering hypnotic drugs far too dangerous because they would have the unwanted side effect of either suppressing his severely depressed heart function or triggering more of the life-threatening arrhythmia that had nearly killed him earlier.

Caught in this dilemma, Pace had to proceed with Barney fully awake. He had decided to substitute words and actions for the usual presurgery medications. In his most reassuring voice, he selected consoling words to describe the events that were about to unfold. He reasoned that a technical blueprint would divert Barney's attention. As a dentist, Barney would be accustomed to focusing on medical procedures. Although in uncharted waters, Pace was confident that he could make this approach work and safely put Barney to sleep.

Pace asked Barney to extend his arm onto the board. Later, he admitted, "That was the only time I became self-conscious. I realized Bill was leaning all the way across the table to watch my hands. And there was the horrible television camera from the university's Channel 7 zooming on my fingers to record what I was doing. This made me very nervous because all attention was focused on me. I was the only one doing anything. The others were waiting for me to get Barney to sleep."

The Calm Amidst the Storm

Pace asked, "Barney, I need to do a few things. Are you okay?"

"I'm okay."

"Good, first I need to place a small catheter in the radial artery. We use this for monitoring your blood pressure and also we can sample your blood. You know that we always need more blood!"

"Yes, I think that you all are part vampire."

"You're probably right. Okay, here we go. All set?"

"All set." So far, so good.

Pace then told Barney, "We are going to give you a drug to put you to sleep."

Barney responded, "All right; go ahead." He seemed confident and well prepared.

The hospital personnel were quite amazed that Barney had arrived in the OR fully awake, had been asked to slide himself onto the table, and had had the arterial blood-pressure line and IVs started without any pre-anesthetics.

Some remarked that Barney was like "the eye in the middle of a hurricane—so calm, given all of the people in the room—photographers, television camera operators, and the entire team, many of them scrubbed and gowned."

Joyce later said, "Barney was remarkably tough, given the commotion in the room." He concluded that either Barney was mentally in control or Pace was very lucky—perhaps both.

Barney was under anesthesia at 11:20 PM. The first challenge had been overcome.

18

The Cutting Edge

I have set before you life and death,
Blessing and cursing; therefore choose life.
—Deuteronomy 30:19

The Implantation

The skill with which surgery is done is a direct reflection of how good the first assistant is. Lyle Joyce and William DeVries had become an extremely well-coordinated team as Joyce began his residency in cardiothoracic surgery in Utah. Don Olsen was also invited to participate in the surgery because he had by far the most experience implanting the artificial heart. He had also taught and worked with Joyce for nearly two years and DeVries for three years implanting artificial hearts. These three men were ready to embark on the most significant surgery they had ever undertaken.

The OR was a whirlwind of activity. Despite its chaotic appearance, this activity was in fact controlled. Each group of nurses, doctors, and technicians was concentrating on the role it played in this medical drama. One group of nurses hurriedly opened large trays of sterilized surgical instruments, meticulously arranging them in an organized pattern that allowed rapid location of a single instrument. This ritual produced a near-constant metal clanging, a noise so familiar that everyone ignored it.

Simultaneously another nurse added to the vast array of multishaped instruments and the growing pile of disposable items—gloves, gowns, sutures, and scalpel blades. Each item was carefully dropped onto the sterile instrument tables from its equally sterile package. Sterility was a high priority for this night's operation. The remainder of the nurses hovered around the patient, strategically replacing EKG patches with sterile ones in a predetermined pattern around his

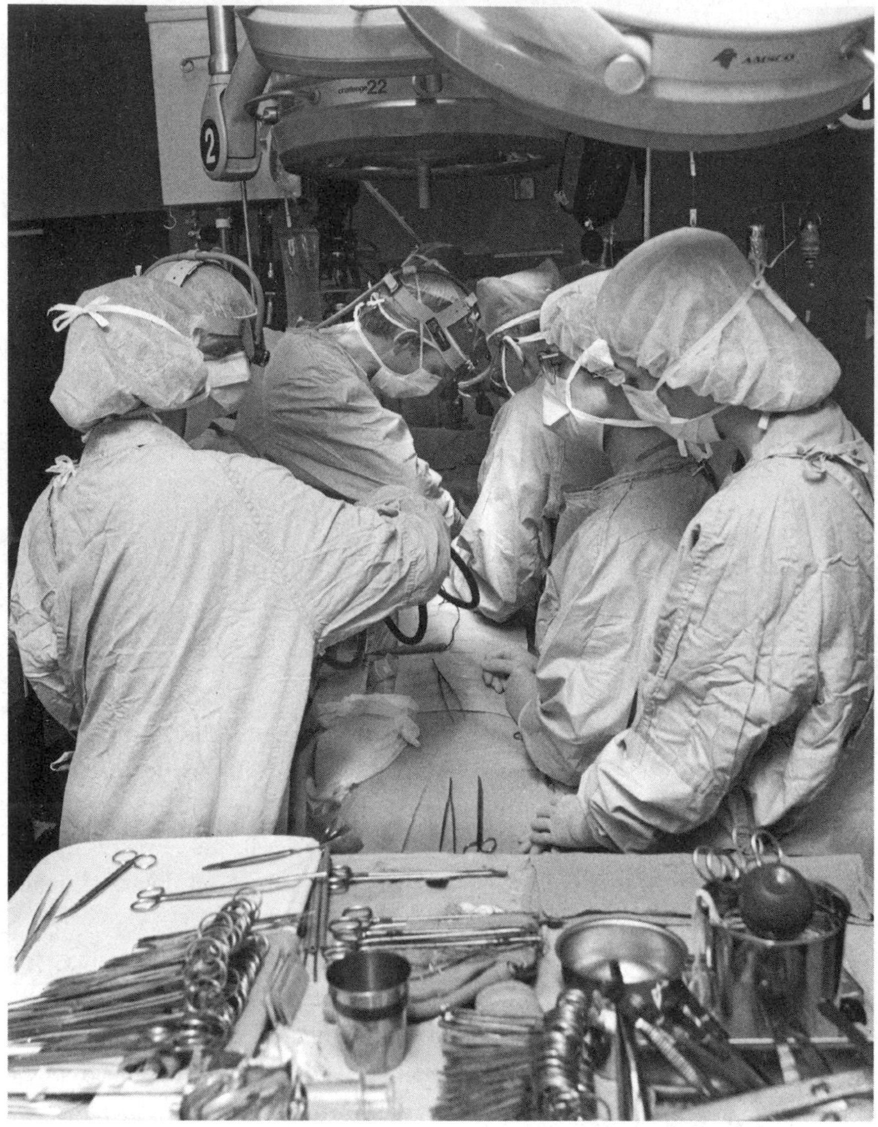

The team was well practiced, and each person had a specific job during the operation.

body. One nurse thoughtfully covered Barney with a warm blanket, a gesture he would have greatly appreciated. The OR was always cold, whether it was July or December.

Adjacent to the operating table was the heart-lung machine, a large, rectangular, stainless-steel device with a dizzying array of knobs, dials, and electronic displays entwined in a spaghetti-like mass of clear plastic tubing. The perfusionists who managed this device watched water flow through the maze of tubing while vigorously hammering randomly with metal clamps to dislodge any trapped air bubbles. When the heart-lung machine was connected to a patient, air was not a friend; it could block blood flow, resulting in a multitude of problems and creating the potential for a stroke. Consequently every bubble had to be fastidiously removed.

Despite its complex appearance, the machine was rather simple. It merely mimicked the lungs by adding oxygen and removing carbon dioxide from the red blood cells and then, like the heart, pumping the oxygenated blood back into the body to nourish the organs. The heart-lung machine, however, would not be used until the moment when DeVries stopped Barney's heart, nearly an hour away. That moment would be very welcome since it would mean that Nathan Pace had successfully coaxed Barney's nearly dead heart to work just a little bit longer to allow implantation of the J-7 heart.

Despite the many similarities to a routine heart operation, the OR on this December night was visibly different. Most obvious was the presence of a cumbersome device pushed to one side of the room. This console contained the crucial components for powering and monitoring the artificial heart. The J-7 heart consisted of two polyurethane pumps, one for the right side of the circulation and one for the left. These were the components that DeVries would sew to Barney's atrial and great vessel remnants after the ventricles—the actual pumping portions of the heart—were removed. By themselves, however, the J-7 ventricles were useless. They required external power and an external control system.

Pulses of compressed air powered the J-7. The air's actual source was a large system outside the OR, where individual pipes directed the highly filtered air to the areas where the artificial-heart recipient would receive his care. The compressed air also had to be regulated to selectively adjust the pressure of the air delivered to the J-7 ventricles based upon the resistance to the pumping of blood.

An additional complication was the significant difference in resistance exerted by the right and left sides of the patient's circulation. The left ventricle, which pumped oxygenated blood via the aorta to all the organs, required a much higher pressure than the right ventricle, which pumped unoxygenated blood to the lungs.

The simple turn of a dial adjusted the pressure of the heart driver to ensure that each ventricle ejected its full volume of blood with each beat, no matter what the resistance was. The heart driver also had a thumbwheel dial to select the number of beats every minute—the J-7 heart rate. The final variable controlled

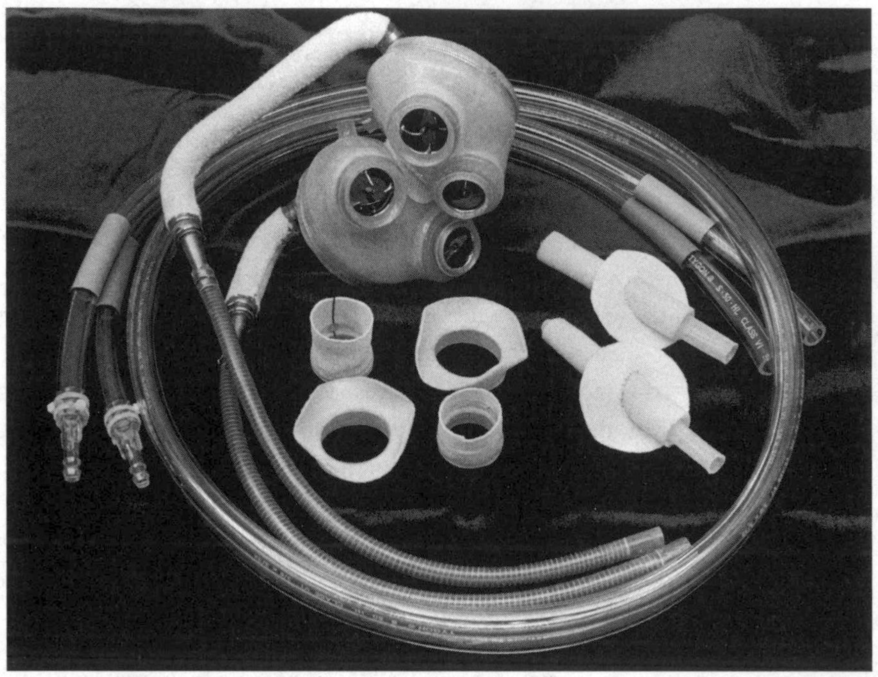

The components of the J-7 artificial heart.

by the heart driver was selecting how much time was spent in ejecting blood with each beat, the systole, and how much time was spent in filling, the diastole.

The artificial heart was in a sterile, double-wrapped package. There was also a second, individually wrapped heart to be used as a backup. Tom Kessler and his assistants had meticulously built, examined, and tested both artificial hearts. Each package contained two ventricles, two six-foot drivelines, size-matched cuffs to be sewn to the atria, and short Dacron vascular grafts for the great vessels. The cuffs had large, nearly flat skirts that would be trimmed on the table to fit the atria after the natural ventricles were cut and removed. The vascular grafts were nearly the same diameter as the aorta and pulmonary artery stumps after they were cut just above the valves.

People and Equipment in the OR

The primary surgical-implantation team consisted of the following people: surgeons Bill DeVries, Lyle Joyce, and Don Olsen; anesthetist Nathan Pace; cardiologists Fred Anderson and Jeff Anderson; perfusionist Doug Smith; heart-driver engineer Steve Nielsen; heart-driver manager Larry Hastings; advisor Robert Jarvik; and nurses Gayle Baldwin and Diane Karsten.

Pace stood at Barney's head behind a low drape in a nonsterile working area. His anesthesia machine required connections to power and gas from the central hospital supply, so lines to the video-monitoring screens threaded among the equipment. Smith positioned the heart-lung machine to Pace's left. The machine had six pump heads that squeezed plastic tubes to move blood and a heat exchanger to cool the blood and then rewarm it during surgery. The heart-lung tubing passed between Olsen and Joyce, who were also on the left.

DeVries was on Barney's right side next to the anesthesia equipment and directly across the table from Joyce. The surgical resident, Chuck Berry, had scrubbed Barney's chest and stood next to DeVries for the short time he was involved. A young female medical student rotating through surgery training was in the OR briefly, prompting DeVries to remark that in medical school, he would have killed to have the chance to attend this kind of surgery. However, she had to leave when Robert Jarvik arrived because there wasn't enough space. Jarvik came in after the surgery had begun and remained for about an hour while the heart was placed inside Barney's chest. The head instrument nurse stood close to DeVries so she could pass him what he needed efficiently.

The heart driver, where Nielsen and Hastings waited, was placed immediately behind DeVries. The sterile heart drivelines passed off the table to Hastings on DeVries's left so that the surgeon would not be trapped. The two cardiologists were there to monitor and advise about the patient's status throughout the procedure. Two photographers recorded the entire procedure on film with both a still and a movie camera.

Very early in the procedure, DeVries—at a nurse's request—announced there were far too many people in the room (twenty-seven by then), which posed an increased threat of infection to Barney. Supported by the head nurse, he asked all nonessential people to leave, and they reluctantly complied.

DeVries then requested that a nurse select some soothing background music. Later he remembered, "Gayle Baldwin played *Fresh Aire* by Mannheim Steamroller." Jarvik, though, later made a big deal of telling a reporter that he had personally selected the background music: *Bolero* by Ravel. Many of those in the OR reported that they were concentrating so closely on shutting out all nonessential sounds that they didn't remember anything about background music.

Initial Incision

After checking that Pace was ready for him to proceed, DeVries picked up the scalpel and boldly made the first long, midline incision, extending from just below Barney's chin to under the sternum, or breastbone. An electrocautery extended the incision and seared the blood vessels, clotting them as it cut. After the incision reached the hard bone of the sternum, DeVries and Joyce stopped all the bleeders with DeBakey forceps, and Olsen touched the forceps with the cautery to seal the cut vessels and minimize blood loss.

DeVries asked for a bone saw to cut through the sternum. When placed close to the underside of the sternum, the shoe on the end of this small jigsaw prevents the surgeon from accidentally cutting too deeply into the chest. "This saw does not work," DeVries exclaimed in frustration. A backup saw was obtained. "This one's good," he said.

As soon as the sternum was cut, the bone marrow was quickly packed with sterile beeswax to control oozing blood, and all bleeders were cauterized. DeVries did one side, and Joyce did the other, based on what each could see best.

A rib spreader gave the surgeons greater vision and access into the chest cavity. They could now see the pericardium that encased the grossly oversized, fatty heart, with the lungs on either side inflating and deflating with each respiration. Barney's heart was so enlarged that only the right ventricular wall was visible, feebly moving with each beat. The left ventricle was pushed so deeply to the left that it was out of sight. Barney's heart was bigger than any Joyce or DeVries had ever seen before, and they realized that neither of them had ever operated on such a sick patient.

DeVries and Joyce both pinched up part of the pericardium with DeBakey forceps, creating a space between the instruments. DeVries used scissors to cut the pericardium between the forceps and continued toward the aorta, then extended the incision toward the diaphragm, exposing the apex of the heart. Sutures placed into the cut edges of the pericardium in four places on each side created a cradle to support the heart and keep the lungs from blocking the view of the surgery field.

Smith was preparing the heart-lung machine as well as the blood-tubing circuit. Three tubes needed to be attached to Barney, two lines to collect venous blood and one to return oxygenated blood from the heart-lung machine. An electrolyte solution and one unit of blood filled the circuit, and this mixture was pumped for several minutes to blend it and remove any trapped air.

In routine cardiac surgery, one sucker picks up all blood that enters the chest during surgery. However, the doctors had learned that much more blood was lost from the heart-lung circuit when the natural ventricles were cut out during artificial-heart implants in animals. A great deal of blood was also lost when priming the artificial ventricles to remove trapped air. Therefore, two high-volume suckers were included in the pump circuit to implant the artificial heart in Barney.

Normally the blood from the suckers runs through a cell saver that rinses away the plasma-free hemoglobin and removes cellular debris and the extra fluids used for irrigation. To assure success in keeping calves alive on the artificial heart, Olsen had developed precise protocols for each step of the implantation. Early on he had purchased a cell saver to attach to the heart-lung machine in the animal implants, so he was surprised to see there was no cell saver attached to the heart-lung machine for the Barney Clark surgery.

Surgeons are always concerned about the bypass time on the heart-lung machine. The longer the time spent on the machine, the more damage is likely to the red blood cells and the greater the loss of blood-clotting ability. Normally a membrane oxygenator is used when the patient is expected to be on the heart-lung machine a long time because oxygen and carbon dioxide easily pass through the membrane.[1] Yet Barney Clark was placed on a bubble oxygenator, which is far more damaging to the blood in longer surgeries.

Both DeVries and Joyce had assisted in numerous artificial-heart implantations in calves, and every one had included a membrane oxygenator and a cell saver. Olsen asked Joyce why the Barney Clark surgery was using a bubble oxygenator and there was no cell saver attached to the heart-lung machine when the doctors knew the pump run would be very long. Joyce said that DeVries had made that decision. Although DeVries often said he welcomed suggestions from the support staff, no one challenged his orders. Barney was his patient, and he was in charge.

Prior to connecting the heart-lung tubing for bypass, Barney was anticoagulated. Protection with anticoagulation was so critical that the surgeons injected heparin directly into the right atrium, and within three minutes, the entire blood system was anticoagulated. Blood-clotting time was periodically measured to monitor and adjust the level of anticoagulation.

DeVries dissected between the aorta and the pulmonary artery and placed a purse-string suture into the wall of the aorta to close it when the ends were tied. The suture only went through the two outside layers of the wall because DeVries knew that putting it all the way through would cause leakage. Then Joyce and DeVries placed similar purse-string sutures in the inferior vena cava and wall of the right atrium for the two venous lines. A catheter was inserted into the distended aorta through a stab wound in the purse-string suture ring and securely positioned by tightening the suture tails. Venous catheters were placed to pick up the blood from both the superior and inferior venae cavae, and tourniquets forced all of the blood into the uptake cannulas to the heart-lung machine and stopped nearly all of the venous blood from entering the right atrium. Suckers picked up the small amount of blood that returned to the right ventricle from the small bronchial and coronary arteries.

On the Heart-Lung Machine

Smith slowly began to circulate some blood outside of Barney's body. After the blood was thoroughly mixed with the machine's electrolyte solution, the flow was increased. The tubing clamps were removed, and Barney was placed on the heart-lung machine. Olsen commented, "It just turned midnight, and Barney's heart simply quit beating." Barney's heart was dead.

Normally a heart transplant is irreversible when the scissors first cut into the heart, but in Barney's case, there was no turning back when his heart stopped beating. There was absolutely nothing to do but implant the artificial heart. Smith quickly increased the flows, taking over completely for Barney's dead heart and quickly cooling the blood and Barney's body.

The heart-lung machine collected the venous blood from the two venae cavae and ran it through the venous reservoir, where all the air bubbles escaped. The two handheld suckers rid the chest of all accumulated blood as the surgery progressed and also dumped it into the pump circuit. All of the blood was then pumped through the bubble oxygenator to rinse out carbon dioxide, and the heat exchanger lowered its temperature.

The heart-lung machine returned the blood to the aorta under a pressure comparable to the patient's normal blood pressure. The amount of carbon dioxide and oxygen in the blood regulated the acidity of the returned blood. Managing and controlling all these factors was Smith's job. DeVries commented, "Doug [Smith] is the one in control, but Barney is my patient."

Jeff Anderson had previously placed Barney on steroids, and their long-term use made his tissues dangerously weak. His heart was now soft and extremely flabby. DeVries took the scissors and prepared to cut the aorta. Joyce realized that in all the excitement, the aortic cross clamp had not been placed. He quickly did that just before DeVries started to cut.

Olsen supported the apex of the left ventricle with a towel clamp. DeVries quickly opened the wall of the right ventricle and vented the septum into the left ventricle with the scissors to protect the lungs from pressure damage from incoming blood. He then cut the ventricles free from the aorta, pulmonary artery, and the right and left atria. A clear groove marked the position for cutting. The aorta was cut just above the openings into the coronary arteries to avoid major blood leaks.

Lifting the Diseased Heart from Barney's Chest

It was now 12:10 AM. Actually lifting the double-sized heart out of Barney's chest was an emotional event. Surgeons normally do not cut the beating heart out of living patients except in cardiac transplants. DeVries said, "I have never seen a heart this large. Those people always die." The heart weighed nearly seventeen pounds. It was covered with clumps of fat and had much damage from blood clots and scarring.

Fred Anderson considered Barney's heart to be valuable and unique and did not want it to be mishandled or lost. The Utah team would lose very important information and suffer serious embarrassment. Anticipating the late hour, Anderson had called the Department of Pathology to ensure that someone would be available. It was important to conduct tests on the fresh heart. Dr. Liz Hammond was the pathologist in charge.

The removed heart was placed in a stainless steel bowl, and Fred Anderson and Jeff Anderson carried it out of the OR. Fred said that felt strange. When he was asked, "What did you think?" he responded, "Well it was a little—first of all it was a new experience for me to be involved in a situation where the heart was cut out of a patient who was still alive. It was a—a—a little peculiar to have a man's heart in the basin and see that it was still fibrillating."

Fred said that the heart was fibrillating, but it had been in total arrest for nearly a half hour before it was removed from Barney's chest. What he saw was most likely the heart muscle twitching due to lack of oxygen. He handed the bowl to Dr. Ron Weiss, the pathology resident.

The mechanical Bjork-Shiley valves in the Utah artificial heart were held in place by compression-fitted, rigid polyurethane parts. The valves were positioned to fill the ventricles from the atria and eject the blood into the great vessels. They were also oriented to provide maximum flow with the least amount of turbulence. The grafts and cuffs had a lid like an aspirin bottle cap that permitted them to be snapped onto the ventricular outflow and inflow ports so the heart could quickly be replaced if necessary. This also permitted the implant team to rotate the heart later to fit the chest better.

After the heart was removed, DeVries and Joyce tailored the aorta, pulmonary artery stumps, and atria to fit the artificial vessels and atrial cuffs. DeVries placed the artificial heart easily into the chest. He determined the length of the grafts by placing the ventricles in the chest after removing Barney's heart to size them. "Two hearts would fit in that large chest," Joyce commented in awe.

Olsen suggested, "Some of the dilated left atrial wall should be removed because it will collapse into the inflow valve, restrict filling the ventricle, and limit cardiac output."

DeVries said he preferred not to cut away the atrial wall. Both atrial cuffs were sewn in place, as well as the aortic and pulmonary artery grafts, and were tested for leaks. The left driveline was positioned so it would fix the left ventricle inside the chest and allow the left heart to be shifted if necessary.

DeVries handed the left driveline to Hastings, who had marked the left line red and the right one blue to avoid mistakes. He then snapped the left heart into place, connecting it to the inflow and outflow.

At 2:20 AM, DeVries told Hastings to slowly start the left heart. The driver was set at 33 percent systole to allow a filling time of 66 percent of the cycle time and forty beats per minute with the driving pressure at 60 millimeters of mercury (mmHg). The driving pressure was increased to unload the ventricle totally at each beat. That setting produced a pulse on the otherwise-flat aortic blood pressure on the monitoring screen. This proved that the heart was pumping and the drive pressure was adequate.

The Left Ventricle Would Not Fill

Hastings followed the same procedures he had worked out in the animal implants. When he started Barney's left heart, it pumped two or three small strokes and then stopped ejecting blood. That was because blood couldn't enter the left ventricle. "Look, that left atrial wall is blocking the inflow valve," Olsen pointed out in concern. He had warned DeVries about that. The blood pressure filled the part of the atria that was held wide, which presented the misleading picture that the atrium was full.

There were three opinions why the blood did not enter the left ventricle. DeVries thought the left inflow valve was sticking shut, so the left ventricle was disconnected and lifted out of the chest three different times. The four people at the operating table carefully inspected the valve; it looked clean and opened and closed with ease.

Jarvik thought the position inside the chest was limiting the amount of blood that could enter the ventricle. The heart was moved around and even removed and replaced three times without correcting the problem.

Olsen repeated that the excessively dilated left atrial wall was being sucked into the valve opening. When the left atrium was filled with blood and the heart driver was turned on, the blood was ejected for two or three beats and then it stopped.

DeVries disagreed with Olsen. He reached his hand behind the heart to determine if indeed the atrial wall was collapsing into the valve. The heart was stopped and started three or four times. It consistently pumped blood for a few beats and then stopped.

DeVries continued to explore the valve and atria with his finger. "Oops," he muttered. His finger had pierced the flimsy atrial wall. Now the ventricle had to be removed and the wall cut away to get rid of the hole and the excess piece of wall. When the ventricle was replaced, the artificial heart pumped blood the way it was supposed to.

When DeVries was interviewed later, he was asked, "Do you remember being damned frustrated that this thing was not working?" He responded,

> Yes, really frustrated. I remember saying to someone—after we got the heart working—if we hadn't [done] all the animal experimentation, we would have just thrown it [the heart] down and walked away, and Barney would have been dead. Because of the animal experimentation, we had seen this before, and we knew that it does occasionally happen, and we knew how to get out of it. And that was to put a new heart in. So that experimentation really helped.

DeVries later said that he had used a new left ventricle, and after he implanted it, the artificial heart worked. He never described the surgical steps of doing this, however. Olsen had worked out a protocol with calves of removing the nonsterile air drivelines without infecting the chest, but DeVries never explained how he accomplished this when he replaced the left ventricle.

It is interesting that neither Joyce nor Olsen remembers these events exactly the way DeVries does. Kessler had delivered two complete heart sets. One set was opened and used in Barney's initial surgery. Eleven days later, the inflow valve had fractured so the second set—the backup one—was opened, and the left ventricle in this set replaced the damaged one in Barney's artificial heart. Kessler repeatedly said, "There was never an additional left ventricle used on Barney."

Kessler and the heart-building team had developed a comprehensive inventory control and tracking scheme. Detailed logs were kept. This well-organized tracking system became a stable component of the program and helped the Utah team get FDA approval to implant the artificial heart in human patients. It is highly unlikely that he could be wrong about the number of hearts used during Barney's surgery.

Pace became concerned with the long time Barney had been on the heart-lung machine because many red blood cells were being damaged and hemoglobin was leaking into Barney's circulatory system. Pace observed that Barney's urine was turning pink, but he did not mention it to the surgeons because he realized that the only way to prevent that was to stop the heart-lung machine, and that was not possible. Because of the damage to the red blood cells, the kidneys were excreting the free hemoglobin into the urine, making it red.

After the surgery, Pace reported that the plasma-free hemoglobin was measured at 585 milligrams, which is exceedingly high. This large amount of free hemoglobin damages the lungs, kidneys, and liver. Barney's system had to remove it from the blood, and the main route was through the kidneys, which were also impaired by the hemoglobin. The hemoglobin limits pulmonary function as well by causing increased pulmonary-artery pressure, which results in "stiff" lungs.

At startup the initial heart rate and the percent systole for the right heart were the same as the left, and the drive pressure was started lower at 40 mmHg to protect the lungs until Pace could get them to inflate and deflate fully. Hastings started the right ventricle at 3:30 AM, and he teamed with Smith to begin to wean Barney off the heart-lung machine. They worked together to get the lungs inflated: Hastings increased the artificial-heart pressures and flows while Smith decreased what was coming from the heart-lung machine.

Meanwhile Pace was facing some complicated problems with Barney's lungs. Barney had a significant amount of emphysema, which is obstructive lung disease where air is trapped. Before the heart-lung machine could be removed, his lungs had to have enough inhale and exhale volume to oxygenate the blood. Pace found that air was entering the lungs, but he could not get it out because Barney's lungs had become very stiff. They were so dilated that his chest incision could not be closed.

Pace inflated the lungs to start Barney breathing. Normally this pushes the air out, but Barney's emphysema limited the rate and volume of his exhalations. Pace recognized bronchial spasms that had to be treated. He had four possible drugs to use. The first two had no effect, but fortunately the third and fourth worked.

After some magic by Pace, the collapsing lungs began working well on the respirator, resulting in a partial pressure of oxygen in the blood of 300 mmHg. Normal breathing of room air produces 85 to 95 mmHg of pressure. Fred Anderson was very pleased with the oxygen levels and said they proved that the artificial heart and Barney's lungs were both working well. Barney could now be weaned from the heart-lung machine, and the artificial heart could take over.

The staff began gradually to shut down the heart-lung machine, a closely coordinated effort among Smith, Nielsen, and Hastings. Hastings slowly increased the cardiac output from the artificial heart while Smith slowed down the heart-lung machine. This process took fifteen or twenty minutes. The surgery staff had learned in the calf experiments not to rush this critical step.

On the Artificial Heart

Hastings adjusted the heart driver to deliver a cardiac output of six and a half liters of blood per minute. Jeff Anderson suggested lowering it to four and a half because Barney had been living on two and a half for some time. A rapid increase like this might harm him, so the cardiac output was lowered. Barney's total time on the heart-lung machine was four hours and nine minutes—much longer than usual and not the best situation for him.

The driving pressures for both the left and right sides of the heart were correlated to the desired blood pressure and flow, and the right and left heart outputs were balanced.

The surgeons explored the chest looking for bleeders with the sucker that removed loose blood. When the sucker did not pick up any blood from the pericardial cradle, DeVries decided to close Barney's chest. Then Olsen reminded him that the left pericardial wall had been opened into the left hemithorax to accommodate the left ventricle. He asked DeVries to place the sucker deeply around the left lung. DeVries found a great deal of blood, and he placed two or three additional sutures on the aortic line to stop the hemorrhage.

Joyce then expressed two major concerns. First he feared postoperative hemorrhaging because of the long time Barney was on the heart-lung machine and the resulting impact on blood clotting. Secondly, he was worried that removing and replacing the left ventricle three times might have caused unknown complications. Was all of the air completely removed from the ventricle each time, or had an air embolus possibly occurred that might result in permanent brain damage? The surgeons had been very careful, but the risks were still there.

It was 4:09 AM, and Barney was off the heart-lung machine. The Utah artificial heart was performing wonderfully.

The heparin anticoagulant was reversed with protamine. Removable monitoring lines were placed into the right atrium, pulmonary artery, and left atrium. Chest drains were placed into the right and left chest to remove any leaking blood and air so the lungs could inflate. Wire sutures were placed around the bones of the sternum, pulled tightly, and twisted. The incision was closed in layers in the reverse order of opening.

Barney was alive with a new heart. There was not a doubt in anyone's mind that he would not have been alive if surgery had been delayed until the next

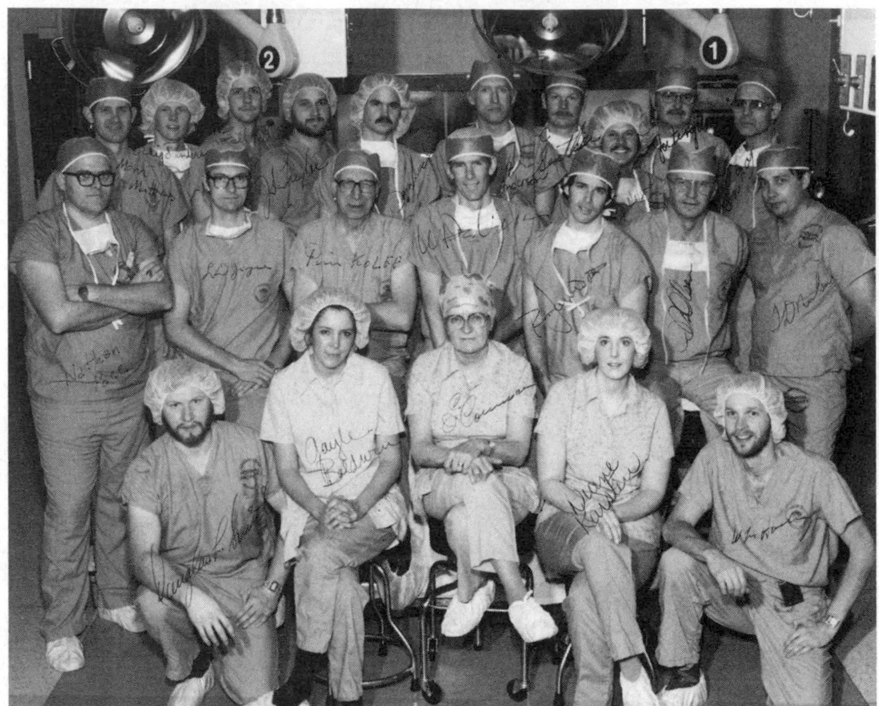

The members of the artificial-heart implant team.

morning. The first patient in the world to receive a permanent artificial heart was alive and progressing well!

The Utah Heart Team Reacts

At 4:15 AM, the surgery finally came to an end. The total operating time was a long five hours. The whole team felt great relief to have succeeded this far. Unheralded men and women of valor in their own right, they were beginning to feel the aftereffects of the long and tense day and night and the letdown after the adrenaline high that had sustained them through the long hours.

Initially the team members said little about their accomplishment, but later—during the postoperative interviews—everyone expressed a great deal of pride. Joyce said, "I guess my feeling at that point was just marveling at how fortunate we had been, how somebody was looking out for us. There was every reason in the world for us to have lost him. He could have died on the table just as easy as anything. When Barney was able to respond to commands such as 'squeeze my hand' or move his leg and wiggle his toe, that was another sense of accomplishment."

Olsen changed and went to the research lab to start a new day of responsibilities. The environment was so electric and intense that he was still full of energy and didn't feel tired the entire day. Chase Peterson called and invited him to participate in the news conference scheduled for that afternoon. Peterson wanted to introduce the entire team to the press. Olsen declined. "Barney is a human patient," he said, "and will be managed by clinical physicians, not a veterinarian. I am very pleased to have had the opportunity to have played a role in the surgical implantation, and yes, I take great pride in our successful achievement."

After the surgery was over and Barney had moved his limbs and blinked his eyes on command, Joyce was asked, "You have been working since seven yesterday morning and then all night. Aren't you tired?" Joyce's response was, "No, I expect it will take me about two more days to unwind."

In a later interview, DeVries was asked what he was thinking when the surgery was over—at 4:15 AM. He answered, "I was very excited that it was going as planned. We always thought that would happen, and this was proof. The observers as well as the workers were relaxed. Everyone seemed to be relieved and happy. No one appeared grim, depressed, or disappointed. They had all shared an exciting event."

Note

1. It is interesting to note that Willem Kolff had actually invented, tested, and perfected the membrane oxygenator.

19

Barney Clark on the Artificial Heart

Valor is a gift. Those having it never know for sure whether they have it till the test comes. And those having it in one test never know for sure if they will have it when the next test comes.

—Carl Sandburg

Implant Surgery Completed

By 4:15 AM on December 2, the implant surgery was complete. While Barney was still under anesthesia, Nathan Pace delayed waking him, waiting for a dentist to arrive to extract an infected tooth. The infection was a great concern because it could spread into his artificial heart. Shortly after the extraction, Barney was wheeled into Room 12 in the Surgical Intensive Care Unit (SICU), where he was allowed to recover slowly from the anesthesia.

Barney opened his eyes and moved his limbs approximately three hours after his chest was closed. Pace said that Barney was slower waking from anesthesia than usual because both his liver and kidneys were impaired from the large amount of plasma-free hemoglobin. His liver could not metabolize (break down) the anesthetic drugs, and his kidneys could not excrete them.

Much later in the day, Barney responded to commands to move his limbs and squeeze a hand. Later that evening—although still on the ventilator with a trachea tube down his throat—he mouthed "I still love you" to Una Loy. Some had speculated—rather facetiously—whether he could still love his wife with an artificial heart.

As was usual for patients in the recovery room, Barney was heavily sedated during the first uneventful night. His blood oxygenation was good, and he had what his doctors felt was acceptable lung function. The mechanical ventilator

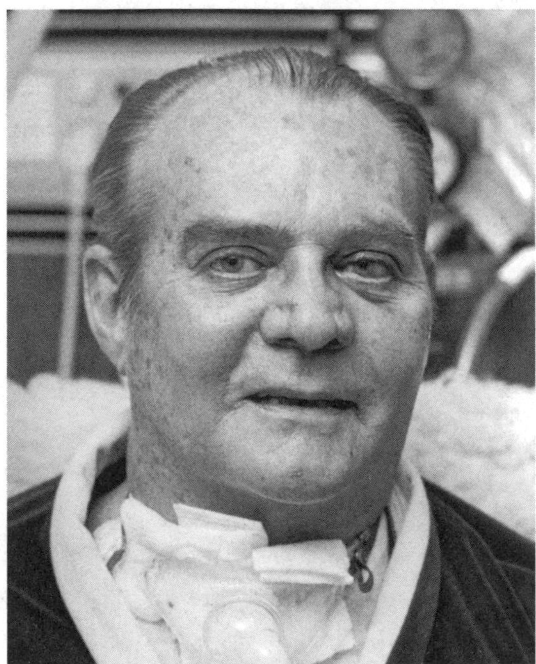

Barney Clark was alert and responsive.

doing most of the respiratory work was occasionally disconnected to see if Barney could breathe independently. When he could move enough air with frequent breaths, Pace ordered the trachea tube removed. Oxygen was delivered to Barney's nostrils, and he maintained acceptable blood-oxygen levels. Unassisted breathing was the third major achievement after getting him successfully on and off the heart-lung machine with his newly implanted heart.

Clark's nurses found Barney with his artificial heart much easier to care for than the usual cardiac-surgery patient. They did not have to monitor heart rate and blood pressure or flow carefully or give a lot of drugs. The heart ran like a machine, they commented, somewhat wryly. They also observed that the technicians overseeing the heart driver made no changes. Everything remained very stable, and Barney rested and recovered from his long, extensive surgery.

Jane Stetich, the intensive-care nurse with Barney just before surgery, commented, "In fact, I heard some things just sitting and watching local television that other people on the case did not know. Before surgery his legs were blue because the circulation was so low. Now they are, like—bright red. Patients feel better when they are shaved and have their teeth brushed." Stetich made sure that Barney received these patient comforts.

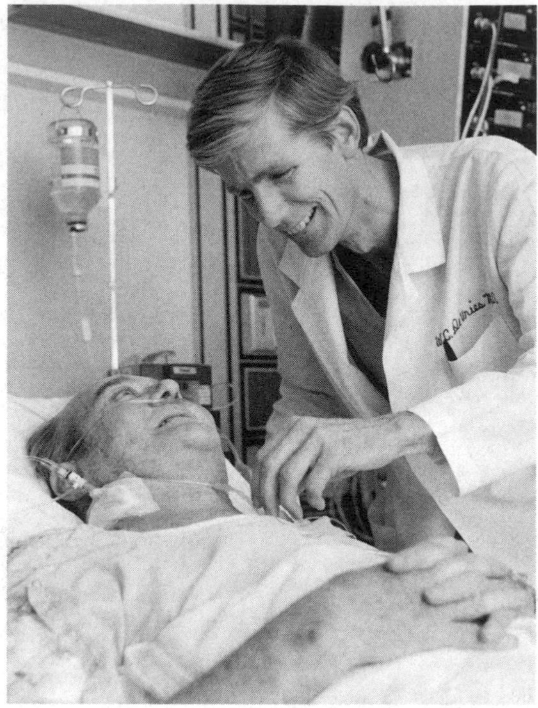

William DeVries checks his patient after the surgery.

On one or two occasions, Barney said, "Let me die; just let me die." Many patients waking up after surgery say that, so Stetich was not surprised. "He had some good days and some bad days. I thought technically the artificial heart was positive," she said.

The Cardiologists and the Patient without a Heart

Barney's cardiologists also found caring for this patient unique. Usually they dealt with patients whose surgically repaired hearts were vulnerable to all sorts of problems that required careful monitoring and judicious administration of cardiac-stimulating drugs. With Barney they did not need a stethoscope or an EKG, their usual tools, because very few concerns were pertinent. Primarily the settings and function of the mechanical heart were the responsibility of Larry Hastings and Steve Nielsen under the direction of William DeVries or Lyle Joyce.

Fred Anderson decided what Barney really needed was an internist to address multiple ailments not related to the implant that showed up during and after the surgery. Many of University Hospital's medical experts in a variety of fields were called in for consultations. Joyce recorded that twenty-one different departments were consulted during Barney's hospitalization. The constant vigilance and curiosity of the press in Barney's case partly dictated the wide use of specialists.

Kolff Shows Emotion

Willem Kolff met with Don Olsen and Una Loy the day following surgery and told them, "This was the realization of a long dream." Overwhelmed, he suddenly teared up. The emotional outburst was short, however. Kolff quickly regained his usual pragmatic composure and offered to make many copies of a letter he had written requesting donations. He was always looking for funding for his projects. He suggested Una Loy sign the letters, and he would send them to all of the people who had written her letters of support. Una Loy thought this was rather insensitive, and she turned him down. She had the social worker, Peggy Miller, intercede with Kolff and also deal with some other issues that made her feel uncomfortable. Miller became Una Loy's advocate and protector.

DeVries was often asked the expected question: "As a physician, what is the first thing you want to know of your patient after extensive heart surgery?" He responded,

> After something like this, I want to know, first of all, is the patient neurologically intact? We know that hemodynamically everything is fine—blood pressure and flow of the artificial heart. We asked... [Barney] to respond to commands such as 'move your arms, your legs, and flex your knees and squeeze my hand.' We asked him to nod or shake his head yes or no to further questions—'Do you hurt?' or, 'Is there pain?' He shook his head no. I was comfortable that Barney was mentally intact with no evidence of... brain function [loss].

Una Loy had informed the hospital when Barney was admitted that he had essentially stopped eating a month before surgery. He was suffering from malnutrition as reflected in a low serum-albumin level. A nutritionist was consulted to reestablish healthy eating.

During the second postsurgery night, attendants attempting to make Barney more comfortable accidentally pulled both drainage tubes from his chest. This accident greatly concerned the heart team. Joyce worried that Barney might still be bleeding from the extensive surgery. Pace and DeVries were concerned that air accumulation in the chest could interfere with respiration. They all took a wait-and-see position.

Surgery Number Two

Two days after the implant, DeVries reported,

> On Saturday [December 4] the trachea tube had been removed, and we talked with him [Barney]. Most surgical patients like this are mildly sedated.... [They] don't wake up and all of a sudden start talking.... [They slowly] realize they have a voice.... [Barney] talked with Lyle, with Doug and Larry. In fact, Doug and Larry were talking, and one of them said he wanted a Coke. Barney overheard them and said, 'Get my trousers over there, and I will buy.' He was spontaneously interacting in the conversation, all of which is really a good sign.

DeVries continued his assessment during an interview:

> Nathan [Pace] saw Barney on Saturday [December 4] and said he was extubated and breathing on his own. He looked pretty good considering how ill he was and how long the surgery and pump run had lasted. The chest drains had extracted about four liters of blood but were dry, with no blood draining, when they were accidentally pulled out. There was a growing concern, however, since there had been a small and persistent amount of air being removed from the chest by the chest drains.... [We hope]...that the source might be...small pulmonary blebs that...[have] ruptured. Such little ruptures in the lungs...seldom leak air unless the patient is on a respirator that fills the lungs with pressurized air, which Barney [experienced].

Air began to collect slowly under the skin at the upper end of Barney's chest incision. It seemed to expand. This subcutaneous emphysema (air under the skin) brought the team to some emergency discussions. What was the source of the air? Was it from leaks in the lung, or was it more serious—an air leak from the artificial heart's pneumatically powered ventricles or drivelines? If the air was coming from the heart or drivelines, it was not sterile and signaled a serious situation. If Barney's chest was infected, corrective surgery would have to take place immediately to replace the leaking heart and/or the drivelines.

Team members did not agree on the source of the air. Kolff argued that it had to be coming from the heart or drivelines. Olsen disagreed: "We have not had any air leaks in the hearts in animals for years." All leaks had stopped when Kessler had found improved adhesives to fasten the parts of the heart together. "My bet is that it is not the heart and drivelines," Olsen said.

After much discussion, Barney was anesthetized and his chest reopened by removing a few of the sutures from the previous surgery near his chin. The leaks were not easy to see until a small amount of saline was poured over the surface of the lung. The team borrowed this technique from the old practice of submerging a car or bicycle inner tube in water to detect leaks. In Barney's chest, fine streams of bubbles indicated three leaks near the medial aspect (middle area) of the right lung, which were closed with two fine staples. Such blebs frequently occur, but nearly all of them seal off when the lung contacts the surrounding lining. Perhaps Barney's had remained open because they rubbed on the artificial heart that moved as it beat.

Two new chest drains were placed, and there were no further air problems. In spite of the extensive implant surgery and now a second one, there was no bleeding. Pace was amazed:

> Three days before, we put this guy to sleep as gingerly and cautiously as possible because we feared that his heart could stop at any second. Now three days later, we take him into surgery, and we don't hook up the EKG because he doesn't have a heart anymore. And we give him any drugs we want to. It doesn't matter what we give him; his heart continues beating at the selected rate. It is amazing and very safe to give anesthetics to a patient with an artificial heart.

Barney and Una Loy were reassured that things were going well. Following the second surgery, Barney quickly recovered, talked, and felt well. In one of his special interactions with DeVries, Barney asked, "Am I doing all right with the experiment? Is everything going okay for you guys? Are you getting the information that you wanted?"

Renal Insufficiency

The day following the implantation, Barney was excreting 100 to 200 cubic centimeters (cc's) of urine per hour while his body removed the excess fluids from his cardiac failure and surgery. This urine was bright red from the relatively high amounts of hemoglobin from red blood cells that had been damaged while Barney was on the heart-lung machine.

On Sunday, December 5, Barney's urinary output dramatically decreased to 20 to 30 cc's per hour, dropping briefly into the teens. His kidneys were not producing enough urine to eliminate wastes. His blood creatinine was high at 2.2, and the BUN (blood urea nitrogen) was nearly five times normal at 105. A check of his fluid intake indicated he was receiving adequate amounts. His blood pressure was checked to ensure his kidneys were being adequately perfused.

Barney was given the diuretic Lasix, which did not work. Immediately the team met. Their choices were dialysis on an artificial kidney, which Joyce preferred and Kolff adamantly opposed, or increasing the heart-driver rate and pressure to send more blood to the kidneys. Increasing the blood flow had worked in animals to increase urine output dramatically. A major concern was that increasing pressure would subject the heart valves to more strain, which could possibly make them fracture.

A reporter later asked DeVries, "Did you consult with other people in terms of whether the heart-driver rate should be increased?"

"Oh, yeah, we were all talking about it," DeVries said. "All of us were there: Lyle, Larry, Don, Rob [Jarvik), and I. We all came to the agreed solution.... [We] decided to increase the heart rate and the heart driving pressure in Barney's [heart], and he immediately started to produce more urine." It was a better option, DeVries said, than subjecting the patient to dialysis.

In the postsurgical period, the heart's output had been adjusted between six and eight liters per minute. The device was turned up to yield a cardiac output of ten to twelve liters per minute. Later, when questions arose about the seizures that Barney suffered, there was no record of how this level of cardiac output had been determined, just that Ted Stanley and some others had been involved.

Increasing the blood flow did the trick. Barney's urine output quickly increased to more than 100 cc's per hour, and within hours, his BUN and creatinine levels became normal.

DeVries told the media that "high concentrations of hemoglobin in the blood stream had to be excreted through... [Barney's] kidneys." Otherwise the inordinate amount of hemoglobin being excreted by the kidneys could damage or perhaps destroy them and result in renal shutdown. DeVries told reporters that it appeared the threat posed by the high levels of plasma-free hemoglobin did not destroy Barney's kidneys because the increased blood supply from adjusting the artificial heart produced much more urine.

Grand Mal Seizures

However, the benefit from the increased heart output was quickly offset by a new problem. Barney experienced grand mal seizures about 6:00 AM on December 7. He suffered general and focal seizures lasting for almost three hours. These occurred after his cardiac output had been increased, sometimes to twelve liters per minute. In one instance, Stanley had even increased it to fourteen liters per minute for a very short time. Joyce was extremely concerned about the possibility of brain damage from blood clots, although CAT scans did not show blood clots or other brain abnormalities.

At this crucial time, Kolff, Olsen, and Jarvik were at an NIH contractors' meeting in Washington, DC. Kolff requested that DeVries immediately turn off the key on the heart driver because he believed Barney's heart had thrown a blood clot to his brain. Olsen argued that turning off the heart driver would be problematic with the entire world watching. Kolff inquired if Barney's blood circulation was normal, and it was. By the time the group returned from Washington, the seizures were over, but mentally Barney was not himself.

The team met and tried to determine the cause of the seizures. What had happened inside Barney's brain? A blood clot from the heart that had caused a stroke was possible, but repeated brain scans revealed nothing. Chase Peterson, a nephrologist and the heart team's official liaison with the media, suggested that a metabolic imbalance may have been the cause, but, again, there was no evidence. The team members were left with nothing concrete, and a month later, they were still reviewing hospital charts. The only consistent, possibly connected event was the increased blood flow. Joyce was among those who did not accept this conclusion, however.

It was a couple of days before Barney became lucid enough to carry on a simple conversation and nearly a week before he could speak intelligently. Hospital charts listed that "on 12/9 he was making appropriate responses to commands and verbalizing." The effects of the seizures were shattering, but the team seemed no closer to finding a definitive cause.

Many of the Utah team finally decided that the convulsions had been caused by the precipitous increase in blood flow. Extensive tests, including CAT scans, encephalograms, and neurological examinations, showed no evidence of a blood clot. Call it what you want, but the origin of the seizures remained unknown.[1]

The Utah team later learned that heart-transplant recipients occasionally had otherwise-unexplained convulsions when the healthier transplanted heart increased cardiac output dramatically. At the time, no one on the Utah team remembered reading anything about seizures in heart-transplant patients. Patients in heart failure are always overloaded with fluid, and the new heart recognizes the increased blood pressure. The new healthy heart can immediately produce nearly three times the output of a sick heart. Whether this relates to Barney's situation remains an unanswered question.

DeVries called Dr. Phil Oyer, a transplant surgeon from Stanford, to ask about seizures in patients in cardiac failure who then received a healthy heart. Oyer told him that transplant surgeons had occasionally noted seizures in patients but had not made the information known. Oyer added, "We have no proof that the increase in blood perfusion was the direct cause of the seizures, only a suspicion."

Olsen tried to replicate Barney's seizures in calves with artificial hearts. He turned the heart driver very low for several days to represent heart failure and then quickly turned it up as high as it would go. Urine production increased a great deal, but the calves had no seizures.

Una Loy also struggled to understand the new development. The university team had explained to her that the heart's blood flow was increased to deal with the drop in urine production and that the technique had been successful, so she understood the rationale for increasing the heart action, but no one was absolutely certain if or how that impacted the seizures. DeVries, at least, seemed convinced that the increased heart output was responsible for the seizures. He was quoted later in the *Journal of the American Medical Association*, "Patient one [Barney] was maintained with high cardiac outputs (10 to 12 L/min) that were related to his postoperative seizures."[2]

Whether Barney ever fully recovered mentally was a question Una Loy was frequently asked. How deeply the seizures affected her as well as her husband is clear from her response to a reporter:

> That was the most difficult thing for me about the whole thing. Barney and I had always been so close and had talked with each other and knew exactly where we stood and what was going on. With me there [during the seizures], it was like I was not myself, like I was playing a role. What was going on inside [me] was not at all like I was appearing on the outside. My whole idea with Barney was to give him my full support—I wanted to appear comfortable and well. I didn't want him to think I was going through a lot of stress because he [had] told me in the beginning of the decision-making process in November that he thought he should let me get on with my life, let everything go and not put me through this. And at one time, I think in the video recorded in the documentary, he said, "No woman should have to...." In other words, what he was trying to tell me and wanted to say in that documentary was that "no woman should go through this." And that part really got to me.
>
> That was really hard for me, watching the documentary about us.[3] I don't know if anybody else grasped that. They were asking him questions, and he looked up at me and said, "I love you," because that was easier for him to say. I could see that he was struggling, so I said, "I love you, too."

Una Loy also told her confidante, Miller, "Barney was concerned about his mental processes, and so when they would want him to perform, it would be very painful to me because I knew how he was struggling. On occasion Barney would say he wanted to die. It was not for himself. He wanted to die because he didn't think he was going to get well, and he did not want to burden me and go on with the expense. And he did not want to put us through the suffering."

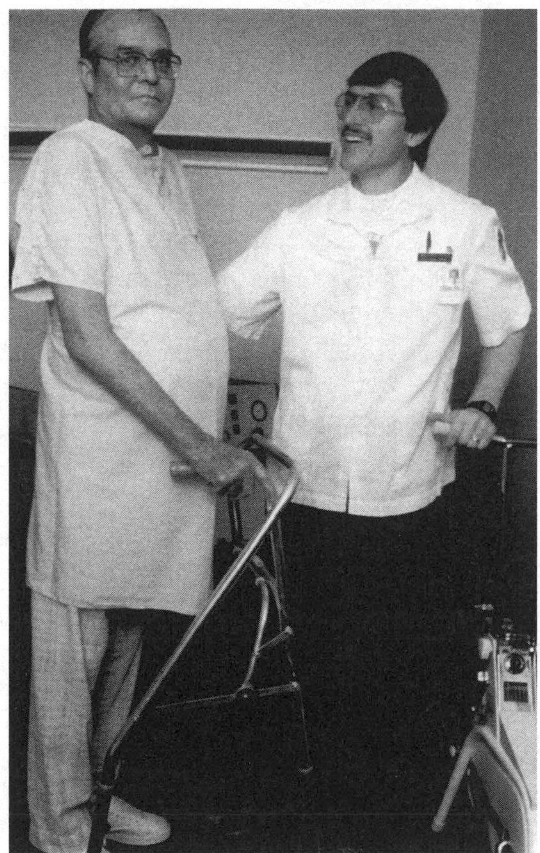

Barney Clark exercising with the aid of a technician.

Fred Anderson did not believe Barney recovered mentally after the seizures. Una Loy and their son, Stephen, shared that feeling.

Peterson continued to tell Barney's story to a world eager for every update. He issued a press release on December 15, following the seizures: "Dr. Clark has had a good day of recovery. His mental status continues to improve. He is brighter and more conversant than before the TAH implant. His blood pressure is 130/80 mmHg, pulse 75/min, and cardiac output of 7 L/min. The team is encouraged with his progress."

A New Problem Surfaces

The implant team had practiced all the possible scenarios that would lead to failure or complications with the heart. Corrective procedures were detailed and rehearsed in the laboratory.

One of the potential emergency situations they were prepared for was valve fracture. Welded struts suspended the heart's Bjork-Shiley pyrolytic carbon disks. Welds like these had broken in calf experiments. A plan to diagnose the problem and act quickly to preserve the life of the calf—or, in this case, Barney Clark—had been practiced in the Artificial Heart Research Laboratory.

On day fourteen (December 16), Joyce visited Barney, talked with him, and evaluated his condition. Reassured that all was well, Joyce left the room. He was still in the hallway when Barney's nurse shouted that something was severely wrong with his blood pressure. It had dropped to nearly zero. Racing back to the room, Joyce noted that the cardiac output on the left ventricle registered fourteen liters per minute, but Barney's blood pressure was very low. If the inflow valve on the left ventricle had broken, the ventricle would fill quickly, but virtually no blood could be pumped into the aorta, resulting in very low blood pressure.

Joyce recognized what was wrong and immediately implemented the corrective measures practiced in the lab. He and Hastings used one pneumatic driver on the right ventricle and one on the left. They increased the heart rate on the left driver to about 180 beats per minute, which moved as much blood as possible from the ventricle into the aorta. On the right side, they turned the rate down to 25 to 35 beats per minute, which ensured that the right ventricle emptied at each systole. The plan was to increase the left ventricular rate to maximize forward blood flow and then match the performance on the right side based on readings from the cardiac output monitor and diagnostic unit.

Joyce was careful not to overpump the right ventricle, which would have flooded the lungs with blood, resulting almost certainly in pulmonary edema and death. The tested emergency procedures worked very effectively. Barney's blood pressure became more acceptable, and he was resting well. Reducing the flow from the right heart protected his lungs from overfilling with blood. Jeff Anderson later commented that Barney appeared in this emergency like a person who was not badly off at all.

DeVries was with his children at a dental appointment when the valve broke. Later he commented, "Barney was looking really…[well]. I had been in to see him about fifteen minutes before the valve broke, and I was happy that everything was going so well. Then I got a beep to call the SICU stat."

The team consulted with Una Loy. "Do we subject Barney to another open-chest surgery and time on the heart-lung machine, or do we do nothing but sedate him and let him die?" Might this patient become the first in medical history to die of mechanical heart failure? They quickly made the decision to replace the left ventricle in Barney as had been done in calves. They then discussed the procedure with Barney, who was lucid and indicated he understood what they proposed.

Failure of the welded struts of the valve disc supports was considered the likely culprit. The heart had probably operated under these conditions for several days before the welded strut had failed and the disc had dislodged. Welds had failed in some of the calf experiments, but the valves had been reused in several surgeries. Barney's heart had completely new, unused valves. The Utah team was aware that Barney's increased heart rate and air-driving pressure could have caused weld failure. This situation had been considered before making changes in driving Barney's heart.

Surgery Number Three

Barney returned to the OR for his third major surgery with anesthesia and was placed on the heart-lung machine a second time. Everyone's thoughts were the same. Could he survive this additional trauma? The original surgical team was again in the OR to replace the left ventricle. This included DeVries, Joyce, and Olsen with Doug Smith operating the heart-lung machine and Pace administrating anesthesia.

Anesthesia was smooth and uneventful. Barney's chest was quickly opened, and he was immediately placed on the heart-lung machine so the artificial heart could be turned off as soon as he was stable. Removing the ventricle with its broken valve required great care. The six-foot-long driveline that extended from inside Barney's chest to the heart driver was nonsterile and could not be pulled back into the chest. The driveline was cut off inside the chest. The air from the driver was not sterile, so as soon as the tube was cut, it was covered with fingers from a sterile glove. The driveline could now be removed safely by pulling it out through the chest wall. A new line was threaded from inside the chest through the original channel. The damaged left ventricle was replaced by connecting a new ventricle to the original aortic and atrial quick connectors. Barney was on the heart-lung machine for thirty-eight minutes, and according to Smith, it took just fifteen minutes to exchange the ventricle.

The removed left ventricle did contain the intact pyrolytic carbon disc that had fallen out when the strut fractured. Barney's recovery from this third surgery was uneventful, and Joyce believed that he was much more lucid and rebounded more quickly than he had after the much-longer first operation.

Peterson passed the word to the media.[4] A press release detailed the removal of the left ventricle, indicating the patient was on bypass for forty-six minutes.

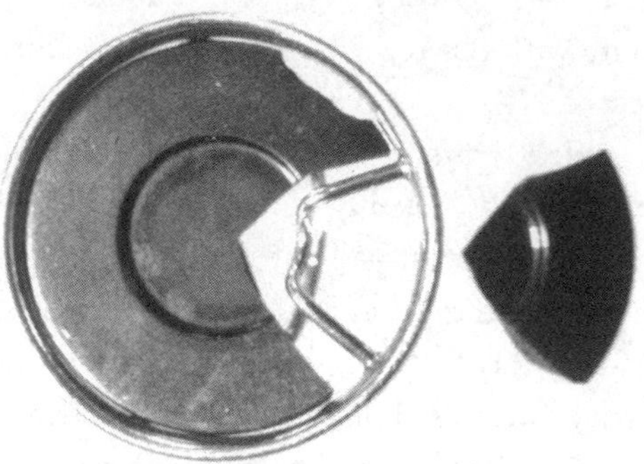

A Bjork-Shiley valve with a fracture.

The new ventricle was in place in just twenty-five minutes. The conflict in times from Smith's assessment shows that the press did not always have all of the correct information. "Barney Clark is awake from the anesthesia and is stable," Peterson told reporters. Now all everyone could do was see how well Barney recovered from this latest surgical assault on his body.

Barney had never met DeVries's wife, so on the following Sunday, he brought her to the hospital. She walked in and said, "Hi, I am Karen DeVries." Barney took her hand.

"I am so happy to meet you," he softly replied, squeezing her hand.

She responded, "We are all praying for you and hope that things go well."

"Thank you," Barney said.

Mending a Broken Heart for Christmas

When Earl Selby interviewed DeVries, he asked about a special holiday that had been planned for Barney. "On Christmas your children and Lyle's kids went in to visit, and how was that arranged?"

"We mentioned to Barney that this was going to be his Christmas and tried to get him excited about things," DeVries said.

> He was over his seizures and was slowly getting back [to normal]. He was a little bit depressed...and it was Christmas time, so it kind of gave him a little bit of support, a little bit of life. I cannot remember who initially suggested it, but we were playing a lot of Christmas music for him.... I think Lyle suggested the kids come in and sing.
>
> As soon as that was mentioned, the wives got into it. They got some costumes, and Ross Woolley stole the piano from the rehab center and brought it up. We got a tree from some other place in the hospital. Presents...were under the Christmas tree, and Barney got excited about Christmas....

> Barney was increasingly excited by 2:00 PM, particularly when the kids came in. He…grinned at them. They all went up and said, 'Merry Christmas.'…It was the first period where he was excited, very happy.… At times he was still having periods of nonlucidity, but they were getting less and less frequent.

Barney's Setback

Barney's Christmas adrenaline rush was short lived. "Christmas night was bad for him," DeVries recalled in his interview with the Selbys.

> He had a real setback. He did well until about ten or eleven o'clock… when suddenly his blood pressure shot up, and his pulmonary artery pressure was also high. Blood pressure in the lungs shot up, and we thought he might have had a pulmonary embolism [from a blood clot]. We had to put him back on the respirator. It took about two days to get him back in the routine. We never were really sure what it was or what caused it, but the day following Christmas was not a good day for him. We were not sure if he was all tired out.

A post-Christmas report in the *Deseret News* said, "Barney Clark is in serious but stable condition on the 27th day on the heart." Soon after, Barney traveled to DeVries's office by wheelchair on a sightseeing tour and visited some personnel on the floor. Peterson's news release stated,

> Barney Clark continues to have periods of mild renal and pulmonary insufficiency and mental confusion. He remains in serious but stable condition. Yesterday Dr. Clark was taken by wheelchair to the sunroom on the west side of the University [Hospital] with a beautiful view of the Salt Lake Valley. Dr. Joyce, his nurses, and his wife, Una Loy, accompanied him. He enjoyed the different surroundings and asked to stay a bit longer, according to Mrs. Clark.

The January 10, 1983, news release reported, "Today is Dr. Clark's 40th day on the Jarvik-7 artificial heart. He had a quiet Sunday. The nurses report he slept very comfortably throughout the night. He continues in serious but stable condition."

For long periods of time, Barney had a nasogastric tube for feeding. He was also taking Coumadin and aspirin to minimize blood clotting, and there were occasional periods when he had nosebleeds. From January 14 through 18, the staff reported moderate to severe nosebleeds caused by the combination of irritation from the nasal feeding tube and the anticoagulant therapy. His nasal passages were packed to control the bleeding, but later Barney had to have surgery to stop the persistent nosebleeds.

On February 14, Barney celebrated his sixty-second birthday a few weeks later than the actual January 21 date. His condition was upgraded to fair, and he was moved into a private room. It was also Dr. Kolff's birthday. Unfortunately, Barney later had to return to the SICU and was placed on a ventilator.

February 22, Barney's 83rd day on the Utah artificial heart, was an exercise day. He pedaled his Exercycle, walked with assistance, and visited his wife and daughter, Karen. Another attempt was made to take Barney off the ventilator and move him from the SICU to a private room.

At this time, the National Conference of Christians and Jews sponsored a formal dinner honoring the Clarks and Drs. Kolff, DeVries, Joyce, Jarvik, and Olsen. Each received a beautiful commemorative plaque. Ironically, the most important player in this unique medical experiment, Barney himself, could not be present.

On March 1, DeVries did an extensive personal interview with Barney Clark on his 90th day on the artificial heart. Devries asked Barney many questions, and the interview was videotaped for a later broadcast. One question was how Barney would respond if someone asked what life was like with an artificial heart and if he felt the experiment had been worthwhile.

Barney replied, "I would tell them that it is worth it if the alternative is they die or they have it done."

DeVries asked, "I know it has been very hard for you at times, hasn't it, Barney?"

"Yes, it has been hard, but the heart itself has pumped right along, and I think it is doing very well."

When the interview was over, Barney was disappointed. He did not think that he had presented himself well. "Oh, I could have done a lot better than that. I could have at least smiled," he said regretfully.

DeVries wrote in *The New England Journal of Medicine* published on March 2, 1984, "The patient's renal function had improved, and his mental status was intact, his physical therapy was progressing, his appetite had returned, his respiratory status had stabilized, and plans for eventual discharge from the hospital were being made."[5]

Aspiration Pneumonia

On March 4, Peterson reported a sudden turnabout: "Dr. Clark suffered a severe pulmonary setback yesterday and was returned to the respirator to treat aspiration pneumonia, which developed following some nausea and vomiting he had experienced."

The next day Joyce said, "Dr. Clark has experienced no nausea or vomiting for more than twenty-four hours, and there is no reason to believe Thursday's gastric upset was anything other than stomach flu." Joyce added, "Barney continues to receive respiratory and antibiotic therapy, and he appears to be slowly improving in his bout with aspiration pneumonia. Dr. and Mrs. Clark celebrated their thirty-ninth wedding anniversary. Dr. Clark watched television of his favorite basketball team, the BYU Cougars, losing to the University of Utah's red team, the Utes. He remarked, 'It's a shame we lost.'"

March 11 marked Barney's 100th day on the artificial heart, and he continued his slow, but steady, recovery from the aspiration pneumonia. On March 15, he had no fever and continued in fair condition. It was his 104th day on the Utah artificial heart.

On March 21, the 110th day into the experiment, Peterson announced that the patient had "showed some deterioration in renal function over the past twenty-four hours and had developed a fever. His physicians looked for a possible source of infection that was causing his increased temperature, and everything was negative."

About this time, Una Loy learned from television that the hospital was covering all its charges. Kolff had donated fifty thousand dollars, and there were two gifts of twenty-five thousand dollars each. The show reported, "Dr. Clark's condition has not improved in the past two hours. He continues to have fever and reduced renal function. His physicians suspect that he has an infection, but all laboratory cultures to date were sterile. It is his 111th day on the artificial heart."

Una Loy asked what was causing the aspiration pneumonia. DeVries told her, "Nausea and vomiting...probably the flu...but we are not sure. Several people in the hospital...[were experiencing the same symptoms and were] nauseated and vomiting at that time."

Barney's Death: The Turn of a Key

The medical staff had decided to take Barney back to the SICU when DeVries looked out the window and saw another phalanx of news trucks driving in. Someone on the staff had notified reporters that attendants were trying to resuscitate Barney. DeVries was furious that Barney had possibly been neglected by one of his caretakers while that person was calling the press. He said he was reminded of vultures clustered in the trees or pacing around an injured animal waiting for their hapless victim to die. These false news reports were most frustrating to the heart team and the hospital administration, but they continued throughout Barney's 112-day stay.

That afternoon Barney started on a steady, progressively downhill course. His blood pressure kept falling, and it did not respond to anything team members tried, such as changes in medication and adjustments to the heart driver. "There were no ups and downs, just downs," DeVries said.

He had long conversations with Una Loy about her husband's impending death. When things began to deteriorate, he took her to another room, so she realized things were serious. He told her the doctors were trying to find out what was going on. Later, he asked Joyce, "Lyle, why don't you go in and talk to Una Loy?" She had become very close to Joyce. Some nurses and Joyce went in to see her while DeVries returned to Barney.

By late afternoon, DeVries told Una Loy he did not know whether her husband was going to make it and that he would be transferred to the SICU where the staff could control things a little better. Una Loy agreed, and Barney was moved into Room 12 in the unit.

At about 6:00 PM, DeVries informed the worried wife that the time had come for a decision. Last-ditch efforts, he said, might include putting Barney on dialysis. "I don't know how you feel about that," he said. Una Loy telephoned her children to discuss the possibility of dialysis. Karen was not excited about the prospect.

As the situation continued to deteriorate, DeVries told Una Loy, "I think he is probably not going to make it to morning; he is slowly going downhill, and there is nothing we can do anymore." Una Loy began to cry. DeVries checked on Barney, then came back and talked to her for more than an hour. She realized the end was coming and again called her daughter, Karen, in Boston. She had talked with her sons Gary and Stephen earlier in the afternoon. Both she and DeVries talked to Stephen, and Lyle spoke with him several times.

DeVries attempted to keep Una Loy posted on Barney's declining condition: "His pressure is now 30 (systolic), and his central venous pressure probably 30 also, and there is no great indication that the artificial heart is doing anything to support his vascular system. His vascular system is dead. He is totally unresponsive. His eyes are not responsive to light—no neurological signs whatsoever. I don't think there is any reason to go on this way. He is essentially dead."

Una Loy knew this, and she nodded. "It's okay."

"Maybe we should stop this," he repeated. She agreed. "Do you want to be in the room?" he asked.

Una Loy shook her head as tears glistened. "No, I would rather not," she said and left.

No one ever divulged who turned off the heart-driver key. During the early deliberations about the consent form, this had been a bothersome issue. The consenting patient had to be offered the opportunity to drop out of the study. This was appropriate when a patient was on an experimental drug. But a patient on an artificial heart could not pull out of the experiment without dying. Kolff had pointed out to the IRB that the patient would have a key that he could merely turn off. That statement prompted a series of lengthy discussions, and it was concluded the patient could not have access to the key.

The Selbys later asked DeVries about this final act. He simply stated, "I don't think it is necessary to know who turned the key off. It was unanimous with everybody that there was no longer any need to keep the driver on."

The key on the Utah artificial-heart driver was turned off at 10:02 PM on March 23, 1983. Barney's passing was described by one person as resembling poet Oliver Wendell Holmes's old one-horse shay. In the poem, a fictional deacon built the wonderful shay so perfectly that it would not break down. The shay endured for a hundred years to the day, then disintegrated all at once "just as bubbles do when they burst."

So it was that within twelve hours or so, Dr. Barney Clark "simply fell apart." He died of circulatory collapse, coupled with multiorgan system failure. He had also contracted colitis. The official word was that he died of pseudomembranous enterocolitis, or antibiotic-associated colitis. The experiment had lasted for 112 days, 2,688 hours, and 12,912,499 calculated beats of his implanted heart.

Notes

1. Dr. Kolff and the Utah artificial-heart team discussed these problems and their solutions in the publication, W. J. Kolff, "Artificial Organs—Forty Years and Beyond," *Transactions—American Society for Artificial Internal Organs* 29 (1983):6–24.
2. William C. DeVries, "The Permanent Artificial Heart: Four Case Reports," *JAMA* 259, no. 6 (February 12, 1988): 849–859.
3. The University of Utah's public-television station, KUED, produced a documentary entitled *The Experimental Heart: 112 Days of Barney Clark* at the time of Clark's surgery and death in 1983; a copy can be found in the archives at the J. Willard Marriott Library.
4. Transcripts of the press releases and press conferences can be found in the Barney B. Clark Collection, Special Collections, J. Willard Marriott Library, University of Utah, Salt Lake City.
5. W. C. DeVries, J. L. Anderson, L. D. Joyce, F. I Anderson, E. H. Hammond, R. K. Jarvik, and W. J. Kolff, "Clinical Use of the Total Artificial Heart," *New England Journal of Medicine* 310 (March 1984): 273–78.

20

Aftermath of the First Permanent Implant

A chief event of life is the day in which
we have encountered a mind that startled us.

—Ralph Waldo Emerson

Barney Clark, Home at Last: The Funeral

With his unique medical interlude at an end, Barney Clark's body was returned to Washington state where he, Una Loy, and their children had made their home for many years. Scores of prominent members of the community, along with family, friends, medical admirers, and media, gathered to pay last respects to this pioneer whose ordinary, quiet life had been capped by a sacrifice of gigantic proportions that had brought him to the attention of the whole world. Some thirteen hundred people attended the funeral held on March 29, 1983, in the LDS stake center in Federal Way, Washington, with interment in nearby Washington Memorial Park, Sea Tac, Washington.

Among the notables in attendance was William D. Ruckelshaus, President Reagan's designated director of the Environmental Protection Agency, who represented the First Family. President Reagan, who was out of the country, sent condolences and laudatory remarks via White House Assistant Press Secretary Anson Franklin. Early in Barney's journey, Reagan had sent a message of congratulations and admiration, and now at the end of the saga, he expressed "deepest sympathy" and extended commendations to "a brave and courageous man."

The Church of Jesus Christ of Latter-day Saints assigned the late Elder Neal A. Maxwell of the Quorum of the Twelve Apostles, one of the church's most sought-after speakers, to address the funeral attendees. Elder Maxwell praised the Clark family and the University of Utah heart team for a "significant adven-

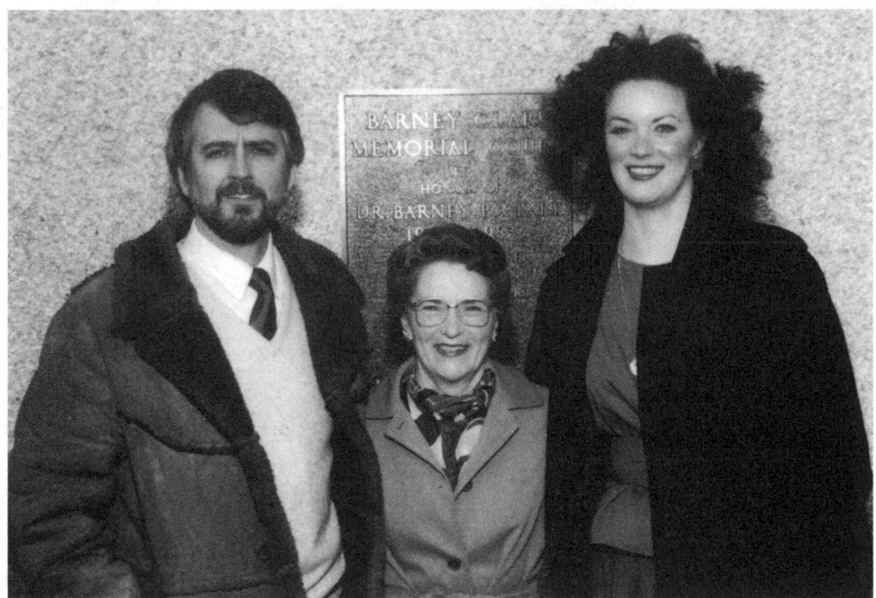

Una Loy Clark at the dedication of Barney Clark Memorial Court in Washington Memorial Park.

ture" and characterized Barney's last weeks of life as "a unique second salute to God, a salute in gratitude for the gift of mortal life." He compared the groundbreaking surgery to the experience of nineteenth-century pioneers, reminding the Clark family that when a group lost a member along the trail, they "picked up their handcarts and headed west." In a message filled with hope for a life beyond the grave, he called on the survivors to prepare for a "glorious reunion with your husband, father, and grandfather."

William DeVries represented the Utah heart team at the service, speaking briefly and emotionally, an indication of the unusually deep ties that had developed among team members and their famous patient.

In Salt Lake City, the flag flew at half staff at the State Capitol from the time of Clark's death until the funeral was completed, as ordered by Governor Scott M. Matheson, who was in Washington DC on state business. He also sent a message lauding Clark as "one of the preeminent pioneers of science."

As Barney's funeral was ending a significant first in artificial-heart research, the University of Utah continued to receive messages from scientists all over the world. They came from locations as distant as Australia, Brazil, Japan, Russia, and South Africa. The messages almost universally hailed the medical center's achievement and recognized the successful use of the artificial heart as another step in the continuing battle to gain control of heart disease, according to a Deseret News report by medical writer Twila Van Leer.

Dr. Christiaan Barnard, who had been in the world spotlight in 1967 when he had performed the first heart transplant, urged the Utah group to continue its work. "Tell those doctors they must not give up," he said.

The atmosphere at the medical center as the high tension of the historic implant wound down was "reflective and subdued," according to Van Leer. Helen Kee, assistant administrator for nursing, was quoted as saying, "I expect we'll remember for a long time to come." She was among those in Clark's SICU room when he succumbed to multiple-systems failure. "He was a kind of a hero and very strong. He knew all along what might happen, but he was fully committed to the whole thing. He said he wanted to make a contribution to science if he could, and his contribution has been incredible," she reflected.

In her first days as a widow, Una Loy also offered personal insights into the remarkable events that had marked her husband's final days. "If Barney Clark were here today, he'd do it again," she said at a news conference held after the funeral. Una Loy praised her husband as an indomitable pioneer. "My husband was happy to do this, even though he suffered greatly," she said. "He never gave up, never stopped trying. Never—even in my presence—was there a word of complaint. He wanted to do what he could to help others. We're very, very proud of him."

She also described the last minutes with her husband. She said she kissed his cheek and had a short private farewell before the final steps were taken to end the experiment. She had spent much of the final evening with a brother and other family members in a room near Barney's SICU room.

Una Loy said that the major bonus resulting from the implant was the outpouring of love and encouragement from thousands of people all over the world. She noted she still had five hundred to six hundred letters she had not yet had time to open. She was determined to answer them all, even those in foreign languages that required translation. She stressed that she had no regrets about her and Barney's participation in what was an untried medical-research project but added she wouldn't want to live through it again. If she was asked to advise another person considering an artificial heart, she said, "I'd tell them to go for it."

She also praised the members of the Utah team. "We went down there total strangers, and after three and a half months, there is not a member of the team that I wouldn't call a brother or a sister. I've never seen more love and care from people.

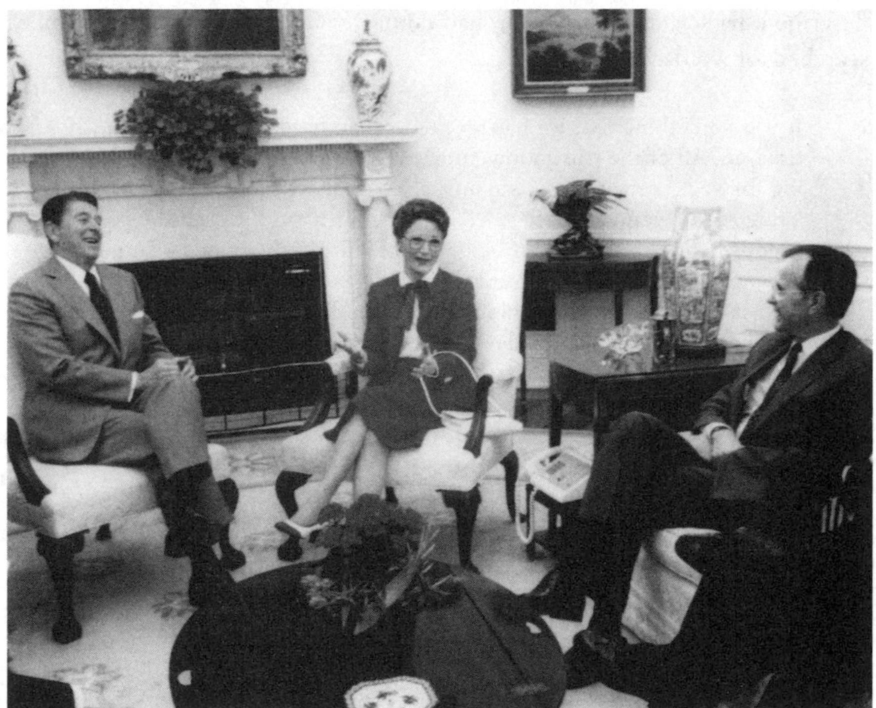

In 1983 Una Loy was honored at the White House by President Ronald Reagan, Vice President George H. W. Bush, and others.

One of Barney's sons, Stephen, a physician as well, also spoke. Although the family's original hopes and expectations for the implant were never achieved because his father could not return home and live a normal life, he said that the implant should not be considered unsuccessful or not worthwhile. The family had many good conversations and happy times when Barney was lucid and ambulatory, Stephen said. "I strongly hope the research continues," he concluded.

Dr. Fred Anderson was one of many who praised Una Loy. Admiration for her steady support of her husband and the medical team was a recurring theme. She had seldom left the hospital and had volunteered to help whenever she could. "I really admire that lady," Anderson said. "Always will. And I think I'll always give her the credit for whatever success we have achieved. I think she has to be given as much credit as anybody else, including Barney."

DeVries was also asked to describe his feelings about the implant. In an interview with Earl Selby, he struggled to describe what he said, in some respects, had been an "almost religious experience" for many of the team members. Trying to describe how science and religion had come together, DeVries rambled as he searched for words:

> It was something that we had worked on so hard and spent so much time on. All of the frustrations of getting all the pieces together, waiting for such a long time, thinking often that we were ready, but not being ready...and another piece comes into it, and just all the pieces suddenly fit together. Then being there during the surgery and seeing in that seven-hour period the influences that came in, it was just almost magical. Just everything all of a sudden fits together perfectly. And remembering that the development was so many times rough and ragged.

As the surgery began, DeVries said, there was a sense almost of euphoria, a feeling that

> aren't we great? We are going to beat disease. By the time it was over, that idea had changed completely. Nobody in the room at all felt that way. Everybody kind of felt in awe. We had seen something that was bigger and better and more eternal—or whatever you want to call it—than we ever deserved to see. We realized at that time the importance of all the training we had undergone. Suddenly, the hours and hours, the days, the years that we spent working with animals—it all meant something. It wasn't how great we were, but how we had been blessed and privileged to take part in something bigger than we were. That is the spiritual concept, I think.
>
> Many of the people there were deeply religious people and, of course, they attributed this feeling to God. Other people there weren't religious at all. Some were agnostic or atheist. But we all knew that something had happened in that room that was more than we could explain. The concept of the spiritual thing was true.

DeVries also talked to the Selbys about his perceptions of the difference between innovation therapies—most often a one-time desperation move to save a patient's life—and the methodical human research that builds progressively toward a desired end. In this case, DeVries said, the goal was to develop a device that could be permanently implanted into a human to extend life after the natural heart had ceased to function.

The Press and Dr. Barney Clark

Although the opinions expressed during and immediately after the Barney Clark experience were mostly laudatory, there were, inevitably, criticisms of the Utah heart team and the surgery. Chase Peterson defended the artificial heart both while Clark was still alive and after his death. "If this country somehow ever got the notion that an idea is dangerous, we would be in the intellectual Dark Ages," he proclaimed.

The internal and external postmortems went on. The success of the first implant had put to rest most of the scientific questions. The Utah team had proved that, in fact, an individual could live with a mechanical device that met the body's circulatory demands. Almost everyone seemed convinced that with a less critically ill patient, the results could be even better. The research to produce a less-onerous mechanical-support system was promising.

Amid all the questions that buzzed around the potential and future of the artificial heart, only one absorbed the members of the Utah heart team: "When can we do it again?" Devries was very anxious to operate on a second patient. The University of Utah had initially given permission to implant two patients, and the FDA had approved seven. After some delay, the IRB approved two additional patients and agreed that the Heimes portable pneumatic driver could be tested on them. The IRB approval came in January 1984, and the FDA gave permission for the second patient in June of that year.

But for reasons that were never clear, Utah did not move ahead. Barney Clark was destined to be the one and only implant patient in Utah during this experimental period. Chafed, Don Olsen specifically asked Peterson, by then president of the university, if decisions had been made in meetings not to go ahead with a second implant. Peterson responded, "I know of no such meetings or administrative decisions."

He suggested, however, that the hospital administration was highly concerned about the mounting costs of the research, and he also conjectured that the long delay in publishing results of the first surgery in medical journals was a factor. IRB members, he said, were upset that they had not received detailed information about the Clark implant though months had passed. Whether through decisions, concerns about costs, or simple inertia, it became apparent the University of Utah commitment to continued human experimentation with the artificial heart had slogged to a halt. A disgruntled DeVries began looking for options.

Enter Humana Hospital Chain

Shortly after the Clark surgery, Humana Inc., one of several large organizations that had blossomed out of the push for managed health care, approached the University Of Utah and offered to cover the complete costs for a hundred artificial-heart-implant patients. After much discussion, some university officials were concerned that having a large insurance company finance the study might raise questions about objectivity. Willem Kolff was very disappointed that the university refused Humana's offer. He felt it would have been advantageous for the university to have financial backing for a period of experimentation that would ultimately prove or disprove the effectiveness of the artificial heart in treating heart-failure patients.

DeVries Moves to Louisville, Kentucky

On Sunday, September 30, 1984, the *Deseret News* printed an article headlined, "Aggressive, Committed Hospital Revives DeVries' Waning Heart." The article read,

> The 40-year-old surgeon who implanted the world's first permanent artificial heart left the University of Utah Medical Center in Salt Lake City and joined an up-and-coming health center called the Humana Heart Institute International at Humana Audubon Hospital in suburban Louisville. DeVries was lured to Kentucky by a commitment for at least 100 artificial heart operations to be financed by the not-for-profit hospital group, Humana Inc. It was a major medical coup for Humana and for the man who started the heart center, Dr. Allan M. Lansing. David A. Jones, chairman of the aggressive hospital chain based in Louisville, is even more enthusiastic. Lansing formed a team of six physicians and other support personnel for the institute.

In October 1983, Lansing had begun training at the University of Utah to implant the artificial heart, where one year before, DeVries had performed his famous operation on Barney Clark. The two hit it off. "DeVries came to Louisville for a social visit, and we talked about some of the problems he had in Utah," Lansing said. "After an hour or so, I made the suggestion he come to Louisville. He paused and answered, 'Maybe I will.'"

DeVries was frustrated. Red tape and other unknown issues had forced delay after delay of a second operation in Utah. Several selected patients had died while waiting for approval from the university's IRB.

Jones was quick to jump at the chance. Having already provided a million of the six million dollars in venture capital needed to get the Utah artificial-heart manufacturer, Kolff Medical, Inc., off the ground, Humana was solidly behind the artificial heart. DeVries was quickly whisked back to Louisville for a meeting with Jones and Wendell Cherry, president and CEO of Humana. "We made a package that was just ideal," Lansing said.

Under the deal, DeVries would join Lansing's team's surgical practice and be affiliated with Humana Heart Institute International and Humana Hospital-

Audubon. In exchange Humana agreed to pay for a hundred operations like Barney Clark's. In July 1984, a few weeks after Humana made its offer and nineteen months after the first operation on Clark, DeVries stepped in front of a group of microphones at the Louisville hospital to announce his move to Kentucky. He cited red tape in Utah and Humana's commitment to meet the cost of the operations as the major factors. Jones estimated the cost for the hundred operations was around six million dollars.

DeVries performed three additional implants at the new hospital. The patients were William Schroeder, Murray Haydon, and Jack Burcham. Schroeder lived 622 days with his heart but experienced complications that severely impaired him both mentally and physically; Haydon lived more than a year but spent most of the time in an ICU attached to a respirator; Haydon died ten days after his implant, and DeVries acknowledged the artificial heart may have speeded his demise.

Although there was a growing groundswell of criticism of the research, DeVries saw the results as amazing. "It is extremely rare—if ever—that clinical research has been so dramatically successful for the initial subjects," he wrote. (He may have been remembering Kolff's sixteen patients who died on kidney dialysis before one survived.) "Because of the artificial heart, these patients have enjoyed their families, births of grandchildren, marriages of their children, fishing excursions and even participated in parades." Only the valve failure in Clark's heart had marred total reliability of the heart, he noted.

In spring 1988, DeVries was declaring that "I intend to go on with the project," but in June, he resigned from Humana. A long-running feud with the institute's director had come to a head, and DeVries was tired of the bureaucratic battles, the frustration of waiting months and years for official approvals, and trying to live with the public looking over his shoulder. He said he was ready to return to private surgical practice. It seems unlikely that he ever implanted another artificial heart or a left ventricular device in a patient.

Not everyone took DeVries's rosy view of the artificial heart. Gideon Gil, a medical writer for Louisville's *Courier-Journal,* has been an outspoken critic. He wrote in an April 1989 article titled "The Artificial Heart Juggernaut" in *The Hastings Center Report* that "permanent implants of artificial hearts have been halted by bad results, but questions about fairness and informed consent have failed to stop manufacturers, surgeons and hospitals from using mechanical hearts as bridges to transplants."[1] A few weeks later, Gil followed up that article with one in the *Courier-Journal,* where he said that "the artificial heart's momentum will be stopped only when results sour and profit-seeking manufacturers, publicity-seeking hospitals and surgeons seeking to stall death at any cost no longer derive benefit from its use. Patients' and the public's benefit will remain secondary."

Over time Gil's doomsday predictions for the artificial heart have proved incorrect. Work continued doggedly on many fronts to carve out the proper niche for the device in the medical arsenal against disease. Utah remained firmly entrenched in the ongoing research, but its involvement in human implantation, for the time being, had ended.

Note

1. Gideon Gil, "The Artificial Heart Juggernaut," *The Hastings Center Report* 19, no. 2 (March–April 1989): 24–31.

21

The Ongoing Debate about the Merits of the Artificial Heart

Perhaps it is not surprising that the world came to associate a seminal piece of engineering—the work of hundreds over a course of years—with one man. After all, it had his name on it.

—Michael Moyer, *Scientific American*, September 2009

Few if any medical research projects have generated more discussion than the artificial heart. Almost everyone conversant with medicine, medical ethics, or the role of government in medical issues has hurried to state his or her position, but the Barney Clark saga intensified the debate.

Over time the critics seemed to have the upper hand. It almost seemed that publishers welcomed authors who focused on apparent weaknesses in the artificial-heart program. Many of them pursued their self-created controversies for months and even years.

Evaluating the Significance of Barney Clark

A Clark implant follow-up conference was held on October 13–15, 1983, in Alta, Utah, one of the popular ski resorts east of Salt Lake City, to address issues related to the first implant, including ethics. The invited participants were primarily individuals who had been in Utah during the Clark surgery. University of Utah President Chase N. Peterson, who introduced the speakers, said, "This conference brings us together to explore our human struggles as we discuss and evaluate the Utah artificial-heart-implant program."

The proceedings of the conference were published in a book titled *After Barney Clark: Reflections on the Utah Artificial Heart Program.*[1] In her introduction, editor Margery Shaw noted the need for openness and honesty in disseminating information about emerging science. "To oppose technology is self-hatred," she said, quoting Joshua Lederberg. The following excerpts from the book reflect some of the issues discussed at the conference.

Albert R. Jonsen, chief of the Division of Medical Ethics at the University of California, San Francisco, wrote in "The Selection of Patients":

> Since the scarce and costly resource cannot come to all in need, should it come to those in need whose personal benefit represents the highest and best use for society? We face a classical ethical problem long familiar to political and economic life, but unfamiliar to medicine—the problem of justice. We are only on the verge of the debate about the ethical use of scarce and costly technology.

Eric J. Cassell, director of the Program for the Study of Ethics and Values in Medicine at the Cornell University Medical College, commented in "How Is the Death of Barney Clark to Be Understood?": "The implantation of the artificial heart into Dr. Barney Clark, his subsequent illness and his death are monuments to biology, human creativity, the dedication to others that marks medicine at its best—the magnificence of the human spirit."

Denise Grady, freelance writer and contributor to *Discover* magazine, asked in "Summary of Discussions on Ethical Perspectives":

> Is the dominant purpose of the experimentation on the human being to benefit the person on whom it is performed, or to gather data that may help future patients? Jonsen maintains that the ethical justification for clinical research in its early stages is aimed at gathering data to improve care for future patients, and not necessarily beneficial to the subjects themselves. Given this utilitarian objective, the subjects must be volunteers in the fullest sense.[2]

Gilbert S. Omenn, dean of the School of Public Health and Community Medicine at the University of Washington, Seattle, observed in "The Role of the Federal Government":

> It is apparent here in Utah, for example, that the team developing the totally implantable artificial heart had to become fully committed to this project and maintain that commitment for many years. It is impossible in such work to be dispassionate about the relative merits of the totally implanted heart, left ventricular assist devices and cardiac transplantation, even for patients for whom medical therapy may no longer be considered effective.

He added that the government, of necessity, must be involved in all stages of the development, promotion, and application of new medical technology because—in this era of extraordinary costs—most research institutions cannot afford to do it alone.

Renée C. Fox, Annenberg Professor of the Social Sciences at the University of Pennsylvania, had visited the University of Utah in June 1983 to study the sociological impact of the Clark implant. She was impressed then that the Utah heart team had "almost nostalgic remembrances of their recent Barney Clark past that had an it-was-the-best-of-times-and-the-worst-of-times feeling about it." She stated in "A Sociological Perspective on the Case of the Utah Artificial Heart":

> Barney Clark, the recipient of the Utah heart, was a person rapidly moving to his inevitable death from a progressive chronic disease condition for which there was no further established effective medical or surgical treatment. The selection of a patient in this state for such a clinical trial was dictated by the uncodified but binding ethical assumption to which medical professionals adhere: namely, that a therapeutic innovation in the earliest stages of moving from the laboratory (or animal barn in this case) to the clinic still fraught with all the uncertainty and risk that this animal-to-human phase of experimentation involves, should only be tried on individuals who are incurably ill, beyond conventional medical help and close to death. Dr. Clark became what the members of the University of Utah Medical Center referred to as a very 'special' patient. In their words, he was a 'remarkable man' of 'great courage,' with a desire to 'contribute to medical progress and to serve mankind. He chose this unpredictable experiment over eminent death,' they said, although 'he knew he might have considerable anguish.' Throughout the experiment (which lasted for 112 days, 2,688 hours and 12,912,499 heartbeats), he displayed what team members described as 'stamina, endurance and persistence, a sense of humor and ability to love most of all his wife and children.' Dr. and Mrs. Clark were regarded as 'co-investigators with the research team in every sense of the word' and as part of the members' professional and personal families. 'Barney Clark is our hero, in this chapter of medical history,' spokespersons for the team declared in their final tributes to him: 'A pioneer to match these western lands.'

Alexander Morgan Capron, professor of law, ethics, and public policy at Georgetown University in Washington DC, wrote in "The Role of the Lawyer and Legal Advice in the Artificial Heart Program":

> There are three issues that have particular legal content: first, the termination of treatment, or the issue of euthanasia; the issue of surrogate decision-making for an incapacitated patient; and the issue of privacy. In paragraph 16 of the consent form, which is quite brief, it states: 'I understand I am free at any time to withdraw my consent to participate in this experimental project, recognizing that the exercise of such an option, after the artificial heart is in place, may result in my death.' Fortunately, this confused statement never became an issue. It is difficult to see why the issue of surrogate decisions wasn't explicitly addressed in the consent document itself. This item never became a point of concern since Dr. Clark remained lucid right up to his death. The final legal issue is the question of privacy, specifically the control over publicity, most obviously as it affected Dr. Clark and his family, but also as it affected the professionals who were involved. Dr. Clark had consented to the sharing of information about (the implantation) with the world at large. It was also agreed what photographs or films could be shown.

Dr. Lawrence K. Altman, medical correspondent and author of "Doctor's World" for the *New York Times*, stated in "After Barney Clark: Reflections of a Reporter on Unresolved Issues":

> The story that dominated news reports throughout the world on 1 December 1982 and in the many days thereafter came from the University of Utah Medical Center. But from the journalistic point of view, the story about Dr. Barney Clark's artificial heart implant operation did not begin in the closing hours of November 1982. It really began several years before, when the University of Utah Medical Center public relations staff announced to medical and science reporters and news organizations the details of the university's progress in the artificial organs program, particularly emphasizing its aim of developing a functional artificial heart.

Altman then outlined a half dozen or so areas of concern from his viewpoint as a reporter. The first was the failure of the Utah heart team to make scientific reports in medical literature or even to the IRB at the university:

> As we approach the first anniversary of Dr. Clark's artificial heart implantation, I am unaware of any scientific report that has appeared in any medical journal. I am astonished. Dr. Christiaan Barnard's first heart transplant operation in 1967 certainly received as much publicity as Dr. William DeVries' first case. Yet it took less than one month for Dr. Barnard's report to appear in a peer-reviewed journal.

He went on to criticize the university's public relations: It is because the taxpayers paid for the development of the artificial heart and the University of Utah is a public institution that public relations is so important in telling Dr. Clark's story as well as other aspects of the artificial heart program. I think many would have difficulty without further explanation of Dr. Bosso's statement that, seven months after Dr. Clark's death, the IRB still does not have sufficient information from DeVries to evaluate a new protocol.

According to the informed consent form that Dr. Clark signed twice, he was responsible for the costs of his hospitalization, which were nearly $250,000. The university covered all of the costs with non-taxpayer funds so the implantation was without cost to the Clarks.

Altman also felt that the information provided to the media was confusing and inconsistent:

> The university announced the operation in advance and reported the complications as they occurred. The information from Utah was lower and may have been filtered. Several of the reporters wondered how the Jarvik-7 model had been chosen. The university did not provide enough information on the development of the artificial heart models and their names and we were further confused by Dr. Clifford Kwan-Gett's dispute over credit for priority in developing the artificial heart.

Finally, Altman criticized the lack of follow-up information from the university: "The essence of good clinical medicine and research is the quality of the follow-up. The university medical center and the heart team have not provided the press with information about what has transpired since Dr. Clark's death."

Altman predicted that there might be even more popular interest in a second implant. He also noted that Dr. Lyle Joyce, second in command at the Clark implant, had left University Hospital. "How can you proceed the next time so shortly after the number-two surgeon has gone?" he asked.

Peterson addressed several of the criticisms that Altman raised. He said the university had expected exceptional media coverage and prepared for a large number of news representatives with extra phones and food service. However, the actual number of news reporters was many more than anticipated, and no one could have predicted so many of them would remain in Salt Lake City for the entire 112 days of Clark's life after surgery. Peterson also told Altman that Dr. Arnold Relman of *The New England Journal of Medicine* had already accepted an article on the Clark surgery and DeVries had a case study in press with *The Journal of Thoracic and Cardiovascular Surgery.*

John A. Bosso, current chair of the University of Utah IRB, talked about the role of the board in "Deliberations of the Utah Institutional Review Board Concerning the Artificial Heart":

> Institutional review boards are charged with the task of protecting the rights and welfare of human research subjects. The University of Utah IRB received the first heart implantation research protocol for consideration in October 1980. After an agreement was reached with the investigators to limit the subject population to those whose hearts cease during cardiac surgery and cannot be restarted and after significant revision of the consent form, this protocol was approved in February 1981. In the following year, several cardiac surgical patients agreed to implantation of the artificial heart under the specified circumstances, but since no complications arose in the treatment of these consenting subjects, no implant operations were performed. The investigators subsequently requested that the prospective pool be expanded to include patients with cardiomyopathy who were in Class IV congestive failure for at least eight weeks, as defined by the New York State Heart Association. A protocol for cardiomyopathy patients was submitted in May 1982. A subcommittee report to the full IRB was generated and submitted in June 1982. Through a series of communications and meetings with the principal investigator, it was agreed that a full, detailed report of the first case should be submitted for full IRB review along with a revised protocol and consent form.

Bosso commented that there were lingering questions about whether sufficient animal research had preceded the move to human implantation but acknowledged that "the answer to this question lies in the first few implantations in humans."

Bosso then defended the board's apparent inaction:

> The IRB has been criticized for the length of time it is taking to reapprove the artificial heart protocol subsequent to the conclusion of the first case. A number of reasons account for this delay. A subcommittee was formed to gather knowledge on the experience of the first case and was to report to the full IRB its findings and recommendations. The subcommittee took several months to complete this task. Its final report was considered to be incomplete by the full IRB, however, largely because the full, written report on the first case had not been received from the investigators. By late November 1982, all requested information and a revised protocol and consent form were received and were under active consideration. The Utah IRB approved these documents and granted permission for a second implant in January 1984. The FDA gave its approval in June 1984.

Besides the extensive review in *After Barney Clark,* articles in many other publications weighed the pros and cons of the artificial heart from a wide range of viewpoints. Here are some excerpts in chronological order:

In "Martyrdom for Scientific Purposes," Dr. Denton A. Cooley wrote,

> Now that the chapter in scientific history provided by the heroic volunteer, Dr. Barney Clark, has ended, an assessment of the episode deserves reflection. With almost full knowledge of the consequences following implantation of a mechanical heart, from his observance of results in living animals and urged on by his own belief in inevitable doom from terminal heart disease, Dr. Clark gave his consent to spend his last days supported by the device. The remarkable survival record of 112 days may stand for many years for a number of reasons, not the least of which may be the failure to obtain a second such ideal volunteer.
>
> ...The renowned French scientist and experimenter of the 19th Century, Claude Bernard, described in simple terms his opinion regarding the ethical nature of such projects: 'The principle of medical and surgical morality, therefore, consists in never performing on man an experiment which might be harmful to him to any extent, even though the result might be highly advantageous to science, i.e., to the health of others.' Perhaps that statement, made more than a century ago, is not wholly transferable to the present, where truly informed consent from the patient provides the experimenter with a less disturbed conscience. Yet its message remains clear and to the point today.
>
> ...I believe that further orderly investigations must proceed.... To sustain the life of the patient by a mechanical heart until cardiac transplantation is possible seems fully justified, whether or not the surgeon has prior formal approval or patient consent.

Cooley then paid tribute to Barney Clark, "to this man, this dentist, this courageous person already described as a martyr for his determined and heroic stand against a meaningless and defeatist's death. He made a contribution to mankind, the value of which may not yet be determined. History reveals that martyrdom is deserved by those who die for a cause."[3] In a later speech, he elaborated, "There are few patients who have been martyrs.... Such patients do not get enough credit for their courage."

In a wide-ranging article entitled "Response of the Human Body to the First Permanent Implant of the Jarvik-7 Total Artificial Heart," Lyle Joyce and his cowriters—all members of the Utah heart team—discussed the extensive selection process for implant patients, the anatomical fit of the artificial heart, and the way the body responded to the presence of a "foreign" material. The article also confirmed the postmortem diagnosis of pseudomembranous enterocolitis as the cause of Barney Clark's death.

The article concluded,

> In summary: The success of the first permanent total artificial heart implant resulted in several major achievements: First, we were able to demonstrate that the total artificial heart will fit within the male chest without causing obstruction to inflow or outflow channels. Second, we were able to demonstrate that the total artificial heart would sustain life on a long-term basis (at least up to 112 days) without any evidence of systemic or local infection and without any untoward systemic effects. Third, we were able to demonstrate that the patient was able to tolerate a total artificial heart without complaint of the noise or the bulk of the drive system to which he required permanent attachment and that the patient could be comfortable and totally free of pain. An additional finding, which could not be assessed in animal experimentations, was the fact that the patient was able to maintain higher central nervous system activity on an undisturbed basis following the implant of the total artificial heart.[4]

In "Experimental Medical Devices, Drugs and Techniques: Their Future Social, Medical and Political Implications" O. R. Bowen reviewed the impact of the artificial heart and discussed the side issues to its advancement, including potential increases in health-care costs. He said, "The principle of the dangerous precedent is that you should not now do an admittedly right action for fear that you or your equally timid successor should not have the courage to do right in some future time.... Every public action that is not customary either is wrong, or if it is right, a dangerous precedent is established. It follows that nothing should ever be done the first time." The reasoning here resembles Colorado Governor Richard Lamb's statement that "everyone has a responsibility to die."

Bowen continued,

> Perhaps the most exciting medical event since the first heart transplant has been the implantation of the world's first artificial heart on Dec. 2, 1982, in Utah. That ranks in importance with man's first step on the moon. But that event, like other organ transplants, be they kidney, liver or heart and lungs combined, creates problems without answers. These problems are ethical, medical, social and economical. When all of these are part of the problem, political involvement soon follows. As sure as night follows day, when political involvement

> occurs, governmental laws, rules and regulations are just a few speeches and votes away.

At this point, Bowen quoted an article from *The New England Journal of Medicine*, which stated, "We are rapidly approaching the point at which modern medicine can offer more than society can afford. New approaches are required to decide how much of our limited resources can be devoted to medical care."[5]

In a newspaper editorial entitled "Cut the Red Tape: Implant at Full Speed," Harry Schwartz criticized the bureaucratic delays that threatened the use of the artificial heart and their frustrating effect on DeVries:

> Congress should hold public hearings on the barriers that, for almost a year and a half now, have prevented further experiments involving implanting artificial hearts in humans. The artificial heart is probably the most important recent medical advance on which experimentation has begun. Yet an absurd mass of red tape and the thinly hidden fears of business and government leaders who would rather save dollars than lives have so frustrated Barney Clark's surgeon, Dr. William C. DeVries, that he has left the University of Utah to join the Humana Heart Institute, a part of Humana Corporation, a private hospital based in Louisville, Kentucky.
>
> ... Dr. DeVries' frustrating experience has also highlighted the cumbersomeness of the whole complicated program for getting permission to do such experiments. Few medical events in the modern world have been so minutely publicized and scrutinized as the experiment to which Barney Clark gave himself. But that did not prevent the bureaucratic nightmare that finally forced Dr. DeVries to leave Utah.[6]

Barton Bernstein, in "The Misguided Quest for the Artificial Heart," wrote,

> The early 1960s constituted an era of euphoria in which federal funds seemed plentiful, social problems soluble and scientific triumphs imminent. Money, technology and prowess, it appeared, would speedily produce any number of medical miracles. Prominent among the expected achievements of medical science was the totally implantable artificial heart. The device would fit neatly inside the chest cavity of human patients with major heart problems, giving them much, if not all, of the freedom and flexibility that they possessed when equipped with their own natural healthy hearts.
>
> Biomedical scientists, heart surgeons and bureaucrats viewed the TIAH [total implantable artificial heart] as a partial response to the scourge of heart disease, which at that time killed about 700,000 Americans each year. 'The artificial heart is feasible now and ripe for

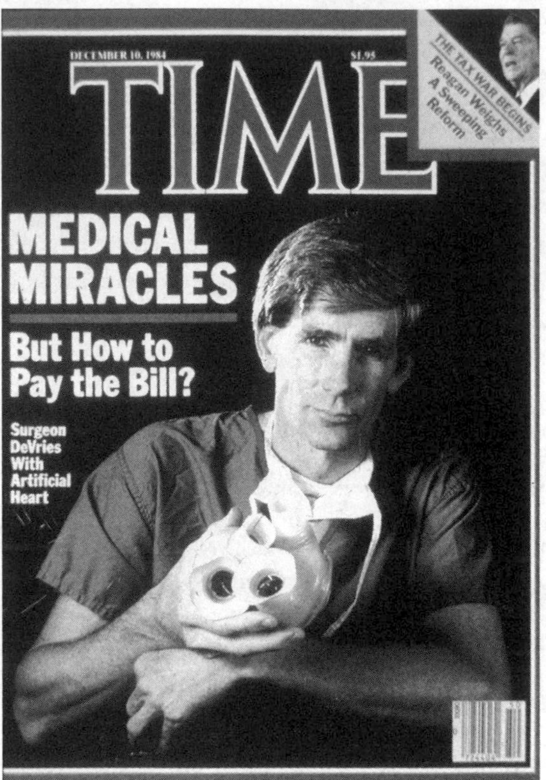

William DeVries on the cover of *Time* magazine.

> development and it can be effectively achieved,' declared a statement by the National Heart Institute (NHI), a federal agency that embarked on the quest to develop a TIAH in 1964.... Today, two decades later, scientists have failed to achieve the lofty goal of a working TIAH.

In his lengthy article, Bernstein minimized the impact of the Clark implant and said the patient had had little freedom because he was tethered to a 350-pound control unit; he "struggled through 112 painful days linked up to the console before he died—hardly a testament to technology triumphant."

Bernstein argued that widespread use of the TIAH would extend the life of millions, swelling the population of the elderly and creating a demand for more costly care. That would strain federal programs, he said. And if the device was not available to everyone, there would be questions about who should receive it, likely involving government bureaucracy. He charged that the University of Utah had carefully orchestrated news about Clark and withheld information to overstate his well-being.

Bernstein quoted Dr. Norman Shumway of Stanford and said he had called the Utah heart "crude and inappropriate." The whole experiment, he said, raised serious ethical and political questions. He suggested Clark's death might have been hastened, not delayed, by the device and questioned the validity of animal research that had preceded the implant.

"Why are technological 'fixes' more attractive than preventive measures?" he asked, suggesting that the drama of implanting an artificial heart eclipsed a preventative approach. Prevention of heart disease would be preferable in the long run, he argued. He also suggested that broader involvement in decision making about finite research funds, including citizen participation, would be helpful.[7]

In a separate letter to Don Olsen, Bernstein, a professor of history at Stanford University, wrote, "Changing the condition of poverty would improve health more than all the medical innovations we are going to get in the next decade."

In "What Are the Ethical and Social Implications of Artificial Organs?", R. Cortesini discussed the responsibility of doctors in using artificial organs: "Let me introduce some basic principles and fundamental justifications for our moral attitude in medicine before discussing the problems of artificial organs. It is clear that the enormous increase of power in the hands of doctors raises many questions that have never previously been posed." Cortesini then quoted the French scientist, Jean Rostand: "Science has made us gods before we are even worthy of being men."

Cortesini acknowledged that the role of a doctor is to help patients live as normal a life as possible and minimize pain. "But when should we give up the struggle?" he asked. "We should, as a rule, fight with all of the means at our disposal as long as we are not convinced that all hope is gone. However, when we have established that the end must soon come... death is a natural phenomenon and should be allowed to run its course."

Physicians are not obligated, he said, to use "all means to prolong life." Only recognition of the inevitability of death can resolve the problems.[8]

In "Early Experience with the Total Artificial Heart as a Bridge to Cardiac Transplantation," Jack G. Copeland and his coauthors described their personal successes using the artificial heart.

> In March 1985 when we implanted the 'Phoenix Heart' in a desperately ill young man, who later died after cardiac transplantation, considerable controversy ensued. Critics and supporters were given much attention by the media, and 'bioethicists' were called upon to provide some 'perspective.' It was clear to those of us directly involved in the care of the young man in question that we had observed and documented a

> definite improvement in his condition during 11 hours of support with the orthotopic [surgically placed in the patient's chest] pneumatic pulsatile biventricular pump. And my greatest regret was that the patient was not supported for a longer period of time, which might have permitted greater recovery prior to his second heart transplant.
>
> ...our next bridge attempt in August 1985 [was] the first to survive total artificial heart implantation followed by cardiac transplantation[. He] remains alive and works full time as assistant manager of a grocery store today. Since then, many bridge-to-transplant procedures with implanted orthotopic biventricular pumps have succeeded and the media and public seem to be less interested in this promising experimental field.
>
> ...From 4 April 1969 to March 1987, there were 61 implants of... artificial hearts. Five of these were 'permanent implants'.... Fifty-six hearts were implanted with the intent to bridge critically ill patients until the time of transplantation. At this writing, 39 patients have had heart transplants, 25 of these (64%) are alive And 18 (46%) have been discharged.
>
> ...There is now 4.1 patient-years experience with the Jarvik devices. There is no doubt that the currently available biventricular pneumatic pulsatile device placed within the chest with transcutaneous drivelines can support life in patients who may then be successfully transplanted.[9]

Finally, S. A. Ruzevich, M. T. Swarz, and J. E. Reedy wrote about the long-term effects of ventricular-assist devices on patients in "Retrospective Analysis of the Psychological Effects of Mechanical Circulatory Support."

> Twenty-seven people, 12 survivors of mechanical circulatory assistance and 15 family members, were surveyed. The twelve survivors (ages 18 to 66 years; mean, 43 years) had ventricular assist devices. Support ranged from eight hours to 90 days. Sixty-seven percent of the patients state that they have returned to a normal life style and 75 percent feel they have a brighter outlook on life. Six patients have returned to work, two are retired, two are disabled and two have physical capabilities to work but choose not to do so. Eighty-nine percent of all those surveyed would recommend an assist device to someone who needed one. Although these procedures are often associated with severe medical and psychological complications, 74 percent of the patients would agree to a second implant.[10]

Dr. Barney Clark Commemorative Symposium

Near the twenty-fifth anniversary of the Clark heart implant, a commemorative program took place in remembrance of the roles Barney Clark and his family had played in the continuing field of mechanical circulatory support for patients with failing hearts. From November 30 through December 1, 2008, meetings were held in the University of Utah Medical Center. The university, Don Olsen, and the Utah Artificial Heart Institute jointly hosted the event. There were scientific presentations and reflections on Barney Clark. Leaders in the field also described some of the most recent therapies and the present status of artificial hearts.

The highlight of the symposium was a short reflection by Dr. Julie Dee, a granddaughter of Barney and Una Loy Clark. She had graduated from the University of Utah's School of Medicine and was then a resident in anesthesiology at the University of Nebraska. She was the concluding speaker. The entire audience stood and applauded when she finished, a most unusual occurrence at a scientific meeting.

Dr. Dee said,

> This symposium is in honor of Dr. Barney Clark. Barney Clark donated his life to benefit artificial-heart technology. Now, twenty-five years later, this and other related technologies are being used to benefit the lives of many people throughout the world. We would like to offer a special thank you to Dr. Barney Clark for his inspiring contribution to the advancement of the field of medical devices and mechanical circulatory support and to recognize Dr. Barney Clark's family for their continued support.

Notes

1. Margery W. Shaw, ed., *After Barney Clark: Reflections on the Utah Artificial Heart Program* (Austin: University of Texas Press, 1984).
2. Grady opened her talk by noting that it had been seven months since the Clark surgery and there appeared to be no movement by the IRB at the University of Utah to authorize a second implant.
3. Denton A. Cooley, "Martyrdom for Scientific Purposes," *Texas Heart Institute Journal* 10, no. 2 (June 1983): 105–106.
4. L. D. Joyce, W. C. DeVries, W. L. Hastings, D. B. Olsen, R. K. Jarvik, and W. J. Kolff, "Response of the Human Body to the First Permanent Implant of the Jarvik-7 Total Artificial Heart," *Transactions—American Society for Artificial Internal Organs* 29 (February 1983):81–87.
5. O. R. Bowen, "Experimental Medical Devices, Drugs and Techniques: Their Future Social, Medical and Political Implications," *Indiana Medicine* 77, no. 6 (July 1984): 450–53.
6. Harry Schwartz, "Cut the Red Tape: Implant at Full Speed," *New York Times*, August 17, 1984.

7. Barton J. Bernstein, "The Misguided Quest for the Artificial Heart," *Technology Review* 87, no. 2 (November–December, 1984): 13–19, 62–63.
8. R. Cortesini, "What Are the Ethical and Social Implications of Artificial Organs?" *Artificial Organs* 9, no. 2 (May 1985): 127–28.
9. Jack G. Copeland, Richard G. Smith, Timothy B. Icenogle, and Richard A. Ott, "Early Experience with the Total Artificial Heart as a Bridge to Cardiac Transplantation," in *Artificial Heart 2: Proceedings of the 2nd International Symposium on Artificial Heart and Assist Device*, ed. Tetsuzo Akutsu (N.p.: Springer, 1988), 217–26.
10. S. A. Ruzevich, M. T. Swarz, J. E. Reedy, et al., "Retrospective Analysis of the Psychological Effects of Mechanical Circulatory Support," *Journal of Heart Transplantation* 9 (1990): 209–12.

22

The Medical Team Twenty-five Years Later

Opportunity is missed by most people
because it is dressed in overalls and looks like work.

—Thomas A. Edison

Those who were involved in implanting the artificial heart at the University of Utah in December 1982 expected to participate in a second surgery in short order. As it became apparent that was not happening, they returned to normal activities or made new career plans.

Dr. William C. DeVries

After his disappointing association with Humana, DeVries continued to follow heart research—now largely out of the public eye—but he did not attend gatherings on the subject after 1988. He declined an invitation to attend or participate in the Barney Clark Commemorative Symposium in Salt Lake City in late 2008. Don Olsen's last contact with him took place during the ASAIO meeting in 1986. According to Wikipedia, the Internet encyclopedia,

> On December 29, 2000, he joined the United States Army Reserve as a lieutenant colonel, becoming at age 57 one of the oldest people to enter and complete the Officer Basic Course.... He was stationed at Walter Reed Army Medical Center in Washington D.C. teaching surgical residents there and medical students from the Uniformed Services University of the Health Sciences and the George Washington University School of Medicine.

Dr. Lyle D. Joyce

With no prospects in sight of a second implant at the University of Utah, Joyce left the state in October 1983, joining the Minneapolis Heart Institute in

Minnesota. He left Utah with the understanding—negotiated with university officials—that he would return to Salt Lake City and assist with additional implants, but none were ever scheduled. He remained involved in research on the artificial heart and ventricular-assist devices that support the heart without removing the organ. He was credited with a series of firsts: establishing the first artificial-heart and cardiac-assist-device program in Minnesota; implanting an artificial heart with the Jarvik 7-70 pump in the first woman; and implanting an artificial heart in the first child. He implanted artificial hearts in nine additional patients, all of them bridges to transplants. Three of his patients were still alive nearly twenty years later.

Joyce was principal investigator in the FDA clinical trials for a number of left-ventricular-assist-device (LVAD) designs and added the Berlin Heart to the Minnesota program to use in children. In 2004 he became director of the cardiac-assist-device program at the University of Minnesota. Within five years, the program was implanting more than fifty ventricular-assist devices (VADs) per year. In March 2009, Joyce joined the Mayo Clinic in Rochester, Minnesota, where he continued work investigating new devices. He also established a pediatric VAD program at the clinic. He remains active in the ASAIO and in 1997 was elected president after having served for seven years on the board.

Dr. Willem J. Kolff

With several others who had been on the Utah heart team, Kolff remained in Utah. Through Kolff Medical, Inc., the company that manufactured the artificial heart used in the Clark implant, he and others of the original group continued work on marketable artificial-heart devices. He was chairman of the board of directors of Kolff Medical and suggested that the board appoint Robert Jarvik as president. The name of Kolff Medical, Inc., was changed to Symbion, Inc., and ultimately Kolff was removed as chairman. After serving as director of the University of Utah Institute for Biomedical Engineering from 1967 until his retirement in 1986, Kolff was continuously involved in work on the artificial heart and other institute projects.

After severing his ties with the university, Kolff and his wife moved to Port Townsend, Washington. Ultimately they separated, and Kolff moved to Villanova, Pennsylvania, to be close to their son, Dr. Jack Kolff. Well into old age, Pim Kolff continued to travel and speak about his lifelong interest in artificial organs. He died on February 11, 2009, three days short of his ninety-ninth birthday.

Dr. Robert K. Jarvik

Actively involved in the development of artificial hearts and LVADs, Jarvik started Jarvik Heart, Inc. He developed an axial-flow rotary VAD, which he named the Jarvik 2000. He and Dr. Howard Frazier of the Texas Heart Institute conducted animal testing that led to an investigational-device exemption from the FDA. This permitted the device to be implanted in humans, and it underwent a limited monitored study. Later, this VAD was approved for use in European patients.

In 2006 Jarvik became a television spokesman for a short time to advertise Pfizer drug company's statin drug, Lipitor. He claimed in the ads to be the inventor of the artificial heart. Many former and present workers in the field found this claim totally unacceptable. Three former presidents of ASAIO wrote a letter to Pfizer CEO J. B. Kindler stating that an artificial heart had been implanted in one of Dr. Denton Cooley's patients years before Jarvik had entered the field. Pfizer immediately changed the ad to identify Jarvik only as the inventor of the Jarvik heart. Even that claim rankled other artificial-heart scientists, who said that Jarvik had only improved models invented by others. However, the J-7 model implanted in Barney Clark was undisputedly Jarvik's work.

The drug company received other letters critical of the ads. John D. Dingell, who represented Michigan in the U.S. Congress, began investigating why a doctor who had never practiced medicine and had no current license to prescribe was indirectly prescribing drugs to a large television audience. Pfizer dropped the ads.

Una Loy Clark

Una Loy continued to serve the interests of artificial-heart development by allying herself with the American Heart Association. She especially focused on the message that heart-healthy behavior—such as avoiding tobacco—is a better alternative than the extreme remedy left to her husband as heart disease overcame him. She remained positive about the family's experience with the Utah artificial heart. Sometime after Barney's death, Una Loy married her widowed brother-in-law, Glen Farrer, of Salt Lake City. They lived until 2007 in St. George, Utah, then moved to Seattle, Washington, to be closer to her family.

Drs. Fred Anderson and Jeffrey Anderson

Both continued their cardiology practices in Salt Lake City. At the time of this writing, Jeffrey Anderson was associate chief of cardiology at Intermountain

Medical Center, a new complex affiliated with LDS Hospital. Fred Anderson remained at the University of Utah Health Care Center until his retirement on June 30, 2004.

Lawrence W. (Larry) Hastings

When DeVries left the University of Utah Medical Center to work with Humana in Louisville, Hastings accompanied him. After DeVries left Humana, Hastings attended medical school at the University of Kentucky in Louisville, specializing in anesthesiology. In 2010 he was in clinical practice in Washington state.

Steven D. Nielsen

Until 1988 Nielsen remained with the University of Utah's Institute for Biomedical Engineering. He then became affiliated with a leading Utah computer-engineering company, Evans & Sutherland, where he remained until his death on April 10, 2006.

Dr. Chase N. Peterson

Peterson remained vice president for health sciences at the University of Utah throughout the Clark implant era, serving as spokesman to the media during and after the historic surgery. In July 1983, he was named president of the university. He remained a strong supporter of the artificial-heart implantation that had occurred in Utah and encouraged continued research. In 1991 he retired as president but remained involved in teaching and patient care as a faculty member in internal medicine in the Department of Medicine. He and his wife, Grethe, resided in Park City for some time but later returned to Salt Lake City. He wrote an autobiography, *The Guardian Poplar*, that described the Clark implant as one of the highlights of his service at the university. Peterson died on September 14, 2014 at the age of eighty-four.

Drs. Nathan Pace and Theodore (Ted) Stanley

Both Pace and Stanley remained in the University of Utah School of Medicine Department of Anesthesiology. Both have been involved in research and development of new anesthetics for surgical patients. At the present time, both are on the School of Medicine faculty and involved in patient care.

23

The Artificial Heart Since Barney Clark

Dr. Barney Clark has taught us that the artificial heart did not hurt, that it caused no pain or discomfort, that the slight noise of the drive system did not worry him, but most of all, that it did not destroy his spirit, his judgment, his desire to contribute to mankind, his considerable sense of humor, and his ability to love.

—Dr. Willem J. Kolff

When the media excitement over the first artificial implants in humans waned, there was a perception among many that the science had died a quiet death and the notion of mechanical hearts had come to an end. Nothing was further from the truth. Research on artificial hearts and LVADs, in fact, went forward unabated.

A timeline of advances since December 1982 is too extensive to detail, but milestones that seem directly attributable to the singular event in Utah include the following:

December 1983: Kolff Medical, Inc., changed its name to Symbion, Inc., and the technology license was also transferred. The FDA approved the use of the Symbion, Inc., Jarvik-7 as a bridge to transplant in University Medical Center (UMC), Tucson, Arizona.

August 29, 1985: Dr. Jack Copeland of the UMC became the first surgeon to use the Jarvik-7 100-cubic-centimeter (cc) model as a temporary bridge-to-transplant successfully. The patient was Michael Drummond, a twenty-five-year-old supermarket manager. The artificial heart supported him for nine days until he received a transplant. He was discharged from the hospital, went back to work and died many years later of cancer.

September 1985 to November 1989: Symbion artificial hearts in two sizes—100-cc and 70-cc stroke volume—were implanted in 192 patients worldwide in more than forty centers. Other artificial hearts designed for permanent use (destination therapy) were also used as temporary devices bridging to transplants. Designs created in Germany, Austria, and Russia were used in a small number of patients, but they had poor results, and doctors stopped using them.

January 8, 1990: The FDA withdrew its investigational-device-exemption (IDE) approval for the clinical studies of the Symbion artificial heart and ventricular-assist device. The withdrawal prevented sales of the products and their use on patients in the United States and Canada. The withdrawal was based on FDA inspections of the Utah manufacturing facilities, which disclosed many shortcomings and led to the conclusion that the manufacturing processes did not have sufficient controls. Symbion spent a great deal of effort and money to resolve the stated shortcomings but was not able to convince the FDA to reverse its decision. Efforts to sell the company to other device producers failed because of the taint from the FDA's action.

September 1990: Symbion, Inc., approached Arizona's UMC about the possibility of transferring the company's assets to Arizona. UMC was interested because it was implanting more artificial hearts that any other hospital in the United States and it feared the loss of the Utah-designed heart. Symbion felt the FDA might look on the company more positively because UMC's program was patient centered.

April 12, 1991: Symbion's licensed technology had reverted to the University of Utah when the FDA edict had prevented the company from marketing its products. Don Olsen and Jack Copeland formed a new company, CardioWest Technologies, Inc., to license the university's artificial-heart technologies and applied to the FDA for approval to market the artificial heart. When the FDA refused to relicense the Jarvik heart, Olsen created a new elliptical one that fit the chest more efficiently. This was possible because of the discovery of new solvents and adhesives that joined the various components of the device more tightly. The heart was dubbed the Utah-100. Olsen became president of the new company during its lengthy negotiations with the FDA. The Medforte Research Foundation in Salt Lake City provided financial support because CardioWest had no income during the two and a half years of meetings with the FDA.

October 17, 1992: The FDA gave conditional approval for an IDE to expand the use of the artificial heart as both destination therapy and a bridge to transplant. The approval added eleven pages of new conditions that took two years to incorporate into the manufacturing and monitoring of the redesigned heart. Initially the approved clinical trial was limited to five centers in the United States.

January 12, 1993: The first CardioWest artificial-heart implant was performed in Tucson. The patient, a forty-six-year-old woman, received a donor heart after 186 days. This was the first of ninety-five bridge-to-transplant surgeries in the IDE study, divided among the five American centers over the next nine years. In France Dr. C. Cabrol and his center in Paris implanted more than two hundred patients with CardioWest hearts over a twenty-five-year period.

October 18, 1998: The CardioWest artificial heart received the European equivalent of FDA approval. Marketing, with guaranteed insurance reimbursement, proceeded in Europe.

March 2001: Faced with financial problems, the UMC announced it had to abandon ownership of CardioWest. The hospital board of directors decided to get out of all areas not directly involved with hospital and patient care.

August 2001: Dr. Copeland in partnership with Dr. Marvin Slepian, a UMC cardiologist, and Richard Smith, a biomedical engineer at the University of Arizona, formed a new corporation called SynCardia Systems, Inc., with a transfer of all licenses and assets from CardioWest. The name of the artificial heart changed to the SynCardia temporary CardioWest total artificial heart.

October 2003: In Bad Oeynhausen, Germany, the Excor portable driver, which was developed by SynCardia but had not yet received approval in the United States, was used on the first patient. The device allowed artificial-heart patients to live at home and be ambulatory while waiting for a donor heart, a much less costly option. The portable driver demonstrated that artificial-heart patients could be safely discharged from the hospital.

March 2004: The FDA panel unanimously recommended approval of the Syncardia heart as a bridge to transplant. This was the first step toward full FDA approval and opened the way to reimbursement from Medicare and health-insurance companies.

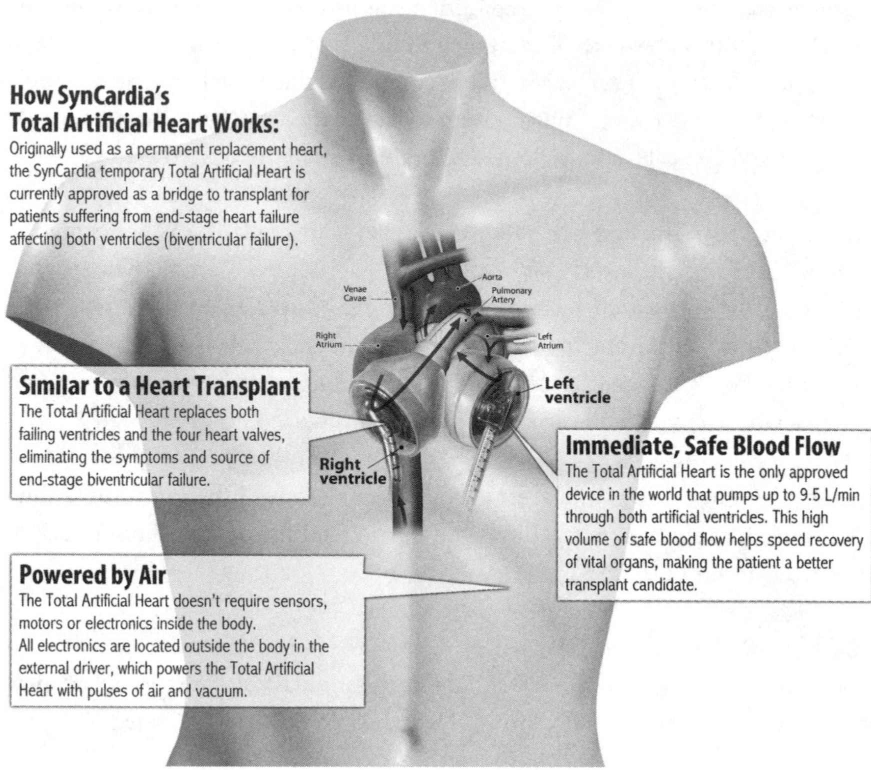

Chart depicting the way the CardioWest bridge-to-transplant temporary total artificial heart works.

August 26, 2004: A *New England Journal of Medicine* article concluded that the one-year survival rate for patients receiving the CardioWest temporary artificial heart was 70 percent, versus 31 percent for control patients who did not receive it. Both one-year and five-year survival rates (86 percent and 64 percent, respectively) were much better. In 2004 the American Heart Association named the CardioWest heart the number-one advance in cardiovascular medicine.

October 15, 2004: The SynCardia heart became the first and only artificial heart approved by the FDA as either a permanent implant or a bridge to transplant.

July 17, 2006: The Excor portable driver received European approval. At the same time, *U.S. News and World Report* included several of the hospitals using the SynCardia heart in its list of 2006's best hospitals.

July 31, 2008: The Companion driver, a simplified, smaller pneumatic driver, received the European mark of approval.

February 2010: SynCardia trained personnel to staff the fiftieth medical center in the world to offer artificial-heart options to patients.

March 4, 2010: SynCardia's Freedom portable driver received the European okay.

March 2010: Reports from around the world noted 890 implants of the Utah-designed artificial heart. Patient 850 was a sixty-year-old woman in Moscow, Russia, implanted in 2010. Having undergone three name changes with only minor design alterations, the Utah-engineered heart has dominated world medicine, accounting for 93 percent of the artificial devices implanted over nearly 180 years of patient experience, 60 years of which have been outside a hospital. At the present time, it is the only artificial heart being implanted in the world. The device implanted in Barney Clark had a 100-milliliter stroke volume with Bjork-Shiley valves. The current SynCardia heart is 70 milliliters with Medtronic-Hall valves. Tables 23.1 and 23.2 document these clinical implants.

SynCardia's Total Artificial Heart Today

Among the hundreds of mechanical heart-replacement devices created, tested, and ultimately shelved over the decades, only the SynCardia heart has withstood the demands of the human body and the maze of regulatory approval. More than a thousand patients worldwide had been implanted as of February 2012. By August of that year, sixty-eight hospitals in fifteen countries, including thirty-four in the United States, had been certified to use the SynCardia heart with many more hospitals seeking certification.

Originally intended as a permanent replacement for the natural heart, the SynCardia heart has proved most useful in extending the life of patients until a donor heart is available. Improvements in surgical techniques, anticoagulation management, and patient care have boosted the success of the heart. Currently at 79 percent, the SynCardia heart holds the highest success rate for bridge-to-transplant implantations of any approved mechanical circulatory-support device in the world.

The growing success of the heart has pushed development of new drivers that allow a patient to live outside a hospital. New models—specifically SynCardia's Companion driver—have replaced the dated Big Blue hospital drivers for use in Europe and are being studied by the FDA. They are designed to power the artificial heart from implant through recovery. Stable artificial heart patients who

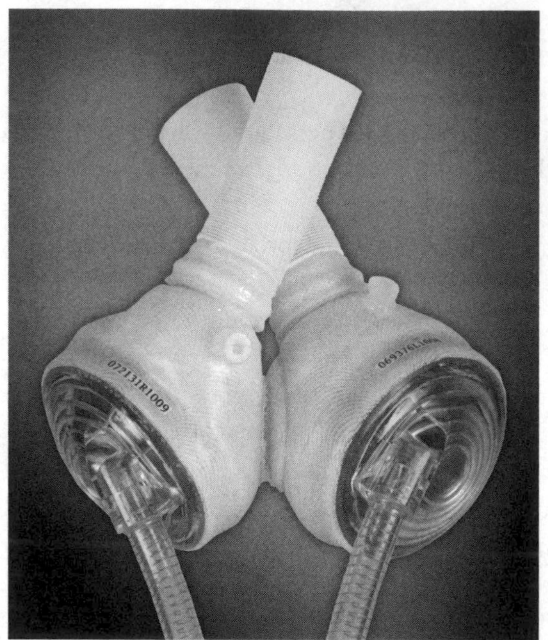

By 2012 the SynCardia temporary total artificial heart reached a thousand implants.

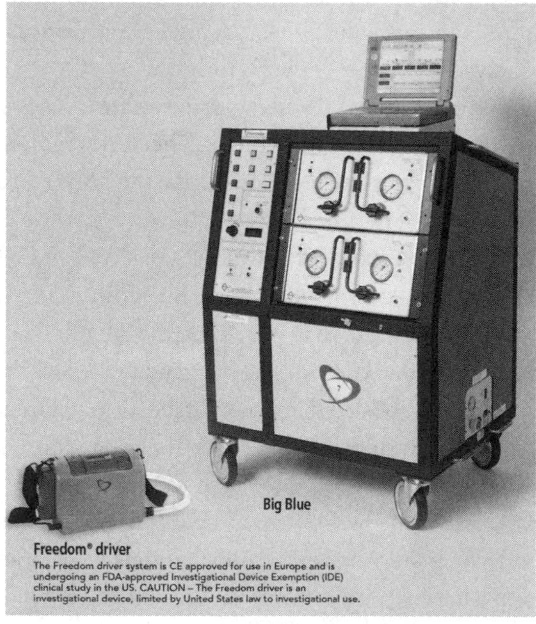

The 13.5-pound Freedom portable driver next to the 418-pound Big Blue hospital driver.

Table 23.1. Number of Human Patients on the Various Total Artificial Hearts

Total Artificial Heart Type	Number of Patients	Years on the Artificial Heart
Akutsu and Liotta	2	80*
Unger (Austria)	6	0.1
Berlin (Germany)	7	0.1
Poisk (Russia)	16	0.3
Abiocor (Abiomed, Boston, MA)	15	5.5
Symbion J-7 100	44	116
Symbion J-7 70	159	11
CardioWest C-70	687	210**

*Average hours to cardiac transplant.
**Some heart patients have been supported on the portable driver at home for an accumulative 55 years.

Table 23.2. Clinical Total Artificial Heart Implants to Date

Total Artificial Heart Type	Number of Implants	Years on the Artificial Heart
SynCardia CardioWest TAH (1993–2010)	950	290
Symbion Jarvik-7-70 TAH (1986–1992)	159	11
Symbion Jarvik-7-100 TAH (1982-1992)	44	6
Abiomed Abiocor TAH (2001-2009)	15	5.5
Nine others (1969–1998)	44	2.5
Total	1212	315

meet proper criteria can now be discharged from the hospital, supported by a Freedom portable driver carried in a backpack or shoulder bag. It is evident that the new drivers replace weeks or months of hospitalization, providing emotional, physical, and financial benefits for patients, their families, and the hospitals.

As successes mount, SynCardia is working to serve a broader spectrum of patients suffering from end-stage biventricular heart failure. Today's 70-cc heart fits approximately 75 percent of adult men and 25 percent of adult women in the United States. A smaller, 50-cc heart is under development to serve smaller women and adolescents.

2011 Notable Total-Artificial-Heart Patients

Among the many patients ranging from twenty to sixty-eight years old who have returned to the comfort of their homes while waiting for a donor heart are these:

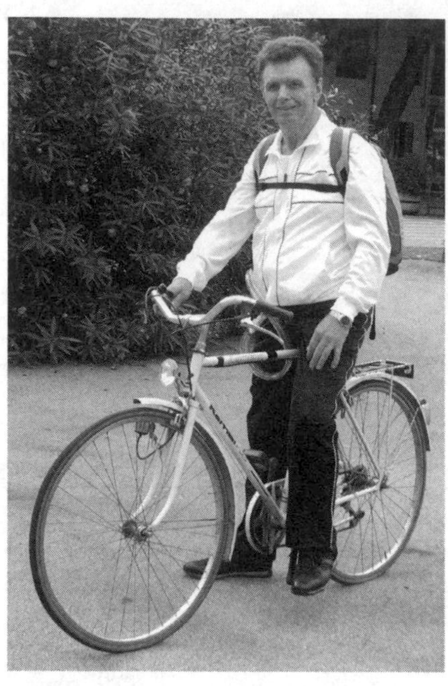

Pietro Zorzetto

As of 2011, the Padova, Italy, man had lived 1,374 days, the longest time any patient has ever spent with an artificial heart. He was admitted to Azienda Ospedaliera di Padova on November 30, 2007, suffering from valvular cardiomyopathy. Two previous operations had failed to repair his failing heart. On December 6, he became the first person in Italy to receive an artificial heart. On September 9, 2011, he finally received his heart transplant from a donor.

Pietro Zorzetto was the current longest-supported artificial-heart patient in the world as of August 1, 2011.

Charles Okeke

Okeke made headlines in May 2010 when he became the first SynCardia total-heart patient in the United States to leave the hospital without a human heart. He was a participant in the FDA-authorized study of the Freedom portable driver. He went home to his wife, Natalie, and their three children, and the driver supported him for 253 days. On January 15, 2011, he received a dual heart and kidney transplant and is doing well.

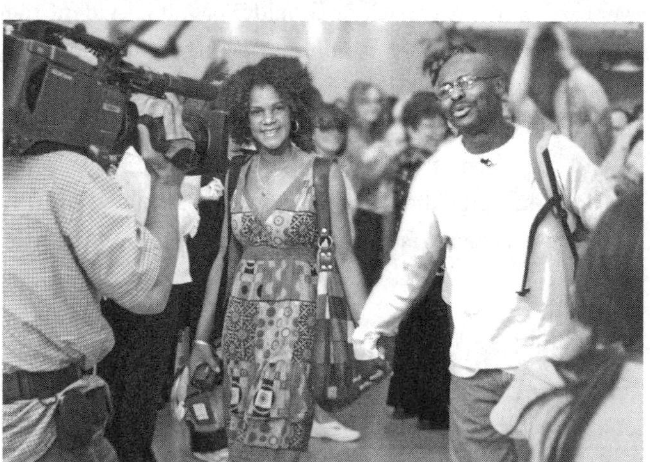

Charles Okeke (here with his wife) was the first SynCardia total artificial heart patient in the United States to be discharged from the hospital using the Freedom portable driver.

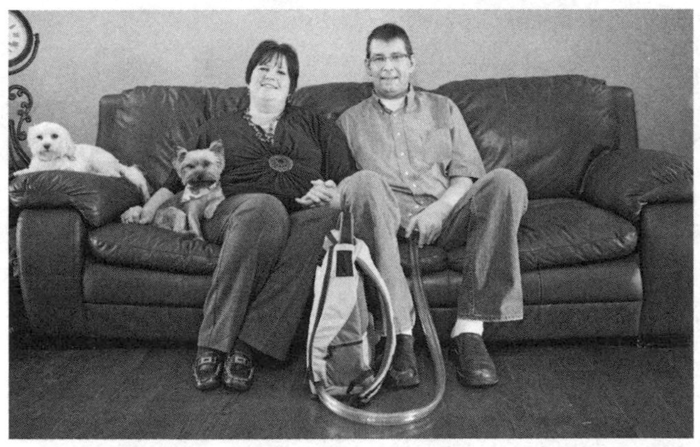

Total artificial-heart patient Troy Golden, the preacher, with his wife.

Troy Golden

Born with a genetic condition that was gradually weakening his heart, Golden was added to a heart-transplant list in January 2010. As his condition deteriorated, he underwent implant surgery on September 15, 2010. On October 18, he was released from the hospital with a Freedom portable driver. Before his implant, Golden, then forty-five, had preached every Sunday for twelve years in the New Life Assembly of God Church in Geary, Oklahoma. After being sidelined for six months, he preached his first postimplant sermon on November 21, 2010. He is still awaiting a transplant but continuing to preach and live a seemingly normal life with his wife and two children.

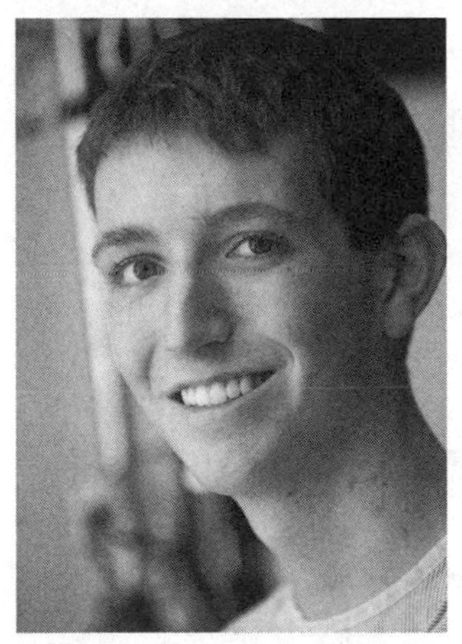

Jordan Merecka celebrated his eighteenth birthday one week after his artificial-heart implant.

Jordan Merecka

Born with multiple congenital heart defects, Merecka grew up significantly impaired. He underwent two open-chest surgeries, a number of surgical revisions, and implantation of a defibrillator. By September 2010, his condition was continuing to go downhill, and at seventeen he was put on a transplant list. By April 2011, he was in Texas Children's Hospital with heart and kidney problems. On May 22, he received the first artificial heart implanted in a pediatric patient. He celebrated his eighteenth birthday a week after his surgery and watched his high-school graduation online as his younger sister accepted his diploma, and he received a long-distance standing ovation.

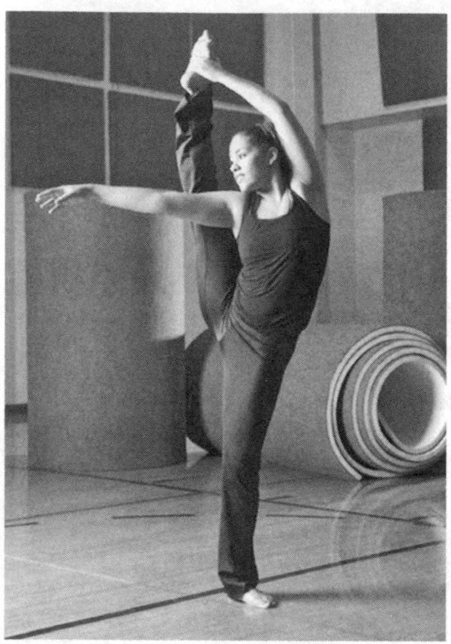

Mia Welch, twenty-one, was bridged to a heart transplant on March 18, 2012.

Mia Welch

While attending Mesa Community College in Arizona, Welch experienced severe heart problems. She was dancing fourteen hours a week with the school's summer dance company when she had to raise her arms and take deep breaths with every exertion. A local hospital's emergency room staff told her its facilities were only for those "with life and death situations" and refused to treat her. In a different emergency room, she finally had a CAT scan that revealed an enlarged heart.

That began a medical odyssey that led ultimately to the implantation of a SynCardia heart in November 2011. About six weeks later, she was taken off the 418-pound Big Blue driver and switched to a 13.5-pound Freedom driver. Although still hospitalized, she began to dance again. On March 17, 2012, the long-awaited donor heart became available. Nine days after transplant, she left the hospital. The interval with the artificial heart and its drivers had improved her health and prepared her for the natural heart to come. It was enough to make someone feel like dancing—and she did.

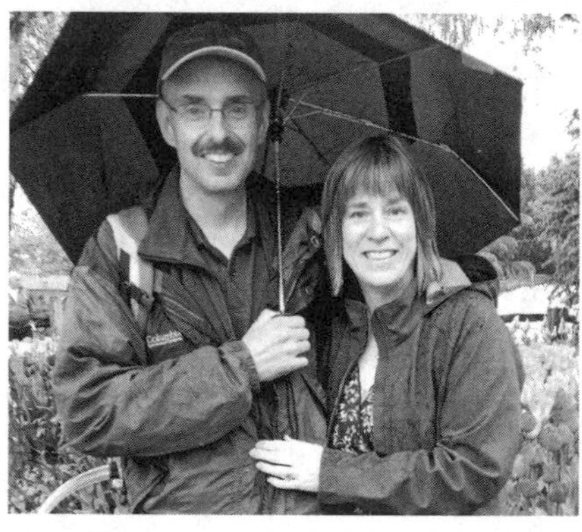

Chris Marshall and his wife, Kathy, explore Seattle. A backpack contains the Freedom portable driver.

Charles Marshall

Marshall was a walker. The Wasilla, Alaska, man had walked for years and continued even after he was hospitalized in a Washington hospital with heart problems. He did up to fifty laps per day through the hospital hallways. When he collapsed on the sixth lap one day, doctors were convinced it was time for implant surgery. His failing natural heart was replaced with an artificial one on February 6, 2012. He was released from the medical center with a Freedom portable driver six weeks later and went back to walking. From late March through mid-August, he added 437 miles to his total. The only addition to his usual equipment was the driver, which he carried in a backpack.

Marshall had battled increasingly debilitating heart failure since 1999 and was excited about his new life. He reported improved color and increased vitality as he walked and waited for the donor heart that is expected to replace the mechanical device. In the meantime, he says, "I really get to go out and live life."

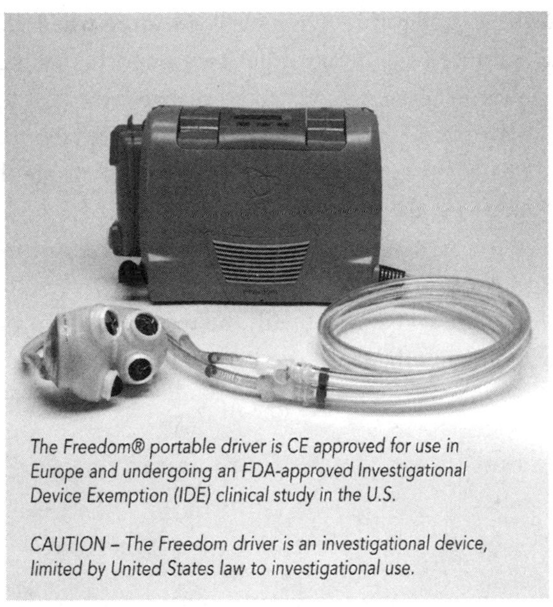

The Freedom driver is designed to power SynCardia's total artificial heart.

Into the Future

The road to success for artificial hearts and their support equipment has been long and filled with obstacles that seemed insurmountable. Dedicated, persevering investigators continue to forge ahead, anticipating new breakthroughs, including new, improved, body-compatible materials to manufacture blood pumps.

One major unresolved problem ubiquitous to all implantable medical devices is the fact that lines to transmit power must pass through the skin to be connected. This includes power lines to all mechanical cardiac devices, colostomy fistulas, and dialysis connections. All of these exit sites are prone to infection, which is the most common reason why these patients die.

The only way to avoid exit-site infections is to stop using leads that puncture the skin. This is not yet possible with pneumatically powered blood pumps. A great amount of work has been done to develop systems that transfer electricity through the skin to drive a pump and monitor and even control it. Transformer coils that transfer power across intact skin to an implanted coil have been designed and tested. These coils have sufficient power to run ventricular-assist devices.

However, the problem is that currently there are no acceptable storage batteries so that the external coil can be temporarily removed when necessary. Battery technology has advanced significantly, but two important things are still lacking: adequate power to allow a patient to be disconnected for a suitable length of time without the need for batteries that are unacceptably large and heavy; and an implantable battery that has a large number of charge-discharge cycles in its lifetime. Otherwise, the battery must repeatedly be surgically removed and replaced.

The challenge of outside-the-body power sources and monitoring devices is one that in the future will, undoubtedly, be resolved. The progress will come because of the foundation that has been laid by the efforts of thousands to this point.

24

Looking Back on a Life

I know in my heart that man is good. That what is right will eventually triumph. And there is purpose and worth to each and every life.

—Ronald Reagan

I did not realize when I was hired by the University of Utah in 1972 that I was launching what amounted to a midlife career that lasted—to date—nearly forty years. I take pride in the role I played in the long-term development of artificial hearts and blood pumps. The Utah team was just one of the national and international groups researching and testing various blood-pump designs, but as the history unfolded, it may have made the most long-lasting contributions. In the past three decades, several artificial hearts from other programs have been implanted into a few human patients, but the Utah-designed heart is the only one with a record of long and continued clinical use, beginning with Dr. Barney Clark, the first permanent recipient, in 1982.

I am grateful to have been intimately involved with a group of remarkable individuals whose contributions were woven into a seamless whole. The list must begin with Dr. Willem J. (Pim) Kolff, who was recognized, with good reason, as the father of artificial organs. His arrival in Utah was a lucky day for the state, the University of Utah, and me. His single-minded devotion to creating artificial organs was the catalyst that ultimately led to the advent of a workable artificial heart. His penchant for working the system until he got what he thought was necessary was legendary. Under his guidance, the university's Institute for Biomedical Engineering, and especially the Division of Artificial Organs, gained international stature.

The first twenty-five years of the forty I spent working on blood pumps were in close cooperation with Kolff. His passion for science was matched with a capacity for loyal friendship and devotion to his family. His son, Dr. Therus Kolff, said, "He was really a great father to his five children." From my perspective, I could not have chosen a better mentor. Scientists throughout the world with an interest in artificial-organ research would have given almost anything to change places with me. Merely associating with Kolff ensured his associates the opportunity to present research findings to audiences worldwide.

The December 2, 1982, surgery on Barney Clark at long last tested what had been our single goal for several decades—to see if our labors had produced an artificial heart that could prolong life in a human being. It was, of course, the highlight of my career. For me—a veterinarian—to be invited by the main surgeons to assist in implanting an artificial heart in a human patient was an unprecedented and rewarding experience.

That same sense of accomplishment was repeated years later when Dr. James Long invited me to assist in implanting artificial hearts in three LDS Hospital patients. Each of these three subsequently underwent transplantation of natural donor hearts, evidence that the artificial heart had found its most useful purpose—preserving a patient's life until a natural heart became available.

Advancing Students' Careers

As exciting and rewarding as these singular events were, the many opportunities I had over the years to help students find and pursue careers in the field overshadowed them. When our research lab was at its busiest, the barn was full of animals implanted with artificial hearts or ventricular-assist devices. We had as many as twenty-five students working as part-time calf sitters. For some of them, this experience led to full-time careers in the field. Individual career paths placed them in graduate programs in science arenas such as bioengineering, chemistry, physiology, and physics. Many went to professional schools—most frequently medical schools. I was often asked to write letters of recommendation for their applications.

Over the years, the fruits of this experience were very gratifying. On one occasion more than fifteen years ago, I spent twenty-four hours as a patient in a Salt Lake City hospital. Five medical doctors on the staff dropped by to visit, including two in radiology, one in anesthesiology, one the head of the hospital's pain clinic, and the fifth a cardiothoracic surgeon. Each had worked in the artificial-heart laboratory, and I had written letters of recommendation to medical school for all of them.

Once when work took me to Charlottesville, Virginia, I met another of my former students. His road into medicine had been rocky. Years earlier he had come to me after twice applying unsuccessfully to medical schools. He was discouraged but determined. We visited for a few hours, and I offered him a part-time job and advised him to apply to graduate school at the university in physiology, which he did. With my letter of support and his own display of determination, he was accepted. When we met in Charlottesville, he was an anesthesiologist on the faculty of the School of Medicine at the University of Virginia and said again how grateful he was for my help.

One year I wrote seven letters for medical-school applicants; five of them were accepted, and the other two enrolled the following year. Utah students were accepted by many of the prestigious medical schools around the country, including Columbia in New York.

Over the years, I traveled to hospitals and research sites around the world, teaching medical personnel about the artificial heart. In the process, I sometimes met former students and biomedical engineers who had started their careers in the Utah heart program. Nearly always they expressed gratitude for the jump start they had received, usually as calf sitters in the old St. Mark's Hospital barn.

At a banquet where I spoke on the artificial heart, I met the owner of a local automobile dealership. Later, he called and asked if I would visit his youngest son, who had just been rejected by a Colorado veterinary-medicine program. It was his second rejection, and he was discouraged. His nonresident status (Utah has no veterinary school) and less-than-spectacular grades seemed to doom his aspirations to be an animal doctor.

I met with the young man and convinced him that he shouldn't give up. I suggested he begin a master's program at the University of Utah and gave him a part-time job in the Artificial Heart Research Laboratory. This approach made the difference. Impressed with his persistence, the administration at Colorado State University reversed its decision. I received a thank-you note from his family for helping the young man achieve his goals. Enclosed with the note was a newspaper photograph of me with a calf that had an artificial heart. The family offered to help in our ongoing heart research.

Taking a lead from Kolff's head-on fund-raising approach, I took a deep breath and dived in. We had an old, worn, almost-junky, Ford pickup truck. Some of the calf sitters refused to drive it, fearing they'd be stranded when it finally breathed its last. With my heart in my throat, I drove to the Hinckley Dodge Chrysler dealership and parked my battered truck directly in front of the showroom.

The father's office was on the second floor, immediately above where I had parked the old pickup. He welcomed me into his office, where I thanked him for the note and subtly reminded him of his offer to help our work. I invited him to look out the window at our sad and sorry old truck. "What an old piece of junk," he said. "I will see that it is removed immediately."

I hurriedly explained that it was our lab truck, used to haul animals, feed, and other items used in our experiments. Then I took the leap. I asked if he could donate a used pickup to the Artificial Heart Research Laboratory, hopefully one in better condition than the pathetic piece of machinery parked under his window.

He equivocated. "The automobile business has been slow," he said. "It might not be the right time for a donation." I all but got down on my knees. He took me to the service area of the dealership and called his shop foreman, who listened to the tale and then pointed to a two-year-old pickup with low mileage that had been used to deliver auto parts around the city. "Will that one do?" he asked. I could not have hoped for more. Two days later we had a newer, much better vehicle. Maybe the Kolff method of begging for support for our research was the right one after all.

Two years later, when I submitted a large research grant application to the NIH, I included a new four-wheel-drive pickup truck in the list of needed items. Of course, we purchased it from the car dealership whose owner had been so generous. His son finished veterinary school with nearly top grades and set up practice in Alaska. This is one of the stories I treasure. These rewarding brushes with students were worth as much as the recognitions members of the Utah team received as we pursued a workable artificial heart.

Interest in the Utah Total Artificial Heart Grows

Most of the personnel who participated in the Barney Clark implant received their initial training in my lab. After the Clark surgery had proved the feasibility of mechanical hearts, hospital groups began seeking training that would prepare them to begin doing human implants. Representatives of some groups seeking approval from the FDA for their own devices also spent time in the Utah laboratory. These included Drs. Denton Cooley, Howard Frazier, Jack Copeland, George Noon, and Bartley Griffith, names readily recognizable in artificial-heart history. As heart implantation became more common, all of these men used the Utah pneumatic heart in patients.

One of the notable physicians who showed interest in the expertise shared in our lab was Dr. William (Bill) Frist, who was finishing his cardiothoracic training with the transplant team at Stanford in California. He contacted me in 1985, asking if he could come to Utah for at least a year to learn about implant surgery and become proficient with using the artificial heart in humans. I was very interested in Frist but had no funds from my NIH grants to pay his salary. I asked if his father and brother could provide financial support for a year. Frist was reluctant. His family already had supported him through college and medical school, and he was anxious to be self-supporting. Regretfully I had to turn him down.

Frist went into cardiac-surgery practice in Tennessee and shortly after was elected to the United States Senate, ultimately becoming Republican majority leader before leaving politics. His financial statement to the Senate showed his personal wealth at fifteen to forty-five million dollars.

A Quick Trip to Tucson

The complexities of obtaining permission to use the artificial heart led to some strange adventures. Protocols often did not match situations. In March 1986, I received an emergency call from Dr. Jack Copeland in Tucson. Earlier Copeland had transplanted a donor heart into a patient, referred to as T. C. in the literature. Initially T. C. did well with only mild rejection episodes.

But on March 6, his cardiac ejection fraction was very low, indicating cardiac failure. Copeland had two choices: to let the patient die or to put him on a heart-lung machine for a second time and seek a second donor heart. He put in an emergency request for a natural heart but also called me. He asked that I bring a Jarvik heart to Tucson in case the patient got worse before a donor heart was found. I chartered a jet and prepared a sterile Jarvik heart that we had in the lab ready for a calf implant. I also invited Steve Nielsen, the electrical engineer developing our support equipment, to go with me.

I didn't want to ask for permission (another trick I had learned from Kolff), but I thought I should inform university officials what I intended to do. President Peterson was out of town, so I called Dr. William Gay, newly appointed chair of the Department of Surgery and my superior. I said, "Bill, I am not asking your permission, but I want to tell you what I am planning to do. Dr. Copeland has a patient on the heart-lung machine, and he has called pleading for help. I wanted you to know so you will not be surprised or embarrassed if newspeople contact you."

Gay wanted to know the possible result of this escapade. I confirmed that the FDA and possibly the NIH could raise objections. However, no federal funds were in jeopardy, I told him. Kolff Medical, Inc., had built the heart with no NIH money. I recalled that Cooley had performed an unapproved surgery on a patient earlier and was only lightly reprimanded by the FDA. So—without official permission—Nielsen and I boarded the jet with our vital equipment and took off for Tucson.

While we were preparing for the trip to Tucson, Copeland's patient had continued to deteriorate. Desperate, Copeland called Dr. C. C. Vaughn in Phoenix and asked him to bring an artificial heart that a dentist, Dr. K. Cheng, had been working on for several years. He used an old pneumatic driver to run the heart in experimental calves.

Nielsen and I were landing at the Tucson airport as the two surgeons implanted the Phoenix heart in Copeland's patient. At the same time, things were stirring in Salt Lake City. Gay had contacted the Salt Lake International Airport and asked the charter jet's pilot to have me call him before unloading the Utah heart. Informed by a technician who had been sent to meet us in Tucson that the Phoenix heart had already been implanted, I immediately called Gay. He advised not to unload the Utah equipment and under no circumstances to use the Utah heart—ironically good advice since the possibility was moot.

Since our earlier discussion, Gay had talked with others who had advised against using the Utah heart in the Arizona patient. Updated on the situation in Tucson, Gay relaxed. The jet pilots agreed to stay a couple of hours, and Nielsen and I unloaded the pneumatic driver and cardiac output monitor and diagnostic unit (COMDU) and were driven to the Tucson hospital. The heart stayed in the plane.

The patient was stable, but the old driver running the Phoenix heart could not monitor the driving pressures of the implanted heart. Nielsen and Rich Smith, a Tucson engineer, switched to the Utah driver and COMDU, a much more informative monitor. The patient's condition was improving as I returned to Salt Lake City. Nielsen stayed in Tucson to operate the support equipment.

A few reporters had met us at the Tucson airport, but Nielsen and I had refused to share any information beyond our identities. However, a gaggle of reporters was on hand as I landed in Salt Lake City, and they were more aggressive. I had learned from an earlier experience with the media, when I had naively shared some information expecting that it would remain confidential. I simply identified myself and carried the packaged artificial heart to my car.

Later that night a donor heart for the Tucson patient was found in Las Vegas. He was transplanted a second time, but he died a few days later from a massive tissue rejection, likely a more fatal version of the one he had experienced earlier.

I had my own aftermath to face. The next morning, I gave Gay a detailed report on Tucson. I assured him the Utah heart had never been unwrapped and was returned untouched. He complimented me on my determination to help in what certainly was a life-and-death situation but rejoiced I had not had to use the Utah Heart.

Robert Jarvik was less sympathetic. About midmorning he was in my office seething with irritation. "You should have done nothing, and you better get a very good lawyer," he warned. It was clear that Jarvik had been the person who had urged Gay to intervene. I dismissed the lawsuit as an idle threat.

Kolff's Retirement Leaves an Opening

Kolff resigned as director of the Institute for Biomedical Engineering (IBE) in December 1983. Dr. James Brophy, the university vice present for research, asked if I was interested in either applying for the directorship or serving on the selection committee. I told him I would serve on the selection panel. I did not bother to add that I had just been diagnosed with coronary artery disease and was facing bypass surgery. I had the surgery in April 1984 in the Cleveland Clinic. After a quick and excellent recovery, I reviewed four applications from individuals wanting to head the institute and concluded I could not work with any of them. None had had experience with blood pumps or biomedical-engineering research. Most of their background was in management.

I met with Brophy and told him that I felt none of the applicants were satisfactory. I asked if I could become an applicant. So I became head of the institute.

However, Kolff had requested that he remain as acting director until after an international meeting honoring him that was planned for his birthday on February 14, 1985. He kept his office, telephone number, and mailing address, leaving me to fend as best I could. Also people who had gone to Kolff for years for advice and help with problems continued to do so. I coped with these irritations, which were quickly resolved when my old friend and mentor actually left.

Refining the Research

Though I moved increasingly into administration, the magnetism of the research lab always lured me. I feel that some of my contributions there will long outlast any I made as an administrator. One of the most important was the method of operating on calves. The surgeons in our animal lab were used to human anatomy, and originally when they implanted artificial hearts in calves, they used the standard approach—splitting the sternum on a prone animal to allow access to the heart cavity. Since the sternum in a calf is much heavier than in a human, that created a deep surgical field. And when the pericardium was released from the sternum, the animal's heart tended to fall, collapsing the atria and blocking the inferior vena cava. Often this lowered the cardiac output and precipitated an emergency.

I modified the implant procedure by removing the fourth rib from the animal as it lay on its left side. This produced a shallower surgical field and improved visualization. The bone covering provided a strong layer for closing the chest. Within six months, a new rib was being formed.

None of the cardiopulmonary bypass lines entered through the incision. The arterial line returning oxygenated blood to the calf was placed into a carotid artery, and a dual-channel venous cannula was threaded through the jugular vein into the superior and inferior venae cavae. Both vessels were repaired at the completion of the surgery. The improved techniques were helpful to the animals and gave us added information that could be applied to humans.

Changes in the Artificial Heart Design

For a long time, there were no solvents or glues that could effectively fasten the parts of the artificial heart together without leaking blood. The earlier Kwan-Gett models and later the Jarvik version included a circular aluminum base with grooves to secure the plastic housing and diaphragm. The inflow and outflow ports were also round and were wired to prevent leaks. A calf had to weigh 150 to 200 pounds to place the two round ventricles into the chest and also have room for the inflow and outflow conduits. Investigators recognized that the two round ventricles did not utilize the space effectively.

I believed that carefully placed inflow and outflow ports on elliptical ventricles would fit calves and—by extrapolation—smaller men. I had Tom Kessler, head of the prosthetics laboratory, make some elliptical models and implanted them in calves as small as 120 pounds. We published the results of our collaborative work in 1983. Dr. Kevin Murray, who had just completed his general surgery training in Chicago, and I wrote a joint NIH proposal that was funded in 1988 for four years in the amount of 2.5 million dollars. Our research was sound enough to obtain FDA approval to test this more efficient heart in humans.

After Dr. Jack Copeland and I set up CardioWest Technologies, Inc., in 1991, it took fourteen months of reports and meetings with the FDA for us to get approval for a successor to Symbion's Jarvik heart. For more than twenty-five years—since the first FDA meetings seeking approval for Kolff Associates, Inc., in 1979—I plodded through the bureaucratic maze. It was 2004 when a successor device was given premarket approval. I had calluses on my calluses from sitting in endless meetings.

Improving the Drive Systems

The ultimate success of the artificial heart seemed contingent on relieving the patient of the huge console that kept the device beating. Any kind of normal life demanded that the patient be mobile and able to live outside a hospital. Though tethering the first human patients to the bulky equipment was necessary, it was a serious deterrent over the long haul. Reliable portable pneumatic drivers needed to be developed.

I was aware of the feasibility of portable pneumatic drivers because we had used them to power the artificial hearts in calves and sheep. We had photos of calves ambling about the yard outside the lab with their artificial hearts sustained by small portable power units even before the 1982 Clark implant.

In 1985 Dr. Bjarne Semb of Stockholm, Sweden, used a portable pneumatic driver to power a Jarvik-7 heart in fifty-three-year-old Leif Stenberg. The patient spent most of his 225 survival days outside the hospital with the portable driver. He told others that he liked to go to the park. "I smell the flowers, listen to the birds, and watch the pretty girls of Stockholm."

But officialdom in the United States was not ready to approve the portable unit, although the Utah heart team had asked permission to test it in the first of an expected series of implant/transplant patients. The University of Utah IRB had approved the portable unit for limited use with "patient number two" after Barney Clark, but no patient number two ever materialized. In Europe patients benefited from consistent portable-driver improvements, but in the United States, the option was unavailable until March 2010.

Human Implants in Utah

I had always hoped there would be additional artificial-heart implants at the University of Utah. When the CardioWest artificial heart was approved by the FDA, several centers were interested in using it. I hoped to revive interest in Utah.

That possibility was renewed when Dr. James W. Long joined the Utah cardiac-transplant program (a consortium of the University, LDS, and Veterans Administration (VA) Hospitals for more effective transplant programs) for his cardiothoracic surgical training. Long originally contacted Gay, then chief of the joint program, in July 1989, but Gay did not have an opening. As an alternative, Long was invited to work in the Artificial Heart Research Laboratory for a year and then join the cardiac-transplant program. During two additional intensive years of surgical training, Long spent what time he could in the lab, working on the artificial heart. He was then offered a position with an LDS Hospital surgical group.

Long's interest in human use of the artificial heart persisted, and he ultimately received approval from the FDA and LDS Hospital's IRB to perform implant surgeries. On April 11, 1995, with Dr. Donald Doty and me as assistants, he implanted an artificial heart in a patient referred to as A. M. The mechanical device supported the patient for 133 days; then he was transplanted. He is alive and doing well twenty years later. A second patient, V. F., was implanted on July 20, 1995, and transplanted after sixty-one days. Though he initially did well, he died of two-vessel coronary disease due to an error in diagnosing the health of the donor heart. A third patient, K. W., was implanted on October 1, 1995, transplanted after seventy-two days, and lived approximately three years. I assisted in the three implant surgeries and the subsequent transplants.

Long began using LVADs in some patients and soon became one of their biggest advocates. He and LDS Hospital participated in the Rematch Trial, the first to compare patients who received LVADs to those who had medical therapy. The two-year study showed the LVAD was far superior to medical therapy. The unreliability of the LVAD's mechanical blood pump, however, was a disappointment. A high incidence of mechanical failures doomed the device used in the study. A new and improved version, HeartMate II, is much more dependable and was in wide use by 2010. Research continues to create even more reliable LVAD devices and alternative power sources.

A Donated Home for Heart Research

When Building 512 on the University of Utah campus burned in 1973, the old St. Mark's Hospital became the new home for heart research. It was a significant step forward but always a bit shaky. Ownership of the building changed hands four times while the heart program was a tenant. In the summer of 1986, the current mortgage holder, Home Savings of America, called to inform me to send rent checks to someone different. The purchasers were well behind in their payments, and their loan was being foreclosed. I met with the Home Savings board and asked that they donate the complex to the University of Utah to support artificial-heart research. That began nearly two years of pleading for a donation.

One member of the board told me the company had never made such a large donation. I was prepared. "On the contrary," I replied, "I know that it built the Los Angeles County Museum of Art." The board member noted that donation had benefited a whole city. I retorted, "I am trying to build an artificial heart for the whole world." I was surprised at my audacity and confident that Kolff would have applauded.

The owners finally buckled to my persistence. A letter containing the specifics of the agreement went to President Peterson at the University of Utah. He thanked me and referred me to his vice president for development. When the vice president had the building inspected, he declared it was more of a liability than an asset and refused to accept the donation.

Stunned, I refused to lose the gift. I formed Medforte Research Foundation to receive the building as a tax-free gift. Many times subsequently I boasted that the university's failure to accept the old St. Mark's Hospital was one the best things the school had ever done for me.

Spaces were renovated and rented as incubator quarters for numerous start-up corporations hatched from university research. Proceeds from rents that exceeded operation costs and limited remodeling supported pilot research and funded related projects such as the Barney Clark Award, given annually to a long-term investigator who has made significant contributions to biomedical engineering. The old hospital became home to a number of devices important to ongoing artificial heart and VAD research. I also am coinventor of three patents covering magnetic bearings in a centrifugal pump.

Outside Research Funds

I gained my first NIH grant for developing blood pumps in 1974 and had continuous funding until my retirement. Millions of additional dollars have flowed into the University of Utah because of the heart-research and device-testing contracts, and significant positive exposure accrues from multiple contributions in medical literature.

When the university was seeking a new head for the Department of Surgery, the magnitude of this federal research became apparent. A brochure with facts about the department was created to facilitate the search. I was one of sixty-one faculty members asked to report on all outside funding for 1996 to 1998. The large Salt Lake VA Hospital reported $6,060,890. The university's Department of General Surgery reported $3,266,057. My personal grants for the artificial heart alone totaled $3,164,100 over the two years.

Among the faculty members, the average was $85,000 for each of the years while my average was $1,054,000 per year. The brochure also cited the number of publications in refereed journals. The overall faculty reported 1.5 per year while I averaged four publications per year.

In May 2005, Columbia University acknowledged me as one of the top NIH grantees in the country. The university asked me how federal infusion of funds had affected the University of Utah. Here is Columbia's letter:

> Columbia University
>
> May 19, 2005
>
> Dear Dr. Olsen:
>
> Joshua Graff Zivin and I are a team of health economists currently doing research on the careers of Top NIH Grantees. Our hypothesis is that prominent researchers positively influence the research productivity of the colleagues around them. We would like to quantify those

impacts. This quantification will provide a more complete assessment of the returns to public investment in biomedical research.

NIH records place you above the 95th percentile of the distribution of extramural NIH grants over the last 25 years (also with 2,500 others.) Would you mind sending us your CV (preferred, it often lists the names of postdocs/fellows) or your NIH Biosketch? All information collected from participants in this study will be aggregated. Thus, your name will not appear in any report, publication or presentation resulting from this study.

If you have any questions, please do not hesitate to contact us. We will be glad to send you a summary report of our findings. We are funded in part by a grant from the Merck Foundation (Columbia-Stanford Consortium on Medical Innovation.) Many thanks in advance.

Sincerely,

Pierre Azouly, Ph.D.

Graduate School of Business, Columbia University

And

Joshua Graff Zivin, Ph.D.

Mailman School of Public Health and College of Physicians and Surgeons, Columbia University

Since the date of that inquiry from Columbia University, I have received additional funding as the principal investigator for research on magnetically suspended impeller blood pumps and other medical devices in the amount of almost thirteen million dollars. Prior to retirement, I was the principal investigator on NIH grants for magnetically suspended rotor blood pumps; harvesting growth factors for surgical use and platelets for wound healing; a point-of-care platelet-function analyzer; and a new, magnetically suspended VAD.

In addition, I have been involved in creating nonprofit foundations, institutes, and corporations spawned by international interest in artificial organs. They share information and create working relationships among nations. Among these are the following:

International Faculty for Artificial Organs (INFA), which was formed on September 18, 1990, at the University of Bologna, Italy. The University of Utah joined with other universities throughout Europe and Japan. There were eight founding members, and I was elected dean of the Americas. The goal was to foster free and effective exchange among disciplines and faculties involved in organ replacement.

American Institute for Medical and Biological Engineering (AIMBE) was created in February 1992 after two years of planning. It has matured into the largest specialty-engineering society in the world.

Dr. Yuki Nosé, Dr. Setsuo Takitani, and I, along with others, created the International Society for Rotary Blood Pumps (ISRBP) in Houston, Texas in 1992. It has become financially stable and sponsors an annual meeting.

Utah Artificial Heart Institute (UAHI) was formally incorporated on October 28, 1998, to provide an independent organization to meet the needs of people whose research results in marketable products. The University of Utah had an employee contract that required all inventions and marketable properties to be filed through the Technology Commercialization Office. When companies approached me to develop or test devices, I wanted to assure them that their new technology belonged to them. Many companies had refused to offer contracted research because of the university requirement. A nonuniversity organization was needed, and UAHI became that organization, eliminating the university's possible claims to royalties.

Other Major Accomplishments

I have published more than 295 articles in refereed medical and biomedical journals, written sixteen book chapters, and made presentations too numerous to count, nationally and internationally.

I hold sixteen United States patents and assorted international ones.

Under my direction, we established a multimillion-dollar base of funding for the Institute for Biomedical Engineering. I also played a significant role in procuring the Biomedical Polymers Research Facility on the University of Utah campus.

I fostered collaborative research arrangements among several engineering and pharmaceutical-science departments.

I was honored as one of the alumni of the year by both of the institutions from which I received degrees—Utah State University and Colorado State University—and was inducted into the Alumni Hall of Honor at Utah State.

Bumps along the Way

Challenges go with the turf. I met some of them as I plodded through scores of years in artificial-heart research. When Dr. Kolff employed me full time in the IBE's Division of Artificial Organs, I also was appointed as a lecturer in the Department of Surgery in the School of Medicine. However, the university provided no financial support or secretarial assistance.

That rankled. The university was collecting nearly 60 percent of additional monies on the NIH grants that funded my research. For the three years from 1996 to 1998, I received $3,164,100 for the direct costs for research, and since I was on the faculty, the institution received the indirect costs to support the research—about $2,000,000—to provide space and facilities and secretarial and administrative support. The university paid very low rent to the Medforte Research Foundation, but I was denied any money for a secretary or administrative costs. I cheated by listing my administrator as my surgical technician. Dr. Richard Kohen, then university vice president for research, claimed that the school had high costs administrating my grants, even though nearly all the research was done in my own lab.

I became very frustrated and felt the university was contributing nearly nothing to support the IBE and my research. That dissatisfaction prompted my resignation from the university in December 2000. I held the rank of tenured professor in the Department of Surgery, an unusual position for someone without a medical degree. The week before I resigned, I sat at my desk or worked in the lab with colleagues, assistants, secretaries, and administrative help. Afterward I worked in the lab with the same equipment and the same personnel, but I had nearly 60 percent more money. The university also had been collecting nearly 60 percent on contracted device testing for corporations. Now these companies came directly to the tax-free Utah Artificial Heart Institute that I had set up.

How Many Animal Implants?

Kolff was always seeking funding from the federal government for his artificial-organs projects. On May 17, 1971, he wrote to Dr. Lowell T. Harmison, acting chief of the Medical Devices Applications program in the NHLBI, complaining that "none of us can even afford to do one experiment a week." The NIH official was not impressed. Kolff's request for money went unheeded.

To back up his claims, I began in January 1974 to record the names and numbers assigned to the calves and sheep implanted with various blood pumps. For sixteen years through December 1989, 856 animals were implanted, an average of one per week (refer to table 24.1). Three years after Kolff wrote Harmison, I had met the target of one implant per week.

Student Scholarships

I never forgot that my ability to go to college after I graduated from a small rural high school in Utah relied on a scholarship. It allowed me to attend Utah State Agricultural College (now Utah State University (USU) and was the foundation for everything that happened afterward. It helped me realize the ambition I had developed as a boy growing up on a farm in Gunnison, Utah, on the edge of the

Table 24.1. Calf and Sheep Totals by Year

Year	Calf	Sheep	Total
1974	46	4	50
1975	40	35	75
1976	28	0	28
1977	38	2	40
1978	30	4	34
1979	15	13	28
1980	36	30	66
1981	21	34	55
1982	26	30	56
1983	32	17	49
1984	76	7	83
1985	57	1	58
1986	103	2	105
1987	74	1	75
1988	22	1	23
1989	22	9	31
Total, 16 years (53.5 surgeries/year)			856

Great American Desert. It set me on my lifelong course focused on agriculture and animals.

My wife, Joyce, and I started a scholarship fund at USU in 1986, and it has grown to $100,000. For several years, I had been trying to convince Colorado State University, where I received my veterinary training, to offer a dual-degree program in the vet school. I pointed out that its graduates knew a great deal about animals but very little about research. They could not develop hypotheses and design experiments to test those hypotheses. There were many employment opportunities for veterinarians who could do research, I argued.

After a few years of wheedling, the school instituted a dual-degree program, and Joyce and I established a $100,000 scholarship fund for students. Then we used money from the Medforte Research Foundation to establish similar financial support at the University of Utah and BYU. We founded the Dr. Don B. Olsen Biomedical Engineering Scholarship and Mentorship at BYU. Then we added another $100,000 for the Don B. Olsen Graduate Fellowship in the University of Utah Department of Bioengineering, where I had been on the faculty for many years.

At a lower level, we provide a scholarship each year to support one graduating senior at Gunnison High School for two years in higher education. We established our own criteria, including the student's need for aid. We also guarantee that no scholarship winner will lose that support if he or she chooses a two-year hiatus for illness or church or military service. I was asked to serve on the selection committee but declined. I don't know the students well enough and cannot gauge relative need. We repeated the scholastic encouragement at Bicknell High School in Wayne County.

A Lingering Question

One of the puzzling questions in the Barney Clark experience—what had triggered the debilitating seizures he suffered—resurfaced in my mind now and again. Ten years later, when Dr. Chris Westenfelder, a university nephrologist, did research that suggested high serum levels of atrial natriuretic factor (ANF) might be related to seizures, I was interested. ANF is a hormone that helps regulate the storage or excretion of salt and water. It has a variety of sources, with atrial muscle cells (myocytes) being a primary one.

Westenfelder asked me questions about the role of ANF in animals with artificial hearts. We knew that we could manipulate renal functions and sodium and water retention in these animals by changing the heart rate and driving pressures. When they were set low, the animals developed symptoms of heart failure with edema, fluid overload, and high atrial pressures. For a time after implantation, the ANF increased or decreased with the salt and water intake, but later it became unresponsive to changes.

I felt Westenfelder's research might hold some clues to the seizures that had set back Barney Clark's recovery. We discussed in depth the posted serum levels in Clark while he was on the artificial heart. Westenfelder found frozen serum samples from Clark and measured the ANF levels in many of them. In general Clark retained excessive amounts of salt and fluids.

Westenfelder also studied Clark's hospital charts and records to see how recorded atrial pressures correlated with serum levels of ANF on specific dates. He found that there were high levels of theophylline in Clark's serum, often exceeding normal amounts. It is a drug often used to treat impaired lung function, for instance in patients with emphysema or other pulmonary diseases. Lower lung function was one of the symptoms of Clark's heart failure. Theophylline may be self-administered in inhalants prescribed for patients.

On day four of Clark's postoperative history, Westenfelder found that his serum level exceeded by tenfold the known seizure threshold of theophylline.

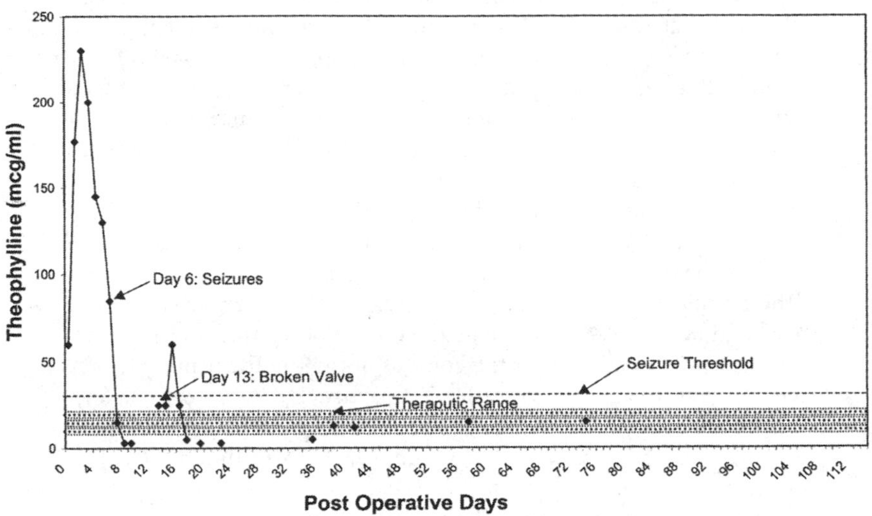

A graph charting serum theophylline levels for Barney Clark.

This was two days before Clark had grand mal seizures. If he had not been on the artificial heart, Westenfelder and some toxicologists conjectured that Clark might have died from theophylline toxicity.

It appeared Clark might have used an aerosol albuterol inhaler at overdose levels to help his breathing before coming to Utah for the implant surgery. No drugs like that and no tracking of serum levels were ordered during his hospitalization. Though Westenfelder's research did not provide conclusive answers, it was food for thought for those who had followed Clark's medical history so carefully.

Dr. Kolff Rarely Gave Accolades

In 1983 Kolff published an article in *Transactions—American Society for Artificial Internal Organs*. It was titled "Artificial Organs—Forty Years and Beyond." The first half page dealt with artificial kidneys, which had set him on the path that earned his reputation as the father of artificial organs. The sixteen subsequent pages focused on the artificial heart. In a subsection titled "CoWorkers in the Experimental Lab," Kolff wrote,

> While the invention, development and manufacturing of the actual artificial heart and assist devices, of course, is very important, one does not get anywhere unless one has an animal laboratory and personnel

> that can implant artificial hearts in animals and can study them without killing the animal. I have been extremely fortunate for the last 10 years to have Dr. Don Olsen as head of our Experimental Heart Research Laboratory. He has implanted artificial hearts in animals in Utah and also Rostock, East Germany; Brno, Czechoslovakia; Lyon, France; Buenos Aires, Argentina; and a few other places. An East German calf named Rosie in Rostock had the impertinence to live longer than any Soviet calf with an artificial heart. Dr. Olsen has had the assistance of a string of excellent and devoted Japanese surgeons. Some of them, like Dr. Hiro Fukumasu, worked with us for three years.
>
> In our calf laboratory, we have the habit of appointing one principal investigator (PI) who is in charge of any calf with an artificial heart. This principal investigator has the full responsibility for the care of this calf, and no one else is to change the course of treatment or the management of the calf without the consent of the PI. The names of some who have served as PIs include Dr. Tet Akutsu, Dr. Yuki Nosé, Dr. Spyros Moulopoulos, Steve Topaz, Larry Hastings, Dr. Clifford Kwan-Gett, Dr. Hans Zwart, Dr. Don Olsen, Dr. Hiro Fukumasu, Dr. Jack Kolff and Dr. William DeVries.
>
> In the case of Dr. Barney Clark, Dr. William DeVries was the principal investigator and Dr. Lyle Joyce was the co-principal investigator. I was extremely happy with the entire team at the University of Utah and particularly with the principal investigators.
>
> We have counted all the scientific co-workers involved with the development of the total artificial heart and assist devices over the years. There were 247 individuals.[1]

Knowing that Kolff seldom waxed sentimental and was reticent with his praise, I valued the accolades he heaped on the artificial-heart workers in his article.

Learning at the Master's Side

I freely give credit to Kolff for having expressed and demonstrated confidence in my abilities in the multifaceted science of mechanical circulation. He had access to and collaborated with hundreds of highly trained and qualified investigators who were eager to work with him. Like a magnet, he drew quality researchers, many of whom came to work with him at their own expense just for the privilege of learning at his side. Our association gave me numerous opportunities for which I feel fortunate. He showed great confidence in me in 1973 in making me the lead surgeon on all blood-pump implantations in animals.

Once I stated that "Kolff was not always particularly easy to work for or with. He was always persistent and driven with ambition. With his personality, these characteristics were contagious. Any success I may have attained I attribute to Dr. Kolff, coupled with my own hard work and, yes, luck."

Some people say the Barney Clark artificial-heart implantation was an expensive failure and did not live up to the hope that launched it. The story seemed simply to fade away, leaving the impression that the artificial heart saga had come to an end. It's true that the number of potential recipients for artificial hearts predicted after Clark's surgery by Kolff and Nosé did not materialize. Getting an artificial heart did not immediately become a panacea for every person suffering from heart problems. But those early trials made the same contributions to the treatment of heart disease that Orville and Wilbur Wright's first feeble flights at Kitty Hawk made to aviation.

The story has by no means ended. The advancements in simpler and more reliable rotary VADs—all incorporating the science developed with those first artificial hearts—has made them far more acceptable to the medical profession and patients. More patients survive the wait for a natural heart transplant because they have been given an artificial heart to tide them over. And because the supply of donor hearts is never likely to equal the demand, it may be that the future will include artificial hearts implanted with the goal of supporting life until natural death. The future indeed looks bright.

In forty years in the field, I have been able to add somewhat to the vast accumulation of knowledge about how to make and operate artificial hearts and how to integrate the timing of blood pumps such as VADs with the naturally beating heart. On a broader plane has been the evolution of materials to manufacture implantable blood pumps. Unique characteristics of materials, methods of manufacture, durability to withstand flexing diaphragms, and the ability to adhere to other plastics or polymers all have contributed to progress. Such victories as learning to minimize clotting when blood is exposed to foreign materials will be written in huge letters in the history of artificial hearts.

The ultimate role of the artificial heart has only begun. The future holds advances that will reduce—if not eliminate—much of the suffering and early death caused by congestive heart disease. Part—if not all—of the progress will be built on foundations laid by the Kolffs, the Olsens, the DeVrieses, the Jarviks, and others who refused to quit when they encountered challenges. They had the courage to look at the possibilities and take each next hard step. They were the vanguard of a medical miracle that has only begun to emerge. They possessed true valor.

Note

1. The article appears in volume 29, pages 6–24. Kolff included an alphabetical list of those 247 people.

APPENDIX A

Giving Credit for Names of Utah Artificial Hearts

The Team: A Loss of Credit

On February 15, 1983, the *Deseret News,* one of Salt Lake City's daily papers, published an editorial entitled, "Giving Credit for Artificial Hearts." A dispute about who should receive credit for inventing the world's first permanent artificial heart is unfortunate because it detracts from the brilliant achievement of the University of Utah medical team. The key word is "team" because dozens of researchers had vital roles in developing the heart known as the Jarvik-7. The device was named after Robert K. Jarvik, who did the principal design work on the heart for several years. But Jarvik did not invent the heart. He built on the work of others who preceded him and was aided by scores of partners and technicians, many of whom made significant contributions.

> This minor tempest of who gets credit began this past week when the National Inventors Hall of Fame honored Dr. Jarvik. This recognition prompted a protest by Dr. Clifford Kwan-Gett, a former researcher at the University of Utah, who said he made the basic design in 1969.
>
> Thus the question of who is the inventor of the artificial heart becomes lost in the outpouring of research from many quarters. It could not have been done without Dr. Kwan-Gett, Dr. Jarvik, and many others whose names will never be known to the public. If anyone richly deserves having the heart named after him, it would be Dr. Willem J. Kolff, Head of the U of U Division of Artificial Organs, who began tinkering with the idea of an artificial heart back in the 1950s, before he ever came to Utah, and was the Chief of the project from the beginning. Perhaps the best solution is one that has already been proposed, one most accurate and most fair to everyone, to simply call it the "Utah Heart."

This editorial was written after an interview with Dr. Don Olsen about the dispute over whether Kwan-Gett's or Jarvik's name should go on the artificial heart. Olsen's idea of not naming the heart after any individual dates way back. In the mid-1970s, he suggested to Kolff that he change one of his long-standing policies: the practice of placing the name of a particular individual on an innovation. Olsen pointed out that frequently a student started working on a device, and after one to two years, left and someone else with a lot of ingenuity came along and made major improvements. A third or fourth person often continued these modifications. Kolff argued, on the other hand, that his approach tapped into pride of ownership and motivated the individual to exert more effort.

Olsen proposed naming the invention the Utah device, which identified it as a team effort. After some discussions, Kolff agreed, and the well-designed artificial heart that Dr. Kevin Murray was then working on was known henceforth as the Utah-100 artificial heart, meaning that it was the team-developed heart with a 100-milliliter stroke volume.

The Winchell Saga

To understand the complete picture, one must listen to a bizarre and intriguing story. It all began when Kolff came across a patent (USP No. 3,097,365) issued in July 1963 to Paul Winchell for an artificial heart. Kolff contacted Winchell and discussed the possibility of a negotiated agreement where Kolff and the University of Utah could further develop the artificial heart without infringing on the five claims in the Winchell patent. An agreement was signed on January 26, 1972, awarding "all right, title and interest" on Winchell's patent to the University of Utah. Winchell was to raise money for research in return. A copy of the drawings for the patent appears in figure A.1.

According to Winchell, a comedian and ventriloquist for a children's television show and later a self-proclaimed doctor, the heart should be known as the Paul Winchell heart. It was clear from the patent's description and drawings that the device would barely fit in a wheelbarrow.

The Kolff-Winchell agreement stated clearly that Kolff had conceived and developed the artificial heart being used at the University of Utah. The agreement also said, "They [Kolff and Winchell] had combined their efforts in the perfection of an artificial heart since December 27, 1971." In return for their collaboration,

> Winchell and his publicity staff was [*sic*] granted reasonable access to the University Laboratory and hospital facilities in order to photograph the same, subject to prior approvals. All publicity and promotional activities

> were to be conducted in a dignified manner. Any party will make no unwarranted promises of success or claims to fame. Publicity must be based upon facts. Winchell, through his contacts and publicity staff, will attempt to arrange for the necessary legal permits to allow for the solicitation of funds through television and other media.

Winchell arrived at the Artificial Heart Research Laboratory in the summer of 1972 with a photographer and two young, very pretty ladies, who posed in photographs with him. He and his entourage returned several times for more publicity shots. In the early spring of 1973, Winchell returned to the laboratory, and Kolff invited Olsen and some other people from the lab to join them for lunch with Dr. Chase Peterson, the vice president for health sciences.

Olsen was running a little late, so he drove to the luncheon by himself. His car radio was tuned to the Paul Harvey lunchtime newscast. Harvey announced, "At this very moment, Mr. Paul Winchell is assisting surgeons at the University of Utah to implant his artificial heart into a patient." Kolff and Peterson could not believe the story when Olsen reported it to them, so Olsen confronted Winchell and demanded that he phone Harvey immediately and have him retract the announcement. At first the ventriloquist smiled and did nothing, but as the infuriated Olsen pushed harder, he became more serious and denied that he had anything to do with the announcement. Olsen refused to be in the laboratory during any future visits from Winchell, which created problems for Kolff because of the agreement.

Winchell appeared on numerous talk shows to describe the way his artificial heart was keeping calves alive in Utah. He also circulated some written statements promoting his involvement with the artificial heart. On August 25, 1975, *Newsweek* printed, "Eventually Winchell joined forces with Dr. William [*sic*] Kolff, head of the artificial-organ division at the University of Utah's School of Medicine, and the two are attempting to perfect the plastic heart pump that Winchell invented. He and Kolff once kept a calf alive for 94 days with an artificial heart after removing the animal's own heart in an operation at which Winchell assisted."

Kolff was away, so Olsen sent a letter to Winchell responding to the article:

> I find the article in Newsweek August 25, 1975, extremely distressing to me and my collaborators in the Division of Artificial Organs. Any further exploitation of the University of Utah by you and the press will elicit immediate response by me to the editors of the publications pointing out the truth of the situation. The calf you referred to as a

> 94-day survivor was operated on and autopsied during the summer of 1974. As my memory serves me, your last visit upon this campus was in the spring of 1973, well over a year prior to this achievement, and the incriminating suggestion that our present artificial heart is resultant from your patent is totally wrong and unacceptable.

The letter did get a response from one person: "Thank you, Don! It was about time he heard this. Janke Kolff."

Winchell also claimed that the Acupuncture and Massage Institute of America in Los Angeles had awarded him a diploma in December 1974. An article in the *National Enquirer* dated January 27, 1976 was titled "Famed Ventriloquist Paul Winchell: I've Successfully Treated a Dozen Patients by Acupuncture." After this he often called himself Dr. Winchell, but he remained a Mr. to us.

On May 12, 1976, a picture in the *Los Angeles Times* was captioned, "Paul Winchell, entertainer and inventor, shows newsmen the artificial heart he patented." What he was holding was clearly a pneumatic pump well known as the Kwan-Gett artificial heart. It bore no resemblance to Winchell's patented heart, which was powered by electricity and never actually built.

On June 14, 1976, Stuart Arden of Parnassus Productions wrote Kolff about a film Winchell wished to have made to raise money for artificial-heart research. Kolff asked Olsen to handle the matter, so he wrote Arden, "Nevertheless, I do not want to find myself and the rest of the laboratory, and particularly Dr. Kolff's fine name, placed in a compromising situation—one of jeopardy and/or ridicule." In the final scene of the script Winchell had submitted to Kolff, Rob Jarvik and a friend were walking across the university campus when suddenly the friend grabbed his chest and fell to the ground. Jarvik just happened to be carrying an artificial heart and implanted it; then they continued quietly on their way. The whole thing was totally ridiculous.

Then Kolff and the University of Utah received the following letter from Winchell on March 18, 1981:

> *Gentlemen:*
>
> *I have honored our agreement in every particular but you have denied me certain contracted rights which you "granted" in exchange for my donating my patent of the artificial heart to you.*
>
> *You are in breach of our agreement and I now insist that you allow me full exercise of same, especially clause #5 which states, "Paul Winchell and his publicity staff shall be granted access to the lab and hospital facilities to photograph same."*

I have been instructed by Melvin Belli, Esq. (the very famous San Francisco litigator) to inform you that unless I receive reconfirmation of my contractual rights; in writing (so that you don't turn down media plans once again after I arrange them), I shall be forced to institute necessary legal proceedings.

Very Truly Yours,

Dr. Paul Winchell

Kolff thought that this threat was nothing but a scare tactic. No one believed that the famous Melvin Belli would take such a case. Kolff, however, was very shrewd and informed John Dwan, the university's public-relations director, about the situation on March 27:

Dear John

We recently sent you a copy of a letter we received from Paul Winchell in which he wants admission [sic] to film a heart implantation. I am enclosing a copy of the contract that was signed by the Provost Tom King and myself in 1972 and a copy of a letter from Don Olsen, which he sent Paul Winchell after he could no longer stand Paul Winchell's claims on Nationwide Television, etc. We also have a copy of the primitive patent of Winchell's artificial heart that would never work, the rights of which were given by Paul Winchell to the University of Utah.

At the time we thought that he might have done some damage with this patent, and it seemed to be more convenient to have him assign it to the University of Utah since our hearts are based on the same principal [sic].

The real reason for the cooperative venture with Paul Winchell was that he promised to collect money and believed that he would be able to do so by Telethons. The success of this venture by Jerry Lewis for another medical project is well known. Indeed, Paul Winchell was allowed to scrub in on some cases, was allowed to have his picture taken with our calves, but the real conflict began when he continued to claim in the press and otherwise, that the hearts that he showed were his hearts where in reality, they were samples that we had provided him. This became so blatantly untrue that my collaborators could no longer stand it and told him that enough was enough. Of his grand fund raising schemes, virtually nothing materialized. Indeed, I received small contributions if I recall well of the order of magnitude of one dollar to twenty-five dollars once in a while after he had given a talk on "his artificial hearts" in various places. (His total contributions amounted to $422 based on the financial records). At the time, I was rather indifferent to his claims of who made the artificial heart, recognizing that comedians often have an enormous ego and hoping that maybe sometime he would bring in some funds at a time that NIH funding was very difficult.

When I was in the apartment where he lived at the time in Los Angeles, I saw a plaque on the wall looking like the kind of plaque that you get for good services for the Boy Scouts. It was a brown wooden plaque with a copper plate on it. The copper plate was engraved something like "In gratitude to Paul Winchell from the University of Utah." I would probably have heard it if any official at the University of Utah would have presented him with such a plaque, which seems unlikely, and my assumption is that he had it fabricated himself....

If my guess is right, then Paul Winchell is broke or nearly so. It seems unlikely that he would hire Melvin Belli as his council. Anyway, Belli did not write this letter. I propose to do nothing for the time being. If any further action is taken, I will take it up with you. If something happens while I am in South America (March 30–April 18, 1981), don't take any hasty action. Be willing to forgive an old actor and comedian a little more than you would forgive somebody else, but he is a fraud....

In response the University of Utah's attorney general, David Wilkinson, sent a letter to Kolff on May 29 in which he noted,

I appreciated the opportunity to briefly discuss by telephone the letter from Dr. Paul Winchell.... I understand that we do not now use or have any interest in his artificial heart patent; and, it does not appear that his letter raises any valid issues of breach of contract. Furthermore, we have not heard from him concerning any previous alleged denial of his rights.

...I agree with your assessment that this is a matter of minimal exposure, if any, and no reply is necessary. Since we have gone this long without a further inquiry from him, rather than stirring up his thinking with a formal response, we should let this matter rest. If we hear any more from Dr. Winchell, I would appreciate your notifying me.

On April 29, 1983, a long article appeared in the *Deseret News* titled, "Winchell Finally Lays Old Ghosts to Rest." The article discussed Winchell's psychological problems and related them to his mother's death and his father committing suicide after that. Winchell had also attempted suicide and been hospitalized.

Winchell was quoted as saying he had been granted a patent in 1963 for an artificial heart powered by an external motor strapped to the patient's chest. He offered it to medical associations, but none were interested because he had not produced a working model.

Winchell then talked about Kolff contacting him and their collaboration. "All through the '70s, it [the artificial heart] was used to keep animals alive. It ultimately led to refinements by [Robert] Jarvik for human application," Winchell said. He added that "Jarvik has always called himself the designer of the heart used by Barney Clark, not the inventor."

Winchell eventually filed a lawsuit against Kolff and the University of Utah for breach of contract in the amount of $500,000. The Utah State Attorney's Office took over the issue, and nothing further happened.

The publicity surrounding the Paul Winchell saga was widely known by artificial heart researchers in other laboratories throughout the United States, and the group in Utah was the brunt of frequent jokes and laughter. The stigma did not go away easily.

Kolff Associates and the Artificial Heart

Kolff formed Kolff Associates, Inc., to market the artificial heart along with its driver and technology. At the initial meeting, Olsen said that because the University of Utah maintained the rights to products developed in its programs, the Artificial Heart Research Laboratory did not own the heart and driver, so they could not sell it.

Kolff, on the other hand, was adamant that he and the lab had developed the heart, and therefore they owned it and could market it. Several years later, attorneys representing potential investors informed Kolff that the company in fact did not own the technology it was selling and needed to license it from the university. Kolff negotiated a royalty-free permanent license for the heart, LVADs, mock circulations, and the drivers. Olsen sold and implanted the hearts in research laboratories around the world for the company, so the heart could just have easily been named the Kolff Associates Heart.

What Is in a Name? The Kolff/Kwan-Gett/Jarvik Quandary

In mid-January 1983, Olsen drove Kolff from the university to the off-campus research laboratory in the former St. Mark's Hospital. When they arrived, Kolff asked, "Can we just sit in the car and talk for a moment?" Olsen always wanted to be able to spend time with Kolff on a personal basis, so he sat and listened.

Kolff told Olsen in a quivering voice, "I have a real problem." Olsen asked if there was something he could do to help. Kolff said, "No. There lies Barney Clark in the hospital on the artificial heart, and it is not the Kolff artificial heart." With tears streaming down his face, he reiterated how many years he had worked on artificial hearts, and now Jarvik was monopolizing the press and exploiting the fact that his name was on the heart. The heart could have definitely been named the Kolff heart. Very few people would have had a problem with that.

In early February 1983—as Dr. Barney Clark was recovering from implantation of the first artificial heart approved by the FDA—the ownership of the artificial heart again was questioned. Dr. Clifford Kwan-Gett asked the University of

Utah to change the name of the artificial heart implanted in Barney Clark from Jarvik to Kwan-Gett. He even threatened to sue the university.

Furthermore, he wanted to have the University of Utah contact all publishers of scientific journals and retroactively change the name of the Jarvik heart to the Kwan-Gett heart. And he requested that all references to the heart developed in the Artificial Heart Research Laboratory should identify it as the Kwan-Gett heart.

His action certainly got the attention of the officials at the University of Utah; they assigned their standing patent committee to investigate what the name of the pneumatic artificial heart should be. The committee interviewed many people involved in artificial-heart research over the years on a fact-finding mission, including Olsen.

After some preliminary questions, they got to the important one: "Whose name should be on the pneumatic artificial heart that is in Dr. Barney Clark?" Olsen told the committee that when he had initially worked for Kolff and Kwan-Gett, the heart was clearly the Kwan-Gett hemispherical, pneumatically powered artificial heart. That was the heart that was used in all of the research when he joined the team full time in 1972, even though Kwan-Gett was no longer affiliated with the program.

Kwan-Gett's contribution to the design and particularly the operation of the artificial heart in calves was tremendous. His observations and teachings on the heart's function and capabilities in human recipients were in many areas astounding. Of particular significance was his seminal paper, "Total Replacement Artificial Heart and Driving System with Inherent Regulation of Cardiac Output" in 1969.[1] His description of the way the pneumatic artificial heart has a Starling-like response to varying atrial pressures was cited in numerous publications over the years and as recently as during FDA approval of the CardioWest (now SynCardia) artificial heart in March 2004. The principle that Kwan-Gett described forty-six years ago has withstood many challenges. His contributions have outshone every other single person's.

However, Olsen pointed out that Kwan-Gett had never raised the naming issue before. He and Olsen had sat on the board of directors for Kolff Associates, Inc., and later Kolff Medical, Inc., and when Olsen reported that he had sold the Jarvik heart and implanted it into calves in many different laboratories around the world, Kwan-Gett never objected to calling it the Jarvik heart. Therefore, Olsen could not really support his insistence on a name change at this late date.

Olsen was well aware that there were numerous previous designs of pneumatically powered artificial hearts. However, the Kwan-Gett heart was by far the most efficient and effective pump.

Jarvik built on Kwan-Gett's design for his early hearts. Shortly after Jarvik graduated from medical school in the spring of 1976, he redesigned the Jarvik-5 (J-5) heart, which had a 150-milliliter-stroke volume, to meet the specifications of the NIH. This design worked well, and the calves in the lab lived longer. However, after trials in human cadavers, it appeared that this size heart only fit large men. So Jarvik designed the Jarvik-7 (J-7) heart with a 100-milliter-stroke volume, and calves were surviving for seven and a half months. The J-7 was the heart implanted in 1982 in Barney Clark and the other permanent recipients. It was also used in some of the earlier calf bridge-to-cardiac transplantations in 1985, but again the device seemed a bit large, so the 70-cubic-centimeter–stroke-volume Jarvik-7-70 (J-7-70) was designed and built for human beings.

The difference between the various heart types was primarily the external geometry. Equally—if not more important—than the geometry, however, was a clear understanding of the heart's function and its characteristics, its limitations and ways to maximize the blood flow without major damage to and loss of red blood cells. Kwan-Gett's early work contributed very much to these issues.

Hank (Hong Kuck) Wong, a Chinese engineering student, designed and built a pneumatic heart driver. Wong was still working on this heart driver when he was tragically killed in a motorcycle accident. Kwan-Gett refined and improved this pneumatic driver.

Kwan-Gett's most significant contribution, however, was his work with his heart in calves, learning the maximum performance and keeping detailed studies. He discovered that the mechanical artificial heart had a Starling-like response to increased venous return or increased atrial pressure, somewhat similar to the natural heart: when the venous return increases, the cardiac output also increases. Basically this meant that when a calf was lying in a cage, it had a relatively low cardiac output, and when it stood, the venous return increased slightly, and its output also increased. When the animal walked on the treadmill, the venous return increased substantially, along with the cardiac output and flow from the heart, without changing the heart rate. Clearly, Clifford Kwan-Gett laid the foundation for virtually all of the subsequent developments in the pneumatic artificial heart.

When Kwan-Gett hired an attorney to look into a suit against the University of Utah over the name of the heart in 1983, Kolff was very concerned, and he had numerous discussions with Kwan-Gett and Jarvik. He went so far as to give a lecture on the artificial heart at the 1983 ASAIO meeting. He dedicated the lecture to Una Loy Clark, whose husband, Barney, had died just five weeks earlier.

Kolff's administrators at the University of Utah, and Olsen as well, strongly suspected that Kwan-Gett's attorney convinced him that he would have a hard time winning the lawsuit, even if he spent a great deal of money, because Kwan-Gett dropped the suit. He had already left the Artificial Heart Research Laboratory to go into cardiothoracic surgery and worked at St. Mark's Hospital in Salt Lake City. He was very successful until his retirement, when he and his wife moved to Southern California.

Symbion, Inc., continued to market the Jarvik 7-70 artificial heart in several hospitals in the United States and some countries in Europe, primarily France, until the FDA rescinded its approval in 1990. The FDA permitted hospitals to use the hearts in their inventory. The last J-7-70 implant in the United States took place on October 19, 1990. There were twenty-two additional implants in Europe and Canada through 1992. The heart designed and built in Utah and named the Jarvik was implanted into a total of 215 patients with full approval from the FDA.

CardioWest to the Rescue

Olsen did not want to see the artificial-heart technology die. He approached Symbion, Inc., to let someone else take over to benefit the small group of patients who could not be saved with any other devices. The Symbion people were reluctant to accept Olsen's offer because they would have to turn over all their files, equipment, and inventory. Olsen also stated that they had messed up relations with the FDA so badly that he needed $400,000 to straighten everything out.

Olsen did not know that Dr. Jack Copeland had also initiated conversations with Symbion to keep the technology available. When Olsen found out about Copeland, they immediately joined forces. They set up a 501-C3 not-for-profit corporation named CardioWest Technologies, Inc., in 1991, located at University Medical Center (UMC) in Tucson, Arizona. Olsen was named president, and CardioWest was financed equally by the UMC and the Medforte Research Foundation that Olsen had set up to receive the old St Mark's Hospital as a gift.

Olsen and Copeland approached the FDA to inquire about getting reapproved to market the J-7-70 heart in the United States. They were informed that the FDA felt that the Jarvik heart was dead. To comply with the FDA, slight modifications were made in the design, and the name was changed to the CardioWest-70 artificial heart. CardioWest assumed that with 215 human implants it would be quick and easy to obtain FDA approval with a newly built building designed to manufacture artificial hearts. Olsen also established improved inspection procedures.

CardioWest hoped to get approval of its new heart without having to do animal implants and reliability testing. Olsen argued, "Surely a well-documented human implant in a German was worth a calf implant in the United States." However, since the company was building the heart in a new facility with newly trained personnel, the FDA demanded that they do the reliability testing. Olsen's group did receive the concession that they did not have to wait for a year for the final results to be presented.

The approval process was much slower than anticipated, and the Medforte Foundation could not continue to support CardioWest. It appeared that the company would have to close. Dr. John Watson of NIH's NHLBI also advised Olsen to abandon the pneumatic artificial heart. However, Copeland offered to have the UMC take over all of the costs, and CardioWest was saved. The FDA approval finally came through in October 1992.

The first CardioWest artificial heart was implanted on January 12, 1993, and successfully transplanted by Copeland and the Arizona team after six months. However, hospitals were not financially healthy, and university teaching hospitals in particular were losing money. The University of Arizona had to reduce costs in 1999–2000 and elected to drop CardioWest. Copeland, Dr. Marvin Slepian, and Richard Smith formed a new for-profit corporation, SynCardia Systems, Inc., in August 2001.

The pneumatically powered artificial heart will continue to be known around the world as the CardioWest. In March 2004, the FDA voted unanimously to approve the CardioWest heart. It was implanted in 2008 in a patient in Australia and continues to be successfully used.

Kolff Continues to Suffer Injustices after a Quarter Century

The controversy about the name on the artificial heart developed in Utah continues to make front-page news. On Sunday, March 10, 2008, the *Salt Lake Tribune* published an article titled "Jarvik's Claims to Credit for Artificial Heart Disputed." The extensive article by Lisa Rosetta and Heather May covered two pages and included numerous photographs. It described the evolution of the artificial heart beginning with Kolff's first implant in 1957 in Cleveland, Ohio. Dr. Kwan-Gett was given a lot of attention for his many contributions to the design and implantation of the Kwan-Gett heart. The article also indicated that Tom Kessler manufactured all of the Utah hearts and Dr. Don Olsen contributed to the long-term animal survival on the artificial heart.

Here are some excerpts from the article:

> "It was a very, very intense time for all of us," said John Dwan, executive director of public affairs for the U's Health Sciences Center from 1978 to 2001.

> Jarvik, who had observed Clark's surgery by William C. DeVries but played no role in it, appeared at the subsequent press conference in scrubs.
>
> While spokesman Chase Peterson, then the vice president of Health Sciences, stood at a podium, Jarvik sat square[ly] in front of it. "You couldn't miss him," Dwan said.... Dwan said he tried to direct reporters to Peterson and the surgeons, feeling Jarvik "was trying to use it to get ahead." Peterson, later the U's president, diplomatically recalls: "It was a job to keep very able people in the same corral."
>
> ...Kolff's son, Jack, said his father's decision to let Jarvik's name stay on the heart—and his efforts to advance Jarvik's career—were among his father's greatest regrets in his life.
>
> ...[Dr. Yuki] Nosé, who worked on predecessor hearts with Kolff at the Cleveland Clinic,...[said that] while Jarvik made significant contributions, his prominence has unfairly eclipsed Kolff's work.

Michael Moyer published an article in *Scientific American* in September 2009 titled, "Artificial Heart: Did the Wrong Man Get Credit for the World's First Permanent Pump?" Moyer wrote,

> Kolff had a tradition of naming new versions of the heart after young investigators in his lab to keep them motivated and prevent them from moving elsewhere. Jarvik was project manager for the iteration that came to be named Jarvik-7. That device was approved for use by the Food and Drug Administration in 1981.
>
> Jarvik was 35 years old when Clark received the heart that bore his name. He appeared at the press conference that announced the implant in scrubs, although he did not take part in the surgery. Jarvik continued to attend press conferences at the center, while Kolff kept a low profile. Perhaps it is not surprising that the world came to associate a seminal piece of engineering—the work of hundreds, over a course of years—with one man. After all, it had his name on it.[2]

Notes

1. C. S. Kwan-Gett, Y. Wu, R. Collan, S. Jacobsen, and W. J. Kolff, "Total replacement artificial heart and driving system with inherent regulation of cardiac output," *Transactions—American Society of Artificial Internal Organs* 15 (1969):245–66.
2. Available online at http://www.nature.com/scientificamerican/journal/v301/n3/fall/scientificamerican0909-75b.html

APPENDIX B

THE DR. BARNEY CLARK AWARD AND ITS HISTORY

Medforte Research Foundation financially supports the Utah Artificial Heart Institute in selecting and awarding the Barney Clark Award. This award was initiated for two purposes: first to acknowledge and perpetuate the important contributions that Dr. Barney Clark and his family made when he became the first recipient of a permanent artificial heart; and second, to recognize and honor special individuals who have made significant, often lifelong, contributions in applying biomedical engineering principles and innovative medicine to alleviate the suffering of patients.

An award committee was formed that accepts nominations and evaluates worthy candidates. One of the most difficult tasks the selection committee faces is condensing the recipient's numerous outstanding contributions into one or two sentences statements to inscribe on a plaque. Here is a list of the recipients and their award citations.

Dr. Barney Clark, implanted with the first permanent artificial heart in humans. Recipient 1982.

An exemplary frontiersman in the spirit of the Barney Clark family.

Una Loy Clark. Recipient 1989.

In recognition of the personal and family sacrifices contributing to numerous advancements in the clinical application of the artificial heart.

Willem J. Kolff, MD, PhD. Recipient 1991.

University of Utah, Salt Lake City.
Recognized throughout the world as the father of artificial organs, he contributed a lifetime of dedicated research, teaching, and leadership in all facets of artificial-organ technology.

Adrian Kantrowitz, MD. Recipient 1993.

New York City. Cardiothoracic surgeon.
He devoted a lifetime of dedicated, innovative research, teaching, and leadership in many facets of artificial-organ technology and played an important role in the clinical application of VADs.

Lyle D. Joyce, MD, PhD. Recipient 1994.

Minneapolis, Minnesota. Cardiothoracic surgeon.
He demonstrated an untiring dedication to patients with surgically correctable heart disease and contributed pioneering efforts to use mechanical circulatory-assist and replacement devices on these patients, in particular the artificial heart.

Horst Klinkmann, MD, PhD. Recipient 1995.

Rostock, Germany. Nephrology.
He devoted years of untiring dedication to research efforts in artificial organs and patient care, applying innovative biomedical devices. As a teacher, the entire world was his campus.

Peer M. Portner, PhD. Recipient 1996.

Stanford, California. Mechanical engineer.
He contributed a lifetime of untiring dedication to alleviation of suffering in patients with cardiac failure through the design, research, development, and clinical use of VADs.

Robert H. Bartlett, MD. Recipient 1997.

University of Michigan, Ann Arbor. Artificial lung.
In recognition of a lifetime of untiring dedication to the alleviation of suffering in patients with respiratory and cardiac failure through the design, research, development, and clinical use of VADs.

Michael E. DeBakey, MD. Recipient 1998.

Houston, Texas. Renowned cardiothoracic surgeon.
Recognized throughout the world as the pioneer of the artificial heart, he provided five decades of leadership, teaching, research, and innovative surgical procedures. He used the first successful VAD and was a champion of federal funding for an artificial-heart program.

Kazu Atsumi, MD, PhD. Recipient 1999.

Tokyo, Japan. Inventor/surgeon.
Pioneer of the artificial heart program in Japan, he initiated and maintained the program for more than forty years, training and being the inspiration for numerous young investigators in the field. He also founded Japanese and international societies of artificial organs.

John C. Norman Jr., MD., DSc. Recipient 2000.

Boston, Massachusetts. Cardiothoracic surgeon.
He had an illustrious career in pioneering and sustaining the abdominal left VAD program from concept, through characterization and validation, to preclinical testing, leading to wide-spread clinical utilization. Everything was done according to the original NHLBI artificial-heart program guidelines of 1964 through 1985.

Jack G. Copeland, MD, PhD. Recipient 2001.

Tucson, Arizona. Cardiothoracic surgeon.
He achieved success in the clinical application of artificial hearts and VADs against overwhelming odds and criticisms, interjecting science into the process. He was also a leader in moving the artificial heart from failure to highly successful clinical application.

Tetsuzo Akutsu, MD, PhD. Recipient 2002.

Osaka, Japan. Cardiothoracic surgeon.
He devoted a lifetime to designing, implanting, and fostering the use of artificial hearts and VADs to alleviate human suffering. The Akutsu heart was implanted into a dog as early as 1957, and an improved version was placed in a man in 1981. He also organized the International Symposium on Artificial Heart and Assist Devices for many years.

Yuki Nosé, MD, PhD. Recipient 2003.

Houston, Texas. Cardiothoracic surgeon.
In recognition of his lifelong dedication, teaching, and mentoring of a very broad segment of biomedical research. As a scientist and inventor on three continents, he founded more national and international societies than any of his peers.

John T. Watson, PhD. Recipient 2003.

Washington, DC. National Heart, Lung and Blood Institute (NHLBI), National Institutes of Health (NIH).

A public servant dedicated to using engineering principles to improve the health of all, he was known for national and international leadership. He contributed to the recognition of bioengineering as a full partner in biological and medical research and was responsible for the NIH programs in assisted circulation and artificial hearts, cardiovascular imaging, and biomaterials.

Karen Burke. Recipient 2004.

Boca Raton, Florida. Executive director, American Society for Artificial Internal Organs (ASAIO).

Wise, skillful, charming, ever tactful, universally respected and admired, she has been the glow and the glue of the ASAIO for forty years. As executive director, she has done as much for artificial organ research as the most accomplished scientific investigator.

William S. Pierce, MD. Recipient 2005.

Hershey, Pennsylvania. Inventor/surgeon.

A lifelong leader in the development of circulatory-support devices and artificial hearts, he exemplifies the ideal balance as clinician/surgeon/researcher and teacher. His contributions to the improvement of the human condition are outstanding.

Yukiyasu Sezai, MD. Recipient 2005.

Tokyo, Japan. Administrator/surgeon.

A pioneer of cardiac surgery in Japan, he established the clinical feasibility of Japanese-developed pulsatile and rotary blood pumps. He was a founder of—and has served as the president of—the International Society of Rotary Blood Pumps (ISRBP), representing Asia. He also contributes to education and was the president of one of the largest universities in the world for nine years.

Paul S. Malchesky, DEng. Recipient 2006.

Cleveland, Ohio. Editor of *Artificial Organs.*

In recognition for his lifelong dedication to the development of various types of apheresis therapy systems, as well as his support of all artificial organs through his initiation of, devotion to, and continuing efforts to maintain the journal *Artificial Organs* successfully for thirty years.

Ernst Wolner, MD. Recipient 2006.

Vienna, Austria. Cardiothoracic surgeon.
For his outstanding contribution in the development and clinical application of the artificial heart and cardiac-assist devices and his dedication to his many patients. He also has steadfastly promoted his field in Europe.

Richard G. Smith, MS, CCE. Recipient 2007.

Tucson, Arizona. Engineer.
He has been a continuing force in using the artificial heart as a bridge to transplantation since the first successful bridge in 1985. As an engineer, his humanistic approach to the artificial heart and device-supported patients has set a standard for others to follow.

Don B. Olsen, DVM, DSc. Recipient 2007.

Salt Lake City, Utah. Experimental surgery. Special Recognition Award celebrating the twenty-fifth anniversary of the Barney Clark artificial heart implant.
In recognition of a lifetime dedicated to designing, investigating, and implanting artificial hearts and cardiac-assist devices. He designed successful surgical procedures to implant the artificial heart and was a master at teaching his techniques to surgeons worldwide. He was also instrumental in reintroducing the artificial heart into the clinical market for patient use.

Victor L. Poirier, BS, MBA. Recipient 2008.

Concord, Massachusetts. Engineer.
For sustained devotion to the design, clinical evaluation, and commercialization of heart-assist systems that improve the health and lives of patients in heart failure.

George P. Noon, MD. Recipient 2009.

Baylor College of Medicine, Houston, Texas. Cardiothoracic surgeon.
In recognition of his lifelong dedication to developing and applying circulatory-assist technology not only for acute but also for chronic heart-failure patients. He also assisted Dr. Michael E. DeBakey in becoming the leader in circulatory-assist technology.

Eli A. Friedman, MD. Recipient 2010.

State University of New York Health Science Center, Brooklyn, New York.
Chief, Division of Renal Disease.
Recognized internationally as a contributing pioneer in dialysis and an inspiring speaker, he served as president of ASAIO from 1987 to 1988 and editor of the organization's journal, *Transactions*, from 1986 to 2003.

O. H. Frazier, MD. Recipient 2011.

Houston, Texas. Cardiovascular surgeon.
Recognized throughout the world as a pioneer in the clinical advancement of cardiac transplantation and mechanical circulatory support and replacement devices, he has dedicated his career to patient care, teaching, and bringing artificial-organ technology from concept to clinical practice.

Illustration Credits

Images, listed by page number, are from the following sources and are used with permission.

Barney and Una Loy Clark Family Collection
v, 140, 144, 162, 168, 190, 193, 203, 207, 339, 341

Don B. Olsen Collection
22, 36, 49, 58, 63, 100, 113, 115, 119, 126, 133, 134, 219, 236, 248, 251, 266, 268, 270, 302, 308, 332, 356, 393

Deseret News
7, 13, 244

Special Collections Department, J. Willard Marriott Library, University of Utah
83, 89, 109, 130, 222, 265, 296, 306, 318, 321, 322, 329

SynCardia Systems, Inc.
124, 368, 370, 370, 372, 373, 374, 375

INDEX

Numbers in *italics* indicate figures.